CASE REVIEW
Brain Imaging

Series Editor

David M. Yousem, MD, MBA
Professor of Radiology
Director of Neuroradiology
Russell H. Morgan Department of Radiology Science
The Johns Hopkins Medical Institutions
Baltimore, Maryland

Other Volumes in the CASE REVIEW Series

Breast Imaging
Cardiac Imaging
Gastrointestinal Imaging, Second Edition
General and Vascular Ultrasound, Second Edition
Genitourinary Imaging, Second Edition
Head and Neck Imaging, Second Edition
Musculoskeletal Imaging, Second Edition
Nuclear Medicine
Obstetric and Gynecologic Ultrasound, Second Edition
Pediatric Imaging
Spine Imaging, Second Edition
Thoracic Imaging
Vascular and Interventional Imaging

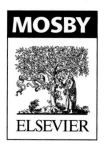

MOSBY
ELSEVIER

Laurie L. Loevner, MD
Professor of Radiology, Otorhinolaryngology: Head
and Neck Surgery, and Neurosurgery
Department of Radiology
University of Pennsylvania Medical Center, Hospital of
the University of Pennsylvania
Philadelphia, Pennsylvania

CASE REVIEW

Brain Imaging

SECOND EDITION

CASE REVIEW SERIES

1600 John F. Kennedy Blvd.
Suite 1800
Philadelphia, PA 19103-2899

BRAIN IMAGING: CASE REVIEW
Second Edition   ISBN: 978-0-323-03179-0

NOTICE

Knowledge and best practice in this field are constantly changing. As new research and
experience broaden our knowledge, changes in practice, treatment, and drug therapy may
become necessary or appropriate. Readers are advised to check the most current information provided (i) on procedures featured or (ii) by the manufacturer of each product to
be administered, to verify the recommended dose or formula, the method and duration of
administration, and contraindications. It is the responsibility of the practitioner, relying on
his or her own experience and knowledge of the patient, to make diagnoses, to determine
dosages and the best treatment for each individual patient, and to take all appropriate
safety precautions. To the fullest extent of the law, neither the Publisher nor the Author
assumes any liability for any injury and/or damage to persons or property arising out of or
related to any use of the material contained in this book.

Library of Congress Cataloging-in-Publication Data

Loevner, Laurie A.
   Brain imaging : case review / Laurie A. Loevner.—2nd ed.
      p. ; cm—(Case review series)
   With cross-references to: Neuroradiology / Robert I. Grossman, David M. Yousem.
2nd ed. © 2003.
   Includes bibliographical references and indexes.
   ISBN 978-0-323-03179-0
   1. Brain—Imaging—Case studies. I. Grossman, Robert I. Neuroradiology. II. Title.
III. Series.
   [DNLM: 1. Brain—Radiography—Case Reports. 2. Brain—Radiography—Examination
Questions. WL 18.2 L826b 2009]
   RC386.6.D52L64 2009
   616.8'04754076—dc22   2008040445

ISBN: 978-0-323-03179-0

Aquisitions Editor: Rebecca S. Gaertner
Project Manager: David Saltzberg
Design Direction: Steven Stave

Working together to grow
libraries in developing countries

www.elsevier.com | www.bookaid.org | www.sabre.org

ELSEVIER   BOOK AID International   Sabre Foundation

Printed in the United States of America.
Last digit is the print number: 9 8 7 6 5 4 3 2

For Steve, Ben, and Alex....
to infinity and back

I have been very gratified by the popularity and positive feedback that the authors of the **Case Review** series have received on the publication of their volumes. Reviews in journals and word-of-mouth comments have been uniformly favorable. The authors have done an outstanding job in filling the need for an affordable, easy-to-read, case-based learning tool that supplements *THE REQUISITES* series, and volumes in the **Case Review** series are ideal for oral board preparation and subspecialty certification tests.

Although some students learn best in a noninteractive study book mode, others need the anxiety or excitement of being quizzed—being put on the hot seat. The **Case Review** format—that is, a limited number of images needed to construct a differential diagnosis presented with a few clinical and imaging questions—was designed to simulate the Boards experience (the only difference is that the **Case Review** books give you the correct answer and immediate feedback). Cases are scaled from relatively easy ("Opening Round") to very difficult ("Challenger") to test the limit of the reader's knowledge. A brief commentary, a link back to *THE REQUISITES* volume, and up-to-date references also are provided.

Because of the popularity of the series we have been rolling out the second editions, with the expectation that the second editions will bring the material to the state-of-the-art, introduce new modalities and new techniques, and provide new and even more graphic examples of pathology.

Brain Imaging by Dr. Laurie A. Loevner is the latest of the second editions. Laurie has labored extensively to provide almost 90% new cases, color images, and examples of the latest imaging modalities. She has worked assiduously for many months to perfect the book in the way that she has said "would earn me an A+ grade." *Brain Imaging* is the best selling of all of the volumes in the **Case Review** series, and I can tell you that the second edition is well worth the wait. Enjoy.

I am pleased to present for your imminent pleasure the latest volume of the second editions of the **Case Review** series, joining the previous second editions of *Head and Neck Imaging*, by David M. Yousem and Carol Motta; *Genitourinary Imaging*, by Ronald J. Zagoria, William W. Mayo-Smith, and Julia R. Fielding; *Obstetric and Gynecologic Ultrasound*, by Karen L. Reuter and T. Kemi Babagbemi; *General and Vascular Ultrasound*, by William D. Middleton; *Spine Imaging*, by Brian Bowen, Alfonso Rivera, and Efrat Saraf-Lavi; *Musculoskeletal Imaging*, by Joseph Yu; and *Gastrointestinal Imaging*, by Peter J. Feczko and Robert D. Halpert.

David M. Yousem, MD, MBA

When I finished the first edition of this book I said I felt a sense of amazement, wonder, and ecstasy. Having finished the second edition, I again feel tremendously amazed, wonderful, and ecstatic too... but I must confess I also feel an extraordinary sense of relief! It is nine years and two kids later, and it has been an equally delightful, crazy, and interesting journey getting here. The completion of this manuscript continues to be among the highlights of my academic career.

This book provides insight into disease processes that affect the brain and the central nervous system through the interpretation of a spectrum of imaging studies. In addition to conventional MR and CT imaging, this edition also focuses on using advanced imaging techniques that have evolved over the last decade, including spectroscopy, diffusion imaging, perfusion imaging, functional imaging, CTA, MRA, and conventional catheter angiography to discriminate one entity from among the other possible diagnoses. In this second edition, close to 90% of the cases are new, and approximately 45 new diseases are presented that were not covered in the first edition. Because the book is organized to present a spectrum of diseases in a case-by-case format, you can pick it up and read it when you find those free moments (without losing your place), or you may read it for hours on end if you choose to (and I hope you do)!

It feels like a million hours have been sunk into the preparation of the images, in the hopes of providing a feast for your eyes! The questions and answers that accompany each case provide insight into the significance of specific imaging findings, as well as the application of advanced imaging techniques in addressing specific questions about disease processes. The questions also provide "pearls of wisdom," as well as pertinent information regarding the clinical, pathologic, and demographic aspects of the diseases covered herein. Following the questions and answers of each case presentation, there is a discussion that provides imaging, clinical, and pathologic information. A cross-reference to the second edition of *Neuroradiology: THE REQUISITES* that refers you to pages in that text and provides additional information about the anatomy, physiology, and/or demographics of the disease process(es) presented in each case is also provided. Lastly, a reference(s) is provided for each case. I have tried either to cite a "classic" article for a particular entity or to highlight current literature that provides new pearls or future directions in developing imaging techniques.

To all of the fellows, residents, and medical students with whom I have studied and continue to study with, your enthusiasm and desire to learn make completing a book like this exciting. Equally paramount in the desire to complete this manuscript, I especially want to recognize all the patients who have allowed me to help in their care. It is through your willingness to share parts of yourselves with me that I learn every day... not just about radiology, but about compassion, humanity, spirituality, and the importance of family and friends. And it goes without saying that David Yousem's relentless nudging, including early morning phone calls while on my family vacation in Lake Placid, kept the midnight oil burning and the early morning coffee brewing when my battery needed charging. Thanks Davey!

This book is intended as an educational tool for a wide spectrum of readers, including radiology residents and neuroradiology fellows (great for exam preparation), practicing general radiologists, neuroradiologists, and medical students. Because of its clinical approach, it is also a focused teaching tool for colleagues and trainees in related fields such as neurology and neurosurgery. I hope you find the pages that follow informative, educational, and fun!

Laurie A. Loevner, MD

I would not have completed this seemingly endless project without the help and support of many people. It has been nine years since the completion of the first edition of this book and when it comes to my husband Steve, some things never change! In addition to successfully running his own demanding business, he still endures my demanding work schedule, which begins before the sun rises and too frequently ends long after it sets. He still endures my scholarly travels that frequently take me cross-country and overseas. And I admit he still endures nights with no planned dinner on the table . . . and accepts the "take-out bring-in" delights from our friendly neighborhood Japanese steakhouse. Furthermore, the kitchen counters and tabletops throughout our home remain cluttered by his standards, and in addition to my computer, the second edition of this book has again taken over his too. But some things have clearly changed! Eight years ago we packed up and left the city for the suburbs, no small task for a guy who spent his whole life in the city! But truth be told, and with cautious optimism, he woke up the first morning in his new country home and declared "I've adjusted!" Our son Ben who was an infant at the time the first edition of this book was published is now a precocious 10-year-old boy, and we had the addition of another bundle of joy, our now seven-year-old son Alex. And not only is Steve a supportive husband, but he is a most devoted and loving father. Parenting in our home is a dual career, and is done with little outsourcing.

As I had mentioned in the preface of the first edition of my book, I was pregnant with my first son Ben while writing it. Because I dictated the first draft of that book, I was concerned that Ben's first words might be "MR imaging" or "signal intensity." I am very happy to report that in fact Ben's first word was "Mom." In utero life for Alex was not too dissimilar from Ben's. He also endured numerous cross-country and overseas business trips, long work hours, and lots of medical jargon. And it only seems appropriate that his first word was "Dad." I want to thank both of my darling sons for all that they have given and continue to give to me. It is not until one sees herself through the eyes of her children that she truly understands the kind of person that she wants to be and should be. I love you to infinity and back.

I want to thank all my students and trainees who make my career interesting and rewarding, and who continue to keep me on my toes! Their curiosity was invaluable in guiding what cases to include in the book as well as in formulating many of the questions. In particular, I would like to thank two medical students who are now blossoming into radiology residents, John Oh and Summer Kaplan, with whom I have worked and continue to work closely. They have been very helpful and understanding, and have so capably worked around my whirlwind days. Special thanks to John Woo, Alex Mamourian, Ronald Wolf, Rajeev Polasani, Ann Kim, James Chen, Jason Sweet, Arastoo Vossough, and the Children's Hospital of Philadelphia for providing some of the interesting and challenging cases in the book.

To my friends and colleagues in the Neuroradiology section at the University of Pennsylvania—Linda Bagley, Nick Bryan, Michele Bilello, Herb Goldberg, Eddie Herskovits, Bob Hurst, Ann Kim, Frank Lexa, Alex Mamourian, Neerav Mehta, Elias Melhem, Paulo Nucifora, Mary Scanlon, Arastoo Vossough, John Weigele, Ronald Wolf, and John Woo—thanks for making life at PENN so interesting. A special thanks to Lori Ehrich who has and continues to be a great source of support. To Bobby G. (Robert Grossman) my close friend and mentor, I finally get it—you

ACKNOWLEDGMENTS

can't please everybody all the time! Accepting this well known fact does make life just a little easier. I thank you and Lissy for your support and friendship. To David Yousem, they say times change and we change with time, but not in ways of friendship. There have been many life and career changes over the last decade, but the basic shared values that define our friendship will never change. Thanks also for your mentorship. I hope I have done you proud again! I thank you and Bobby G. for my academic roots and my academic wings. To my devoted administrative assistants, Carol and Sebrina, I thank you for allowing me to live on the edge. I want to thank the Elsevier staff, in particular Elizabeth Hart, Rebecca Gaertner, and Nancy Lombardi thanks for your patience (really!) and enthusiastic support. I know I can be a tough nut to crack, but this project could not have made it without your extraordinary efforts.

And where would I be without my family and friends. To my parents and the entire Loevner gang, you continue to support and take pride in my crazy existence! And you continue to journey with me each step of the way in my medical odyssey. To Jon Goodman and Hilary, Sandy and Arnie Galman, Rebecca and Ted Perkins, Donna and Jerry Slipakoff, and Lori and Rich Kracum—thank you for hanging with us, and for taking care of Steve and the boys when work takes me away. And I think it is safe to say that while Steve's handicap used to be golf, he has turned into a respectable player. Arnie, the money he won from you should buy some seriously fine wine! Thank you! To Cindy Urbach, Natalie Carlson, and Lynne Secatore, I may not see or speak to you nearly as often as I should, but your friendship over the years has been very important to me, and I think about you and yours often. To Ella Kazerooni—girl we do have fun! I thank you again for your strong friendship, support, inspiration, and wisdom. And a very special thanks to my loving and devoted husband Steve, and our beautiful sons Benjamin and Alexander, I couldn't have done this without you. Your support and understanding have been nothing short of spectacular.

To the readership, a very special thanks. I hope you enjoy this second edition of *Brain Imaging Case Review*!

Opening Round

Mod lentadstrate A

A_2

lot l lentadstrate

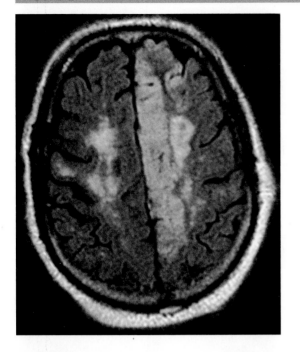

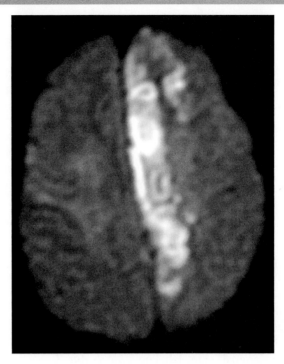

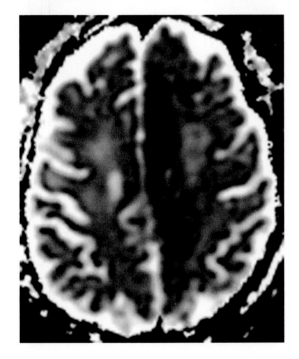

1. From which segment of the anterior cerebral artery do the medial lenticulostriate arteries arise?

2. Which structures does the recurrent artery of Heubner supply?

3. The lateral lenticulostriate arteries arise from which major vessel?

4. What is the major cause of cerebrovascular ischemic disease?

Acute Anterior Cerebral Artery Infarct

1. The A1 segment.   *Med lenticulostriate A.*

2. The head and anteromedial caudate nucleus and the anterior limb of the internal capsule. *A₂*

3. The middle cerebral artery.   *lat lenticulostriate*

4. Atherosclerosis.

References

Kazui S, Sawada T, Naritomi H, Kuriyama Y, Yamaguchi T: Angiographic evaluation of brain infarction limited to the anterior cerebral artery territory, *Stroke* 24:549–553, 1993.

Naidich TP, Firestone MI, Blum JT, Abrams KJ, Zimmerman RD: Zonal frequency analysis of infarct extent. Part II: anterior and posterior cerebral artery infarctions, *Neuroradiology* 45:601–610, 2003.

Taoka T, Iwasaki S, Nakagawa H, et al: Distinguishing between anterior cerebral artery and middle cerebral artery perfusion by color-coded perfusion direction mapping with arterial spin labeling, *AJNR Am J Neuroradiol* 25:248–251, 2004.

Cross-Reference

Neuroradiology: THE REQUISITES, 2nd ed, pp 86, 88, 174–187.

Comment

This case shows the characteristic appearance of an acute anterior cerebral artery territory infarct. On FLAIR imaging, there is hyperintensity in the medial left frontal lobe extending to the parietal lobe, with corresponding restricted diffusion demonstrated on diffusion-weighted imaging and apparent diffusion coefficient imaging.

The major cause of ischemic cerebrovascular disease is atherosclerosis. There are several reasons for performing an unenhanced head computed tomography (CT) [and, when necessary, MR imaging] in the setting of an acute stroke. Among the most important are to exclude acute hemorrhage before treatment and to exclude a nonischemic cause for the patient's symptoms. Other lesions may occasionally present with symptoms that mimic a stroke. In patients with a clinical presentation characteristic of an ischemic event, CT is performed to determine whether there is evidence of an acute infarction (early loss of gray–white matter differentiation or sulcal effacement) or associated acute hemorrhage. There has been an increasing role for the use of lytic therapy (intravenous systemic or intra-arterial). Relative contraindications to this treatment include the presence of acute blood and hypodensity on CT in the setting of an acute stroke.

Conventional diagnostic angiography has a secondary role in the evaluation of acute stroke unless intra-arterial thrombolytic therapy is going to be performed. CT angiography or MR imaging or angiography is frequently helpful in answering specific questions, such as whether a hemodynamically significant stenosis is present in the cervical internal carotid artery to determine whether corrective surgery is needed; in younger patients, these modalities may be performed to determine the cause of a stroke (premature atherosclerosis, arterial dissection, or an underlying dysplasia of the vasculature).

Notes

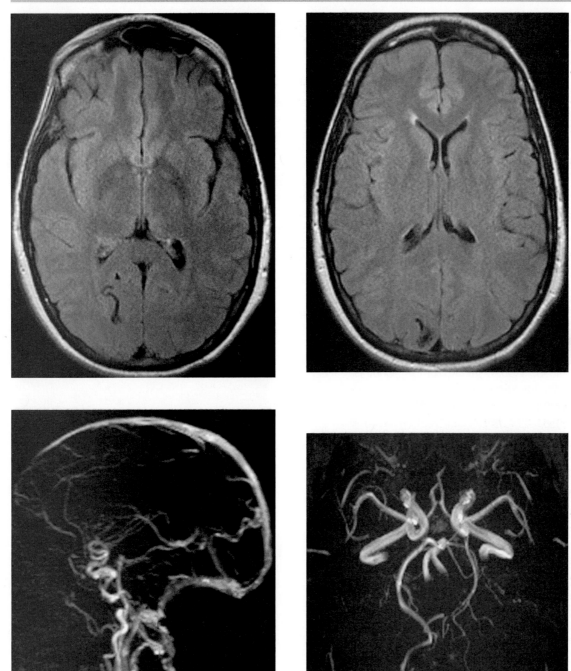

1. What pathophysiology explains why brain tissue around these lesions may be atrophied?

2. What are causes of false-negative findings on angiograms in patients with surgically proven arteriovenous malformations (AVMs)?

3. What is the major vascular supply to the lesion in this case?

4. Where is the venous drainage?

Cerebral Arteriovenous Malformation

1. The "steal" phenomenon, in which there is parasitization of the blood supply from the normal brain preferentially to the AVM. Gliosis in the affected brain may result in focal neurologic symptoms or seizures.

2. Lack of angiographic visualization of a surgically proven AVM may be due to a very small AVM, thrombosis of the AVM, or mass effect related to an associated parenchymal hemorrhage that compresses the AVM and prevents its filling.

3. The posterior cerebral artery.

4. The deep and superficial venous systems, confirmed by conventional angiography.

References

Nussel F, Wegmuller H, Huber P: Comparison of magnetic resonance angiography, magnetic resonance imaging, and conventional angiography in cerebral arteriovenous malformations, *Neuroradiology* 33:56–61, 1991.

Suzuki M, Matsui O, Kobayashi K, et al: Contrast enhanced MRI for investigation of cerebral arteriovenous malformations, *Neuroradiology* 45:231–235, 2003.

Cross-Reference

Neuroradiology: THE REQUISITES, 2nd ed, pp 234–238.

Comment

An AVM is a vascular nidus made up of a core of entangled vessels fed by one or more enlarged feeding arteries. Blood is shunted from the nidus to enlarged draining vein(s), which terminate in the deep or superficial venous system. This case shows a right occipital lobe AVM. Phase-contrast MR venography shows veins draining both deep and superficially, and time-of-flight MR angiography shows that the right posterior cerebral artery is enlarged because it supplies feeding arteries to the small AVM.

Spetzler and Martin have proposed a grading scheme for AVMs that accurately predicts outcome after surgical resection; however, its application to radiosurgery is limited because it does not accurately reflect lesion volume and location. AVMs are graded on a scale of I to VI, determined by size (<3 cm, 3–6 cm, >6 cm), pattern of drainage (superficial or deep), and involvement of the cortex (noneloquent or eloquent). Grade I lesions are small and superficial, and do not involve eloquent cortex. On the opposite end of the spectrum, grade VI lesions are usually inoperable.

On unenhanced CT scans, the vascular nidus of an AVM and the enlarged draining veins are usually isodense or hyperdense to gray matter as a result of pooling of blood. Calcification may be present. AVMs enhance and have characteristic serpentine flow voids on MR imaging related to fast flow in dilated arteries, and arterialized flow in dilated draining veins. The estimated annual hemorrhage rate of cerebral AVMs is 2% to 4%. The mean interval between hemorrhagic events is approximately 7 to 8 years.

In lesions associated with an acute parenchymal hemorrhage, phase-contrast magnetic MR angiography best demonstrates the AVM (it subtracts out the signal intensity of the blood products in the hematoma, in contrast to time-of-flight MR angiography). Cerebral angiography shows enlarged feeding arteries, the vascular nidus, and early draining veins. In cases of very small AVMs, early venous filling should be sought on careful evaluation of the angiographic images.

Notes

I   VI

<3   3-6   >6

deep   Super

cortex .   ∅

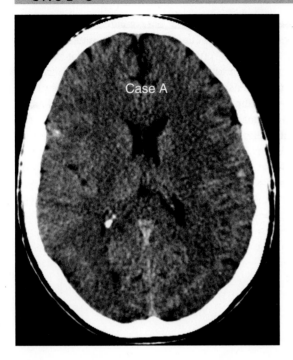

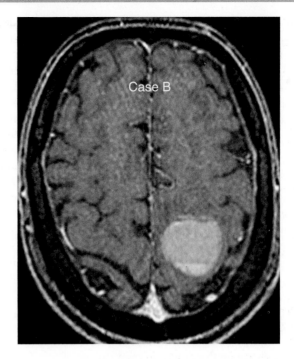

1. What is the most likely diagnosis in both of these cases?

2. What factors may contribute to a lesion appearing hyperdense on unenhanced CT and hypointense on a T2W MR image?

3. How often is metastatic disease to the brain a solitary metastasis?

4. What type of metastases may be associated with little or no edema such that they are missed on T2W imaging, and only readily identified on gadolinium-enhanced images?

Hemorrhagic Metastases—Melanoma

1. Hemorrhagic metastatic disease.

2. Acute hemorrhage, high cellularity, high protein concentration, and the presence of calcification.

3. Approximately 30% to 50% of patients with brain metastases have an isolated lesion on imaging.

4. Cortical metastases. *p edema*

References

Gaul HP, Wallace CJ, Crawley AP: Reverse enhancement of hemorrhagic brain lesions on postcontrast MR: detection with digital image subtraction, *AJNR Am J Neuroradiol* 17:1675–1680, 1996.

Cross-Reference

Neuroradiology: THE REQUISITES, 2nd ed, pp 148–152.

Comment

Metastatic disease is among the most common causes of intracranial masses in adults. Metastases are frequently multiple; however, in 30% to 50% of cases, they may occur as an isolated lesion on imaging. Enhanced MR imaging is clearly more sensitive than CT in detecting cerebral metastases. Metastases are typically circumscribed masses that demonstrate variable enhancement patterns (solid, peripheral, or heterogeneous). Metastases are often associated with a disproportionate amount of surrounding edema, manifested on T2-weighted (T2W) images as increased signal intensity in the adjacent white matter.

Metastases typically occur at the gray–white matter interface because tumor cells lodge in the small-caliber vessels in this location. Metastatic deposits may also involve the cortex. With cortical metastases in particular, edema may be absent such that metastatic lesions could be missed on T2W imaging. Therefore, it is essential to give intravenous contrast to patients with suspected brain metastases. Studies examining the role of double- and triple-dose gadolinium have shown that although higher doses of contrast reveal more lesions than does a single dose, this often occurs in patients whose standard-dose study already shows more than one metastasis. Therefore, management in these patients is not affected, and multidose gadolinium is neither indicated nor recommended. In patients with no or a single metastasis on single-dose gadolinium, higher doses of contrast material yield additional metastases in fewer than 10% of cases.

Hypointensity (T2W shortening) may be seen with blood products, as a result of the paramagnetic effects of melanin, and when lesions have calcification, hypercellularity, or proteinaceous material. In both cases seen here the patients have hemorrhagic metastatic melanoma. Case A has multiple small metastases at the gray–white junction, and Case B has a solitary large hemorrhagic metastasis with a fluid-hemorrhage level. Even though vascular tumors, such as renal and thyroid carcinoma, and melanoma have a propensity to bleed, because breast and lung carcinoma are much more common, a hemorrhagic metastasis is more likely to be related to one of these cancers. In the case of a single cerebral hemorrhagic mass, primary brain tumors, such as glioblastoma multiforme, should be considered.

Notes

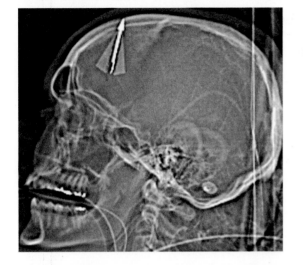
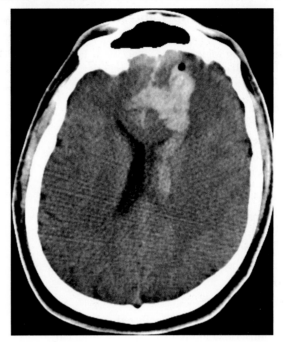
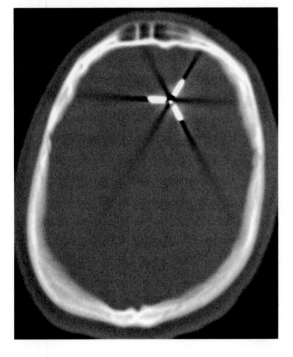

1. What are the imaging findings?
2. What would Quincy, MD, say about how this injury occurred?
3. What is the most effective, efficient way to work up a penetrating head injury?
4. What are the potential causes of the intracranial air?

Penetrating Brain Injury—Bow and Arrow Injury

1. There is a penetrating injury to the head, with frontal lobe hemorrhage and intraventricular extension, and there is a retained bow and arrow.

2. I may be dating myself (Quincy, MD, was a famous TV forensic pathologist), but he would say that this was a self-inflicted injury. The trajectory was entrance under the mandible (submental) and then through the anterior cranial fossa.

3. Computed tomography: short and sweet!

4. Intracranial air may be due to a communication with the extracranial compartment (open fracture) or may indicate an associated fracture through an adjacent paranasal sinus or the temporal bone.

Reference

Kriet JD, Stanley RB, Grady MS: Self-inflicted submental and transoral gunshot wounds that produce nonfatal brain injuries: management and prognosis, *J Neurosurg* 102:1029–1032, 2005.

Cross-Reference

Neuroradiology: THE REQUISITES, 2nd ed, pp 255–256.

Comment

Penetrating injuries cause lacerations of the brain and its coverings (dura), and these are associated with gunshot wounds, stab wounds (in this case, a self-inflicted bow and arrow injury), or displaced bone fragments. With penetrating wounds, there is a risk of injury to critical structures that are in the trajectory of the penetrating object. Brain injury may result in functional and cognitive losses, depending on the region of the brain injured. Injury to the intracranial arteries may result in dissection, occlusion, hemorrhage, or pseudoaneurysm formation. Pseudoaneurysms must always be considered because they have a very high incidence of delayed hemorrhage. Occasionally, arteriovenous fistulas may occur intracranially, although these are more common with penetrating injuries to the neck. Computed tomography is the most efficient and effective way to assess a penetrating brain injury rapidly. It can determine whether a surgical emergency is present, such as an acute hemorrhage with mass effect necessitating acute surgical decompression. It also shows the location and extent of retained foreign bodies. Computed tomography also identifies intracranial air that is due to communication with the extracranial compartment (open fracture) or may indicate an associated fracture through an adjacent paranasal sinus or the temporal bone. Trapped intracranial air may result in tension pneumocephalus related to a one-way ball valve mechanism that causes gradual expansion of the intracranial air and mass effect on the adjacent brain.

Notes

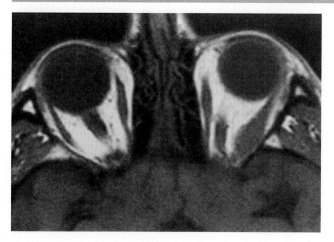 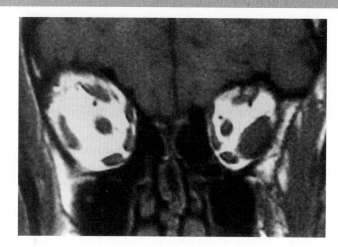

1. What is the most common cause of nontraumatic proptosis?

2. What extraocular muscle is not involved in isolation in thyroid ophthalmopathy?

3. What is the typical clinical presentation of orbital pseudotumor?

4. What structure runs between the superior rectus muscle and the optic nerve?

Orbital Pseudotumor

1. Thyroid ophthalmopathy.

2. Isolated lateral rectus muscle involvement does not occur in thyroid ophthalmopathy.

3. Pain, decreased ocular motility, and proptosis.

4. The superior ophthalmic vein.

Reference

Jacobs D, Galetta S: Diagnosis and management of orbital pseudotumor, *Curr Opin Ophthalmol* 13:347–351, 2002.

Cross-Reference

Neuroradiology: THE REQUISITES, 2nd ed, pp 504–505.

Comment

Orbital pseudotumor, also known as idiopathic orbital inflammatory syndrome, is a nonspecific inflammation of unknown etiology that involves the contents of the orbit. Clinical presentations include proptosis, pain, and decreased ocular motility. This disorder is usually unilateral, but may be bilateral in fewer than 10% of patients. Orbital pseudotumor should be considered a diagnosis of exclusion, with evaluation directed at eliminating other causes of orbital disease. Underlying systemic disorders should be considered, including sarcoid, lymphoma, connective tissue disease, Wegener's granulomatosis, and autoimmune disorders. In the early stages of orbital pseudotumor, histologic features are characterized by inflammation and edema, with an abundance of lymphocytes, plasma cells, and giant cells. In the late stages of disease, fibrosis may be abundant. Orbital pseudotumor may present with a spectrum of manifestations, including myositis (as in this case), dacryoadenitis (lacrimal gland involvement), periscleritis (uveal and scleral thickening), or retrobulbar soft tissue abnormality. In myositis, pseudotumor may involve one or more muscles, and unlike thyroid ophthalmopathy, it often involves the tendinous insertion of the muscle as well as the muscle bellies. When idiopathic inflammation primarily involves the cavernous sinus and the orbital apex, it is referred to as Tolosa-Hunt syndrome. Ophthalmoplegia is secondary to involvement of cranial nerves III through VI in the cavernous sinus.

Because orbital pseudotumor radiologically may appear similar to a variety of disease processes, patient history is important (pseudotumor is classically associated with pain and acute onset). Importantly, there is usually a dramatic response to steroids that may be useful in confirming the diagnosis of pseudotumor.

A small percentage of patients do not respond to steroids and may require radiation or chemotherapy.

Notes

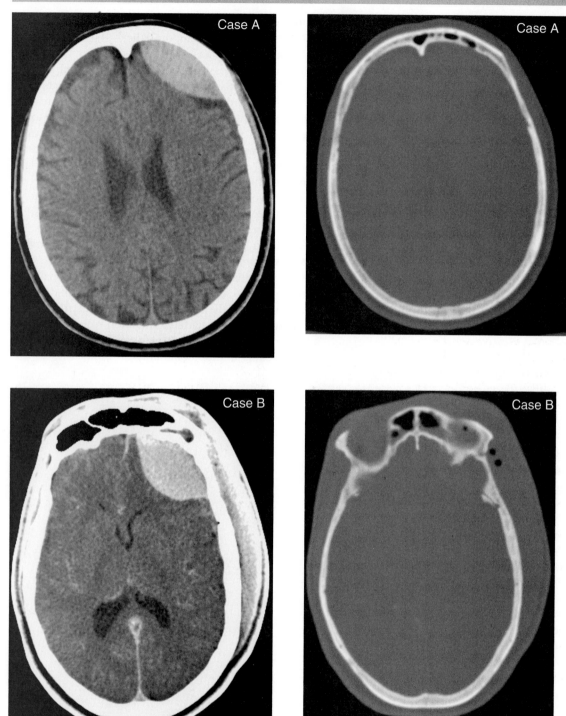

1. What is the cause of a heterogeneous or "swirling" appearance of an acute extra-axial hematoma?

2. What type of extra-axial hematoma is most commonly associated with a skull fracture?

3. What type of extra-axial hematoma runs between the periostium of the inner calvarium and the dura mater?

4. What is the most common cause of an epidural hematoma?

C A S E   6

Acute Epidural Hematoma and Associated Linear Fracture of the Frontal Bone

1. Leakage of serum from the epidural clot or active bleeding. This may also be seen in coagulopathic patients or in patients receiving anticoagulation therapy.

2. Epidural hematoma.

3. Epidural hematoma.

4. Arterial laceration (usually middle meningeal artery) related to an overlying calvarial fracture. Venous tears can result in epidural hematomas in fewer than 20% of cases, and are more common in the posterior fossa.

Reference

Hamilton M, Wallace C: Nonoperative management of acute epidural hematoma diagnosed by CT: the neuroradiologist's role, *AJNR Am J Neuroradiol* 13: 853–859, 1993.

Cross-Reference

Neuroradiology: THE REQUISITES, 2nd ed, pp 247–248.

Comment

There are two anatomic types of extra-axial collections or hematomas, namely, subdural and epidural. On CT imaging acute epidural hematomas are hyperdense extra-axial masses that can usually be distinguished from acute subdural hematomas based on their shape and location relative to the calvarial sutures. Epidural hematomas are usually confined by the cranial sutures because the dura is adherent to the periostium of the inner calvarium. This results in the biconvex or lenticular shape of these collections, which occur between the dura and the periostium. In comparison, subdural hematomas cross sutural boundaries because they occur deep to the dura, occupying the space between the dura and pia arachnoid along the surface of the brain. As a result, subdural collections or hematomas tend to be crescentic in shape, similar to a sliver of the moon.

In the vast majority of cases (80%–90%), epidural hematomas are secondary to a direct laceration of the meningeal arteries (most commonly the middle meningeal artery) by an overlying skull fracture. In a small percentage of cases (<20%), epidural hematomas occur due to tearing of meningeal arteries in the absence of a fracture. This is most commonly seen in children and may be related to transient depression of the incompletely ossified soft calvarium, resulting in laceration of a meningeal artery. Most arterial epidural hematomas occur in the temporal region, although they may be seen in the frontal or temporoparietal regions.

Epidural hematomas due to venous rather than arterial injury are much less common. Venous epidural hematomas are usually due to tearing of a dural venous sinus related to an underlying calvarial fracture. They are most common in the posterior fossa as a result of injury to the transverse or sigmoid sinuses, and are most frequently seen in the pediatric population. Unlike arterial epidural hematomas and subdural hematomas, venous epidural hematomas may extend across the tentorium cerebelli and involve both the supratentorial and infratentorial compartments. These may also occur in a paramedian location over the cerebral convexities or in the middle cranial fossa as the result of a tear in the superior sagittal or sphenoparietal sinus, respectively.

Other traumatic sequelae that may occasionally be seen in the setting of epidural hematomas include pseudoaneurysms of the meningeal artery (most commonly the middle meningeal artery) and arteriovenous fistulas if a fracture lacerates both the middle meningeal artery and vein, resulting in their communication.

Notes

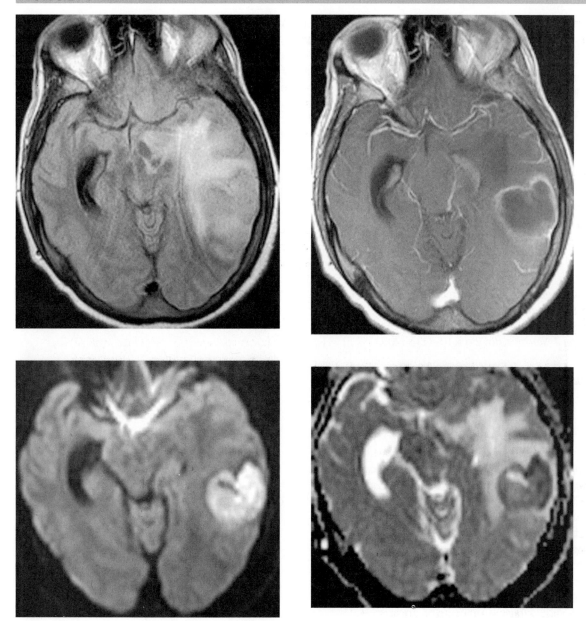

1. What is the differential diagnosis of a ring-enhancing mass?

2. Regarding necrotic metastases, what is the most common cell type to result in this appearance?

3. Pyogenic brain abscesses are most commonly acquired through what routes of transmission?

4. What are the most common cerebral locations for pyogenic brain abscesses?

Pyogenic Brain Abscess

1. Primary brain tumor, metastatic disease, pyogenic brain abscess and other infectious processes, demyelinating disease, a maturing hematoma, and radiation necrosis.

2. Metastatic adenocarcinoma.

3. Either by direct spread from otorhinologic infections (sinusitis, otomastoiditis), or more commonly by hematogenous dissemination from a systemic source.

4. The frontal and parietal lobes in the distribution of the middle cerebral artery.

References

Nowak DA, Rodiek SO, Topka H: Pyogenic brain abscess following haematogenous seeding of a thalamic haemorrhage, *Neuroradiology* 45:157–159, 2003.

Tung GA, Rogg JM: Diffusion-weighted imaging of cerebritis, *AJNR Am J Neuroradiol* 24:1110–1113, 2003.

Cross-Reference

Neuroradiology: THE REQUISITES, 2nd ed, pp 282–284.

Comment

The development of a pyogenic brain abscess may be divided into four stages: early cerebritis (1–3 days), late cerebritis (4–9 days), early capsule formation (10–13 days), and late capsule formation (14 days and after). The length of time required to form a mature abscess varies from approximately 2 weeks to months. In the mature abscess there is a collagen capsule that is slightly thinner on the ventricular side than on the cortical margin (this may be related to differences in perfusion). The presence of a dimple or small evagination pointing toward the ventricular margin from a ring-enhancing lesion should raise suspicion for an abscess. This is also important because intraventricular rupture and ependymitis may occur and are associated with a very poor prognosis. In the presence of a mature abscess, there is relatively little surrounding cerebritis and edema compared with the early stages of abscess formation. A circumferential rim that is isointense to slightly hyperintense to white matter on unenhanced T1-weighted (T1W) images and hypointense on T2-weighted (T2W) images may be present around a brain abscess. This appearance may be related to the presence of collagen, free radicals within macrophages, or small areas of hemorrhage. Diffusion-weighted imaging may be very helpful because the high signal intensity of the pus-filled necrotic center may show restricted diffusion (low apparent diffusion coefficient), differentiating an abscess from a necrotic neoplasm, as in this case.

The management of a mature brain abscess is surgical drainage and antibiotic therapy. Cerebritis and early abscesses may be managed with antibiotics and should be followed closely both with MR imaging and clinically for signs of improvement or deterioration. Successful management monitored with serial MR imaging examinations will show a decrease in the surrounding edema, mass effect, and associated enhancement. It is important to remember that radiologic findings lag behind clinical improvement, and enhancement may persist for months. Resolution of an abscess may result in an area of gliosis with small calcifications.

Notes

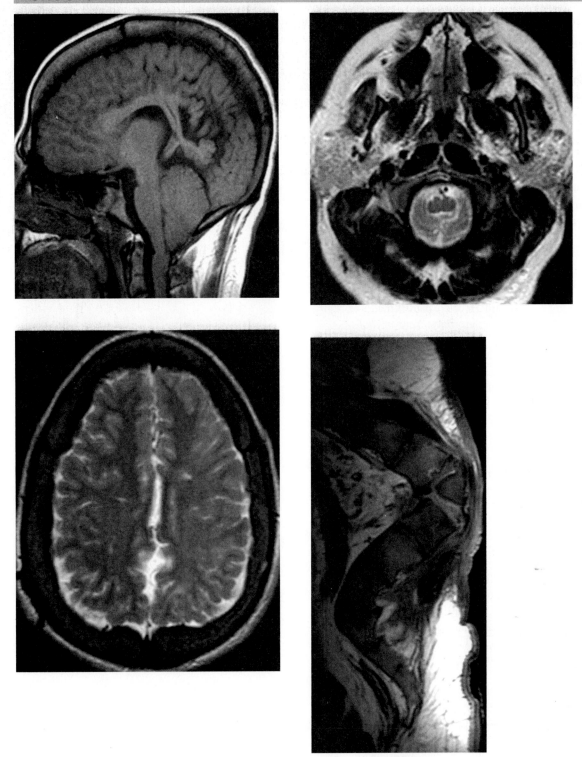

1. What is the in utero abnormality that results in these malformations?

2. What cervical spine anomalies are frequently associated with these malformations?

3. Which type of Chiari malformation is associated with a myelomeningocele?

4. What are the accepted normal limits in children and adults for the inferior position of the cerebellar tonsils relative to the foramen magnum?

Chiari II Malformation with Associated Anomalies

1. Dorsal induction–neural tube defects.

2. Klippel-Feil syndrome, partial fusion of C2 and C3, occipitalization of the atlas (partial or complete fusion of C1 with the occiput), and a hypoplastic ring of C1.

3. Chiari II malformation.

4. Cerebellar tonsil position relative to the foramen magnum varies with age. In children younger than 10 years of age, 6 mm or less is considered within normal limits. In adulthood, 3 mm or less is within normal variation. Typically, low-lying tonsils that are within normal variation are rounded in contour.

References

Naidich TP, McLone DG, Fulling KH: The Chiari II malformation: part IV. The hindbrain deformity, *Neuroradiology* 25:179–197, 1983.

Royal SA, Tubbs RS, D'Antonio MG, Rauzzino MJ, Oakes WJ: Investigations into the association between cervicomedullary neuroschisis and mirror movements in patients with Klippel-Feil syndrome, *AJNR Am J Neuroradiol* 23:724–729, 2002.

Cross-Reference

Neuroradiology: THE REQUISITES, 2nd ed, p 437.

Comment

Chiari malformations typically occur during the first 3 to 4 weeks of gestational life and are dorsal induction–neural tube defects. Chiari II malformations are the most common symptomatic form. This case illustrates all of the findings of Chiari II malformations, which are reviewed later. In Chiari II malformations, the vermis, cerebellar tonsils, and medulla herniate into the foramen magnum and upper cervical canal. The cerebellar hemispheres wrap around the brain stem, the cerebellar vermis herniates up through the tentorial incisura ("towering cerebellum"), and the tectum is "beaked." The fourth ventricle is elongated and displaced inferiorly. Chiari II malformations are associated with a spectrum of supratentorial anomalies, including dysgenesis of the corpus callosum (most commonly splenial anomalies) and heterotopias or sulcation abnormalities, as illustrated in this case. Myelomeningoceles are seen in virtually all Chiari II malformations, and more than 50% of cases are associated with syringohydromyelia.

In Chiari I malformations, there is herniation of the cerebellar tonsils, which are pointed (peg-like) in configuration into the cervical spinal canal. The remainder of the cerebellum, brain stem, and fourth ventricle are normal in location. Syringohydromyelia is frequently seen in Chiari I malformations; myelomeningoceles are not.

Chiari III malformations have the same findings as Chiari II malformations, but also include herniation of the posterior fossa contents into a high cervical or occipital encephalocele. There is no associated lumbosacral myelomeningocele.

Notes

II Myelomeningocele
III

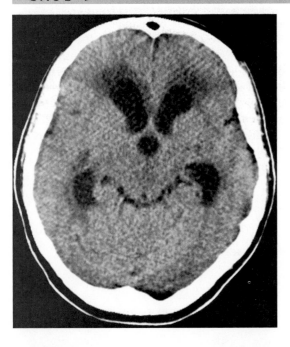

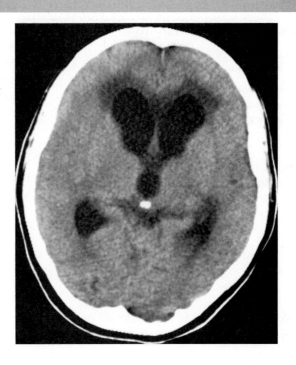

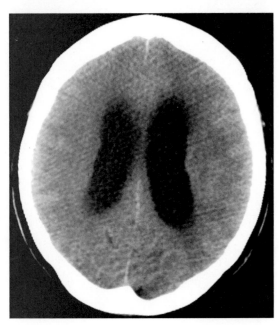

1. What is the primary imaging finding?

2. What secondary imaging findings in this case indicate that this condition is acute?

3. Is this communicating or noncommunicating?

4. What is the management of communicating hydrocephalus?

6mm

Acute Hydrocephalus Secondary to Meningitis

1. Marked hydrocephalus.

2. There is hypodensity in the periventricular white matter consistent with transependymal flow of cerebral spinal fluid. There is effacement of sulci.

3. Communicating.

4. Typically, shunting and management of the underlying etiology of the hydrocephalus. In this case, the patient has acute bacterial meningitis.

References

Daoud AS, Omari H, Al-Shayyab M, Abuekteish F: Indication and benefits of computed tomography in childhood bacterial meningitis, *J Trop Pediatr* 44:167–168, 1998.

Gammal TE, Allen MB Jr, Brooks BS, Mark EK: MR evaluation of hydrocephalus, *AJR Am J Roentgenol* 149: 807–813, 1987.

Cross-Reference

Neuroradiology: THE REQUISITES, 2nd ed, pp 374–377.

Comment

Obstructive hydrocephalus can be categorized as communicating or noncommunicating. Noncommunicating hydrocephalus is usually related to obstruction of CSF flow at some level within the ventricular system and is commonly related to neoplasms; however, infection, hemorrhage, cysts, or congenital lesions (synechiae, webs, arachnoid cysts) may be responsible. Communicating hydrocephalus typically results from obstruction of the arachnoid villi, foramen magnum, or tentorial incisura. Common causes of communicating hydrocephalus include inflammation of the meninges, or meningitis (as in this case; the patient has bacterial meningitis); ventriculitis; subarachnoid hemorrhage; and carcinomatous meningitis. Obstruction of the arachnoid villi in these situations is usually related to high protein concentrations, hemorrhage, or hypercellularity of the CSF. In bacterial meningitis, purulent exudate in the subarachnoid spaces over the cerebral convexities and in the basilar cisterns, where CSF flow is more sluggish, results in impairment of CSF absorption by the arachnoid villi.

On imaging, dilation of the anterior third ventricle in particular is most indicative of hydrocephalus and should not be present in normal subjects or in patients with atrophy. Elevation and thinning of the corpus callosum, best appreciated on sagittal MR imaging, is present in more than 75% of cases of hydrocephalus. Acute hydrocephalus may manifest with hypodensity around the ventricles on CT scans or hyperintensity on MR T2W images in the periventricular white matter due to transependymal flow of CSF. Compensated long-standing hydrocephalus usually does not present with this finding. Treatment of noncommunicating and communicating hydrocephalus is different. Noncommunicating hydrocephalus often requires surgery (e.g., resection of a neoplasm), whereas communicating hydrocephalus is usually treated with shunting.

Notes

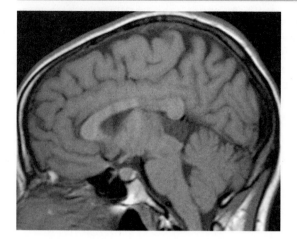

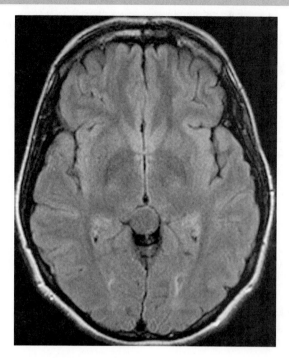

1. What is the finding on these MR images?

2. What are the symptoms and signs of Parinaud's syndrome?

3. What is the anatomic relationship of the pineal gland relative to the velum interpositum?

4. What is the primary cell of the pineal gland?

Pineal Cyst

1. There is a homogeneous cyst of the pineal gland.

2. Parinaud's syndrome represents paralysis of upward gaze, lid retraction, and abnormal pupillary reactions.

3. The pineal gland is directly below the splenium of the corpus callosum. The velum interpositum is rostral and dorsal to the pineal gland and contains the internal cerebral veins, which join to form the vein of Galen.

4. The primary cell is the pineal parenchymal cell, or pinocyte, a specialized neuron related to retinal rods and cones. The pinocyte is surrounded by fibrillary astrocytes.

Reference

Barboriak DP, Lee L, Provenzale JM: Serial MR imaging of pineal cysts: implications for natural history and follow-up, *Am J Roentgenol* 176:737–743, 2001.

Cross-Reference

Neuroradiology: THE REQUISITES, 2nd ed, pp 161–162.

Comment

The pineal gland develops during the second month of gestation as a diverticulum in the diencephalic roof of the third ventricle. Pineal cysts are common incidental findings on MR imaging of the head obtained for unrelated indications, seen in 1% to 4% of patients. In autopsy series, cystic lesions of the pineal gland have been found in 20% to 40% of specimens. Masses of the pineal gland may cause mass effect on the tectum and the aqueduct, resulting in paralysis of upward gaze (Parinaud's syndrome) and hydrocephalus or headache, respectively. However, even large pineal cysts rarely are symptomatic. Pineal cysts are variable in size, and 50% of cysts identified on MR imaging are larger than 1 cm. Studies have shown that, overall, the majority of cysts do not change in size; however, small changes in size (increases and decreases) have been noted. Enlargement of these cysts may be due to increased cyst fluid or intracystic hemorrhage. Rare cases of pineal apoplexy have been reported in which there may be sudden death as a result of intracystic hemorrhage and acute hydrocephalus.

Pineal cysts are less common in young children and are usually seen in middle-aged adults, suggesting that these cysts may develop in late childhood or adolescence and later involute. Pineal cysts are homogeneous on MR imaging. They are typically well demarcated and round or oval, and have a thin or imperceptible wall. On proton density–weighted and FLAIR imaging (as in this case), the cyst contents are frequently hyperintense relative to cerebrospinal fluid. Nodular enhancement of the wall should not be present with cysts. Asymptomatic, larger cysts may cause tectal deformity.

Notes

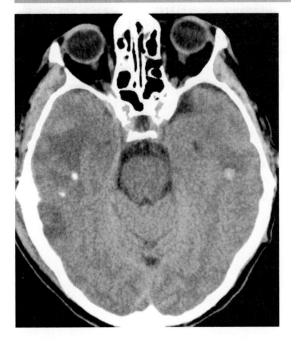 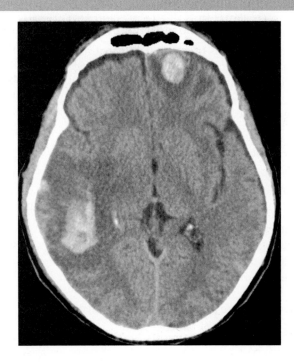

1. What are the findings and what is the diagnosis?

2. What are characteristic locations of cortical contusions in the setting of acceleration–deceleration injuries?

3. What are potential causes of blood–fluid levels in a traumatized brain?

4. What structures on a head CT normally enhance after intravenous administration of contrast material?

Hemorrhagic Contusion—Closed Head Injury

1. There are multiple regions of intraparenchymal high density consistent with hemorrhage, and associated surrounding edema. The pattern of intracranial hemorrhage is consistent with multiple contusions in the setting of closed head injury.

2. The anterior and inferior temporal and frontal lobes, as well as the posterolateral temporal lobes and the occipital poles.

3. Hemorrhage into injured necrotic brain or blood dyscrasias (abnormal coagulation).

4. Structures without a blood–brain barrier (choroid plexus, pituitary stalk, pineal gland, mucous membranes, extraocular muscles), and the blood vessels of the cavernous sinuses. It is important to be able to determine whether images are contrast enhanced because acute hemorrhage has a similar density to iodinated contrast material.

Reference

Oertel M, Kelly DF, McArthur D, et al: Progressive hemorrhage after head trauma: predictors and consequences of the evolving injury, *J Neurosurg* 96: 109–116, 2002.

Cross-Reference

Neuroradiology: THE REQUISITES, 2nd ed, pp 254–255.

Comment

Hemorrhagic contusions are among the most common traumatic brain injuries. Contusions represent petechial hemorrhages in the cortex that may extend into the adjacent white matter and are frequently associated with adjacent subarachnoid blood. They tend to occur along the superficial surfaces of the brain and are the result of acceleration (boxing) and deceleration forces (motor vehicle accident with head impact, such as against the steering wheel or side window) that cause the brain to rub along surfaces where there are prominent osseous ridges or dural reflections. The anterior and inferior portions of the temporal and frontal lobes, the posterolateral temporal lobes, and the occipital poles are typically contused in acceleration–deceleration injuries, as in this case. The surfaces of these portions of the brain rub against the floor and anterior walls of the anterior and middle cranial fossae, sphenoid wings, temporal bones, and petrous ridges. Hemorrhagic contusions may also occur in the setting of penetrating trauma (gun and knife club-type injuries, depressed skull fractures, or iatrogenic causes). Contusions may also occur along the convexities of the cerebral hemispheres adjacent to the midline as a result of the brain rubbing against the rigid falx or the surface of the inner table of the calvaria.

Imaging findings will depend on when the patient is imaged relative to the time of injury. In the acute setting, hemorrhages are hyperdense and are frequently associated with surrounding hypodensity that represents edema. Acute hemorrhagic contusions are hypointense on T2W, FLAIR, and gradient echo MR imaging, with surrounding high signal intensity due to edema. Long-term follow-up shows resolution of the hemorrhage, encephalomalacia in the area of traumatized brain, and hemosiderin in the contusion bed.

Notes

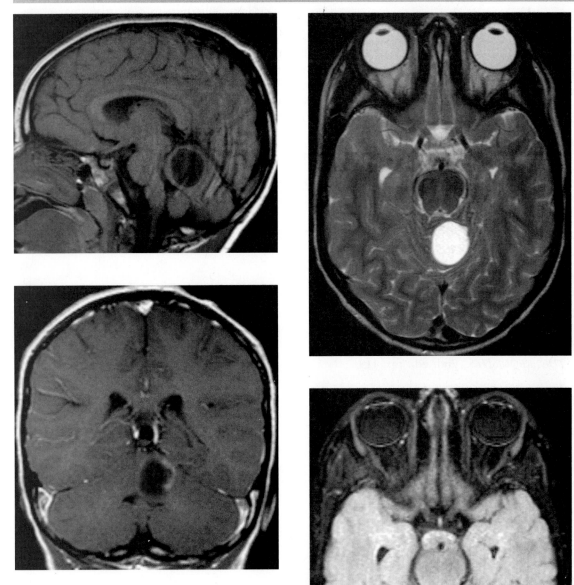

1. What is the typical clinical presentation of pediatric posterior fossa masses?

2. In a pediatric patient, what is the most likely diagnosis?

3. How do you distinguish this neoplasm from a hemangioblastoma?

4. What disorder is associated with pilocytic astrocytomas involving the visual pathway?

Juvenile Pilocytic Astrocytoma of the Cerebellum

1. Symptoms related to mass effect and hydrocephalus, including headache, vomiting, and ataxia.

2. Pilocytic astrocytoma.

3. Age is the best predictor, with juvenile pilocytic astrocytomas usually presenting before the age of 20 years and hemangioblastomas after the age of 20 years. If there are multiple lesions or abnormal vessels or vascularity associated with the enhancing portion or nodule, hemangioblastoma is more likely.

4. Neurofibromatosis type 1.

Reference

Viano JC, Herrera EJ, Suarez JC: Cerebellar astrocytomas: a 24-year experience, *Child Nerv Syst* 17:607–610, 2001.

Cross-Reference

Neuroradiology: THE REQUISITES, 2nd ed, pp 119, 121–123, 132.

Comment

Astrocytomas are the most common intracranial tumors in children, accounting for up to 50% of such neoplasms. Approximately two thirds are located in the posterior fossa. Cerebellar astrocytomas and medulloblastomas are the most common infratentorial neoplasms in children. Approximately 80% of all cerebellar astrocytomas in children are of the pilocytic variety. Most patients with pilocytic astrocytomas have normal karyotypes; however, long arm deletions of chromosome 17 have been associated with them as well. It is important that both radiologists and neuropathologists be able to distinguish pilocytic astrocytomas from the less common but more aggressive anaplastic fibrillary types because prognosis and management are distinctly different. Pilocytic astrocytomas represent one of the more benign forms of glial neoplasms and are classified as circumscribed gliomas by the World Health Organization. Histologically, tightly packed, piloid processes arising from tumor cells are typical, as are microscopic and macroscopic cysts. Eosinophilic granular bodies and Rosenthal fibers (astrocytic processes) are also present. The prognosis is usually excellent after surgical management. Conversely, higher-grade infiltrative astrocytomas have a poor prognosis.

Pilocytic astrocytoma has a characteristic appearance. Typically, these tumors are well-circumscribed masses that usually arise within the cerebellar hemisphere (but may arise in the midline or vermis, as in this case), with a unilocular cyst and an enhancing solid mural nodule.

Usually the cystic component follows the signal characteristics of CSF on all MR imaging pulse sequences. The wall of the cyst does not usually enhance; however, rim enhancement of the cyst can occur and may be related to enhancement of normal adjacent cerebellar parenchyma. Calcification and hemorrhage are uncommon in juvenile pilocytic astrocytomas.

Notes

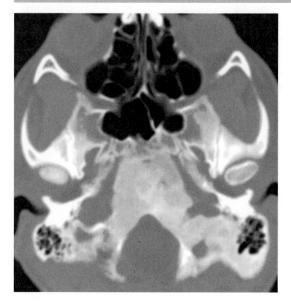 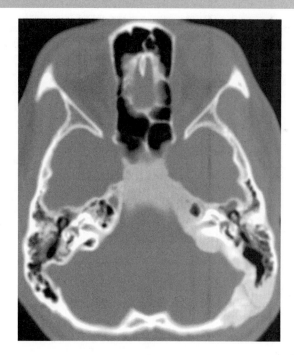

1. What is the most common extraskeletal manifestation in this disorder?

2. What laboratory abnormality is often seen in fibrous dysplasia and Paget's disease?

3. What are the clinical manifestations of McCune-Albright syndrome?

4. Which bones are most commonly affected in polyostotic fibrous dysplasia?

Fibrous Dysplasia

1. Cutaneous pigmentation (café-au-lait spots).

2. Elevated serum alkaline phosphatase levels.

3. This is a form of polyostotic fibrous dysplasia that occurs in girls and is typically associated with precocious puberty and cutaneous hyperpigmentation.

4. The skull and facial bones (as well as the pelvis and spine).

Reference

Chong VF, Khoo JB, Fan YF: Fibrous dysplasia involving the base of the skull, *AJR Am J Roentgenol* 178: 717–720, 2002.

Cross-Reference

Neuroradiology: THE REQUISITES, 2nd ed, pp 513, 662, 864.

Comment

Fibrous dysplasia is a nonhereditary developmental disorder of the bone forming mesenchyma in which osteoblasts do not undergo normal differentiation and maturation. Medullary bone is replaced with fibrous tissue. Trabeculae of woven bone contain fluid-filled cysts embedded in a collagenous fibrous matrix. The etiology is unknown. Fibrous dysplasia may be monostotic (a solitary lesion) or polyostotic (lesions in multiple bones or multiple lesions in one bone). The majority (approximately 75%) of cases are monostotic. Polyostotic fibrous dysplasia more commonly involves the skull and facial bones, pelvis, spine, and shoulder. Polyostotic disease more commonly is unilateral in distribution. Common areas of calvarial involvement include the ethmoid, maxillary, frontal, and sphenoid bones. Involvement of these bones may result in orbital abnormalities such as exophthalmos, visual disturbances, and displacement of the globe. Involvement of the temporal bone may result in hearing loss or vestibular dysfunction. Although Paget's disease may occur in these same locations of the calvaria, unlike fibrous dysplasia, concomitant involvement of the facial bones is less common.

Cutaneous pigmentation is the most common extraskeletal manifestation in fibrous dysplasia. It occurs in more than 50% of cases of the polyostotic form. Cutaneous pigmentation is ipsilateral to the side of bony lesions, a feature that differentiates this disease from pigmentation in neurofibromatosis. The pigmented macules, or café-au-lait spots, are related to increased amounts of melanin in the basal cells of the epidermis. They tend to be arranged in a linear or segmental pattern near the midline of the body, usually overlying the lower lumbar spine, sacrum, upper back, neck, and shoulders.

This patient has features typical of fibrous dysplasia. There is a "ground glass" appearance of the involved clivus, occipital bones, and left temporal bone. There is relative preservation of the cortex and expansion of involved bones that maintain their normal configuration.

Notes

Mandible + maxilla cherubism
facial leontiasis
Myxoma maxabral

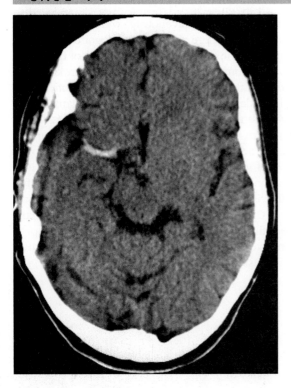 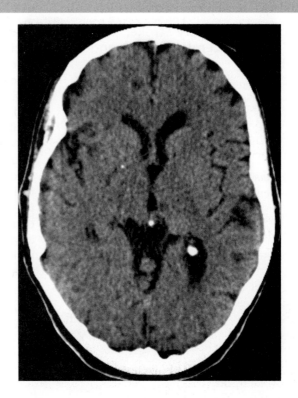

1. What is this patient's clinical presentation?

2. What do these unenhanced CT images show?

3. What is meant by "penumbra" in the setting of acute stroke?

4. What are relative contraindications to thrombolytic therapy?

Acute Middle Cerebral Artery Stroke: "Hyperdense" Middle Cerebral Artery and Insular Ribbon Sign

1. Acute, dense left hemiplegia.

2. Hyperdense middle cerebral artery (MCA) sign (clot in the artery), and early loss of gray–white matter differentiation in the right insula (compare with the normal left insular cortex).

3. "Penumbra" refers to the brain tissue at risk for irreversible ischemia.

4. Acute hemorrhage and a large CT-evident infarction with mass effect.

Reference

Lev MH, Farkas J, Gennete JJ, et al: Acute stroke: improved nonenhanced CT detection—benefits of soft-copy interpretation by using variable window width and center level settings, *Radiology* 213:150–155, 1999.

Cross-Reference

Neuroradiology: THE REQUISITES, 2nd ed, pp 86–88, 183–187.

Comment

An unenhanced head CT scan is the first imaging study for the emergent evaluation of acute stroke because it is readily available, rapidly performed, and sensitive in identifying acute intracranial hemorrhage. Specific imaging findings in the assessment of acute stroke include focal parenchymal hypoattenuation (in the insular ribbon or basal ganglia for MCA infarcts), cerebral mass effect manifested as sulcal effacement, and the "hyperdense" MCA sign. Initial unenhanced CT scans show hypoattenuation in up to 80% of patients with acute MCA strokes, some degree of brain swelling in one third of cases, and hyperattenuation of the MCA in 10% to 45% of patients. In early strokes, thrombolytic therapy may be used either intravenously or intra-arterially with angiographic guidance. Before interventions with clot busters, detection of acute hemorrhage or infarction is important because these conditions are relative contraindications to such therapy.

Ischemic changes on CT scans may be predictive of outcome, response to thrombolytic therapy, and regions likely to become infarcted. In the European Cooperative Acute Stroke Study there was an increased risk of fatal parenchymal hemorrhage in patients with hypoattenuating areas greater than one third the MCA territory or mass effect. Hence, these findings are considered by some to be contraindications to thrombolytic treatment. The National Institute of Neurological Disorders and Stroke (NINDS) Study showed a benefit from thrombolytic agents administered intravenously within 3 hours of stroke onset, and there was a trend toward improved outcome despite initial CT-observed regions of hypoattenuation. The European Cooperative Acute Stroke Study suggested that the subgroup of patients with acute stroke and without demonstrable ischemia on CT scans is also unlikely to benefit from intravenous thrombolysis.

Magnetic resonance imaging is more sensitive than CT in detecting acute infarcts. MR imaging has also shown extension of infarctions on follow-up examinations. It is identification of this "penumbra" (brain tissue at risk for irreversible ischemia) that is at the heart of further development of CT and MR imaging techniques. It is important to protect this tissue from ischemia by applying appropriate interventions. Furthermore, to deliver protective agents, perfusion to this tissue is necessary.

Notes

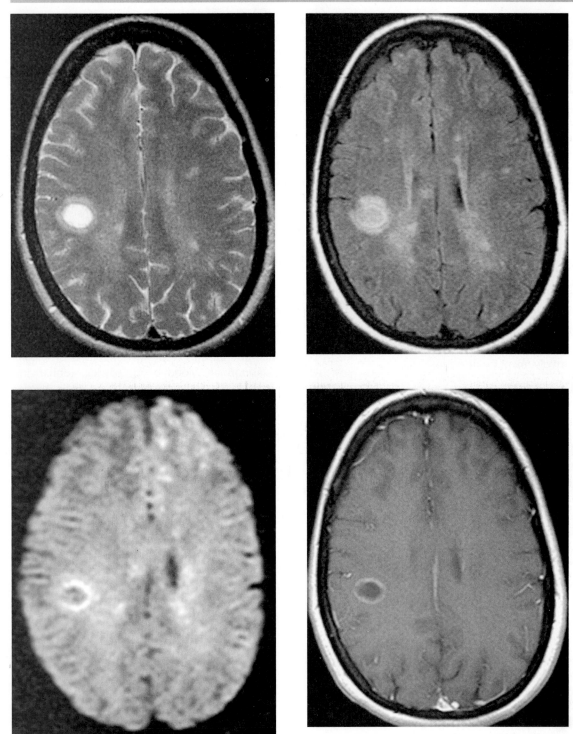

1. What is Balo's concentric sclerosis?

2. What is the pathologic hallmark of an acute, active demyelinating plaque?

3. What percentage of patients with multiple sclerosis have isolated spinal cord disease?

4. What is Devic's disease?

Multiple Sclerosis

1. Balo's concentric sclerosis is an uncommon demyelinating disorder characterized on MR imaging and pathologically as lesions with a laminated appearance that reflect alternating regions of demyelinated and myelinated tissue. Concentric or laminated contrast enhancement is noted around the lesion with a core that is more similar to CSF in signal. This may represent a rare demyelinating disorder separate from multiple sclerosis, but such lesions may be seen in patients with multiple sclerosis.

2. Perivenual inflammatory changes.

3. Approximately 8% to 12%. In patients presenting with myelopathy and an MR imaging study that reveals a cord lesion, multiple sclerosis should be considered. Evaluation should include complete spinal cord and brain MR imaging.

4. Involvement of the spinal cord and/or optic pathways (this may be simultaneous or separated in time) without brain involvement on imaging.

References

Loevner LA, Grossman RI, McGowan JC, Ramer KN, Cohen JA: Characterization of multiple sclerosis plaques with T1-weighted MR and quantitative magnetization transfer, *AJNR Am J Neuroradiol* 16:1473–1479, 1995.

Rovaris M, Comi G, Ladkani D, Wolinsky JS, Filippi M, European/Canadian Glatiramer Acetate Study Group: short-term correlations between clinical and MR imaging findings in relapsing-remitting multiple sclerosis, *AJNR Am J Neuroradiol* 24:75–81, 2003.

Cross-Reference

Neuroradiology: THE REQUISITES, 2nd ed, pp 332–347.

Comment

This case shows numerous white matter lesions with a periventricular predominance. Lesions are also noted in the body of the corpus callosum and the subcortical white matter. The largest lesion in the right frontal white matter has a demarcated central region that follows the signal characteristics of CSF on all pulse sequences, with a peripheral rim, or "halo," that has restricted diffusion (image 3) and enhancement consistent with active demyelination.

Most acquired diseases involving the white matter have similar MR imaging findings. Patient age, history, and physical examination are of paramount importance in limiting the differential diagnosis, which may include vasculopathies (small vessel ischemic disease, vasculitis, hypertension, migraines), demyelinating disease, and inflammatory processes (Lyme disease, sarcoid).

Multiple sclerosis is a chronic inflammatory disease characterized by relapsing or progressive demyelinating plaques in the brain and spinal cord. Multiple sclerosis affects the oligodendrocytes. In the acute stage, plaques have an inflammatory reaction with edema, cellular infiltration, and a spectrum of demyelination. Plaques tend to be in a perivenous distribution. Chronic lesions show astrocytic hypoplasia, resolution of the cellular infiltration, and loss of myelin. The diagnosis of multiple sclerosis is a clinical one; however, MR imaging may be extremely helpful in supporting the diagnosis. On T1W images, plaques may be isointense to hypointense to the brain. Hypointense lesions are chronic and most likely are associated with gliosis and significant myelin loss. FLAIR imaging is particularly helpful in identifying lesions in the periventricular white matter or along CSF interfaces because suppression of water results in increased lesion conspicuity. Lesions at the callosal–septal interface are highly suggestive of multiple sclerosis. Contrast administration allows separation of lesions with an abnormal blood–brain barrier (enhancing lesions) from those with an intact blood–brain barrier (nonenhancing lesions). A lesion that has restricted diffusion also indicates active demyelination. MR imaging is also more sensitive than clinical examination in detecting active disease in clinically silent areas of the brain.

Notes

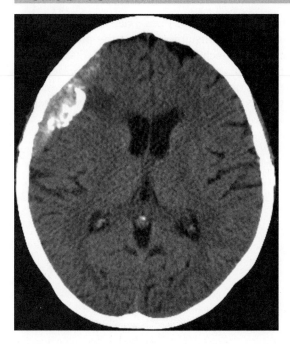
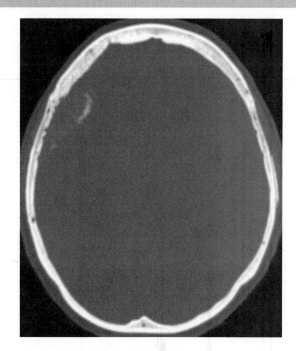

1. Is this mass intra-axial or extra-axial in location?

2. What findings on MR imaging are indicative of an extra-axial mass?

3. Approximately what percentage of meningiomas have calcification?

4. What percentage of meningiomas undergo cystic or fatty degeneration?

Meningioma

1. Extra-axial.

2. A cleft or "pseudocapsule" (composed of CSF, dura, or vessels) that separates the mass from the brain (as in this case); buckling of the gray matter; a mass that is broad-based against a dural surface.

3. Approximately 25% are associated with calcification.

4. Approximately 5% to 10%.

References

Alvernia JE, Sindou MP: Preoperative neuroimaging findings as a predictor of the surgical plane of cleavage: prospective study of 100 consecutive cases of intracranial meningioma, *J Neurosurg* 100:422–430, 2004.

Sheporaitis LA, Osborn AG, Smirniotopoulos JG, et al: Intracranial meningioma, *AJNR Am J Neuroradiol* 13: 29–37, 1992.

Cross-Reference

Neuroradiology: THE REQUISITES, 2nd ed, pp 98–105.

Comment

Meningiomas are the most common intracranial, extra-axial neoplasm. Although there are a variety of histologies, including fibroblastic, angioblastic, syncytial, and transitional types, prognosis is not primarily dependent on the histology but rather on the location of the meningioma. Large meningiomas occurring over the cerebral convexities may be treated with embolization when necessary, followed by surgery without neurologic deficit; in contrast, meningiomas as small as 1 cm involving the cavernous sinus may be very symptomatic and present a more challenging treatment dilemma. Meningiomas occur most commonly in middle-aged women; however, they are also found frequently in men. Most meningiomas are sporadic, isolated lesions. Multiple meningiomas may be familial or may be seen in patients with a history of radiation therapy to the brain, neurofibromatosis type 2, and basal cell nevus (Gorlin-Goltz) syndrome.

On unenhanced CT, more than 50% of meningiomas are hyperdense (as in this case). Approximately 20% to 25% are associated with calcification or a reaction in the adjacent bone (hyperostosis is more common than osteolysis). The bone window in this patient shows that the mass is calcified, but close inspection of the inner cortical table shows secondary "blistering." On MR imaging, meningiomas are often isointense to gray matter on T1W and T2W sequences; however, they may be hyperintense on T2W imaging. Meningiomas typically have avid, homogeneous enhancement. The most important clue to making the diagnosis of a meningioma is in establishing that the mass is extra-axial. One finding consistent with an extra-axial location is the presence of a pseudocapsule, which may represent CSF, dura, or vessels along the pia-arachnoid. Although the presence of an enhancing dural tail is highly suggestive of meningioma, this is a nonspecific finding and may be seen in other disease processes.

Notes

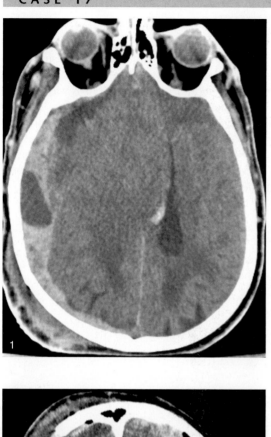

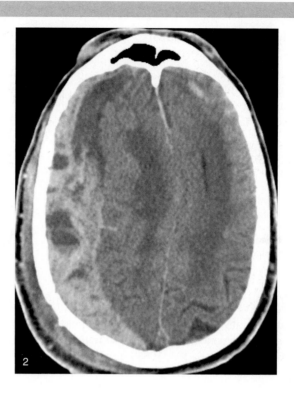

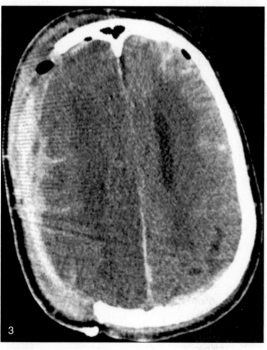

1. What are the most important imaging findings in this patient's presenting head CT (images 1 and 2)?

2. What are the imaging findings in subfalcine herniation?

3. What new finding is evident on this patient's postevacuation head CT (image 3), obtained 6 hours later?

4. What are causes of subacute and chronic subdural hematomas in infants?

Acute Actively Bleeding Subdural Hematoma—Subfalcine Herniation and Stroke

1. There is a large, actively bleeding right convexity subdural hematoma with mass effect including right-to-left subfalcine herniation.

2. Herniation of the cingulate gyrus beneath the anterior free edge of the falx.

3. An acute right anterior cerebral artery infarct secondary to compression of the anterior cerebral artery from subfalcine herniation.

4. Birth injury, child abuse, and coagulopathies (eg, vitamin K deficiency).

Reference

Gentry LR, Godersky JC, Thompson B, Dunn VD: Prospective comparative study of intermediate-field MR and CT in the evaluation of closed head trauma, *AJNR Am J Neuroradiol* 9:91–100, 1988, and *AJR Am J Roentgenol* 150:673–682, 1988.

Cross-Reference

Neuroradiology: THE REQUISITES, 2nd ed, pp 86, 88, 152–156, 174–177, 248–251, 261–262.

Comment

Acute subdural hematomas in young patients are usually the result of closed head injury (eg, motor vehicle accident), as in this case. This case shows a large right convexity, acute, actively bleeding subdural hematoma with right-to-left subfalcine herniation complicated by an acute right anterior cerebral artery infarct due to compression of this vessel. The heterogeneous "swirling" appearance within the subdural hematoma is due to active bleeding in this case, but such an appearance can also be related to leakage of serum from the clot in coagulopathic patients or patients receiving anticoagulation therapy. Also noted is subarachnoid blood and left frontal contusion.

Subdural hematomas are typically caused by tearing of the bridging veins that cross the subdural compartment, extending from the pia to the venous sinuses. Tearing of these veins is due to motion of the brain relative to the fixed dural sinuses. Most subdural hematomas are located along the supratentorial convexities; however, they may also occur in the posterior fossa and along the tentorium cerebelli.

Imaging features of subdural hematomas on CT scans depend on their age. Acute (hours to days old) hematomas are typically hyperdense "crescentic" extracerebral collections. Subacute (days to weeks old) hematomas tend to be isodense to gray matter; therefore, it is easy to miss them on a quick glance at a CT scan. To avoid missing this finding, compare the size of the sulci over the left and right cerebral convexities. Absence of sulci or asymmetric sulci should raise suspicion. Always check that the sulci extend to the inner table of the calvarium, and evaluate the gray–white matter interface for inward buckling. Chronic (weeks to months old) hematomas are usually hypodense. Fluid levels within these hematomas may be caused by interval bleeding. Calcification along the dural membrane may also occur.

Notes

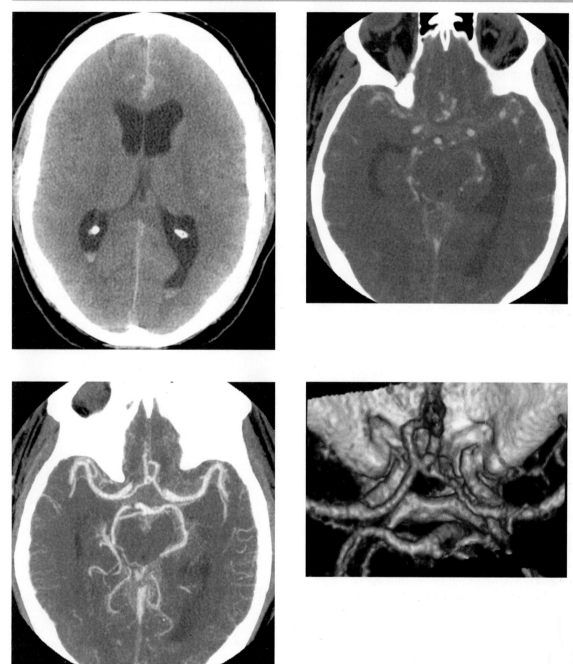

1. What is the diagnosis?

2. What are common anatomic variants associated with aneurysms arising from the anterior communicating artery?

3. At what time after an acute subarachnoid hemorrhage is symptomatic vasospasm most likely to occur?

4. Aneurysms arising from what arteries may be associated with an acute-onset pupil involving third nerve palsy?

Acute Subarachnoid Hemorrhage—Rupture of an Anterior Communicating Artery Aneurysm

1. Acute subarachnoid hemorrhage with rupture of an anterior communicating artery aneurysm.

2. A hypoplastic A1 segment is most common. Other anatomic variants include duplication or fenestrations of the anterior communicating artery and azygous variation of the anterior cerebral arteries.

3. Between the fifth and twelth days. *vaso spasm*

4. The posterior communicating artery, and less frequently, the superior cerebellar artery. Pupillary dilation, ptosis, and strabismus may be present due to compression of cranial nerve III.

References

Jayaraman MV, Mayo-Smith WW, Tung GA, et al: Detection of intracranial aneurysms: multi-detector row CT angiography compared with DSA, *Radiology* 230:510–518, 2004.

Klisch J, Weyerbrock A, Spetzger U, Schumacher M: Active bleeding from ruptured aneurysms during diagnostic angiography: emergency treatment, *AJNR Am J Neuroradiol* 24:2062–2065, 2003.

Cross-Reference

Neuroradiology: THE REQUISITES, 2nd ed, pp 227–230.

Comment

Saccular (berry) aneurysms represent focal vascular dilations most commonly found at branching points of parent vessels. They are the result of a congenital weakness or deficiency in the elastica and media of the arterial wall. The most frequent sites for ruptured aneurysms include, in descending order of frequency, the anterior communicating artery complex, the origin of the posterior communicating artery, the middle cerebral artery, and the vertebrobasilar circulation. Multiple aneurysms may be present in up to 15% to 20% of cases. Although most aneurysms are sporadic in nature, there is an increased incidence in certain conditions, such as connective tissue disorders or collagen vascular disease (fibromuscular dysplasia, moyamoya disease, Ehlers-Danlos syndrome, and polycystic kidney disease).

The most common clinical presentation of acute subarachnoid hemorrhage is "the worst headache of my life." Acute high-density subarachnoid blood is present on CT in 90% to 95% of cases in the first 24 hours. The sensitivity of CT in detecting acute subarachnoid hemorrhage decreases with time. Detection drops to 80% within 3 days, and to only 30% by 2 weeks. If CT is negative and acute subarachnoid hemorrhage is suspected, a lumbar puncture is performed. Evaluation of a patient with suspected acute subarachnoid hemorrhage should always begin with an unenhanced CT head study.

Patterns of intracranial hemorrhage seen with rupture of anterior communicating artery aneuryms include bilaterally symmetric subarachnoid hemorrhage, hemorrhage within the interhemispheric fissure, frontal lobe hematoma, or septal or intraventricular hemorrhage. This case shows bilaterally symmetric diffuse acute subarachnoid hemorrhage, most notably in the sylvian cisterns and basilar cisterns in a pattern consistent with rupture of an anterior communicating artery aneurysm. There is intraventricular blood and early hydrocephalus. The CT angiography source and maximum intensity projection images show a small aneurysm arising from the anterior communicating artery arising from the junction with the left A1 segment.

Notes

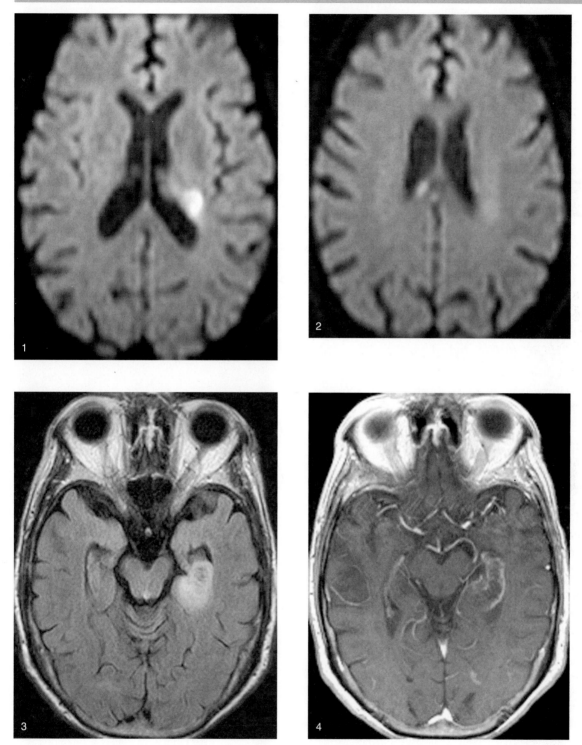

1. What are the imaging findings?

2. What are the types of ischemic stroke?

3. What is the most common type of infarct?

4. What are some hypercoagulable conditions that can cause thrombotic strokes?

Embolic Infarcts (Acute and Subacute)—Atrial Fibrillation

1. Diffusion-weighted images (1 and 2) show acute infarcts and FLAIR and enhanced T1W images (3 and 4) show a subacute infarct in the proximal left posterior cerebral artery territory.

2. Embolic, thrombotic, and lacunar strokes.

3. Embolic infarct.

4. Antiphospholipid antibody syndrome, severe dehydration, oral contraceptives, and protein C or S deficiency, to name a few.

Reference

Min WK, Kim YS, Kim JY, Park SP, Suh CK: Athero-thrombotic cerebellar infarction: vascular lesion-MRI correlation of 31 cases, *Stroke* 30:2376–2381, 1999.

Cross-Reference

Neuroradiology: THE REQUISITES, 2nd ed, pp 174–176.

Comment

Approximately 80% of strokes are ischemic. They can develop in major blood vessels, referred to as "large vessel infarcts," or in small blood vessels, perforating arteries deep in the brain and referred to as "lacunar infarcts." Types of ischemic stroke include embolic infarct, thrombotic infarct, and lacunar infarct. Infarcts of undetermined etiology may account for as many as 30% of cases of stroke.

Cardiac embolism, in which a blood clot forms in the heart and travels to a vessel supplying the brain, accounts for about 20% to 30% of ischemic strokes. Recurrent strokes are most common in patients with a cardioembolic source, and these strokes have the highest 1-month mortality rate. Thrombotic infarcts account for 10% to 15% of strokes and occur when a blood clot forms in an artery that supplies the brain, causing tissue death. These usually occur as a result of plaque buildup from atherosclerosis and develop over time. Lacunar infarctions account for 20% of strokes, and usually occur as a result of small arterial blockage, most often caused by high blood pressure. Lacunar infarcts have a predilection for the basal ganglia, internal capsule, thalamus, pons, and corona radiata. This type of stroke has the best prognosis.

A transient ischemic attack (TIA), defined as a transient neurologic disturbance that usually persists for less than 15 minutes and resolves within 24 hours, is a risk factor for ischemic stroke. In a TIA, arterial blockage occurs briefly and resolves on its own, without causing tissue injury. Approximately 10% of ischemic strokes are preceded by a TIA, and approximately 40% of patients who experience a TIA will have a stroke.

Notes

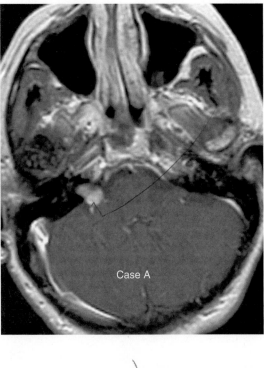

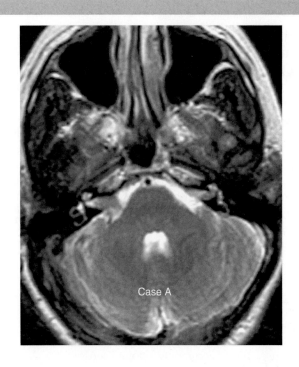

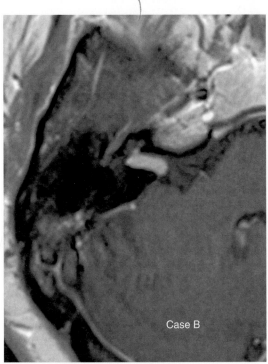

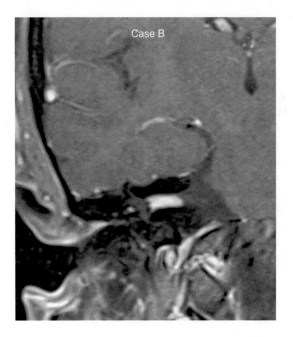

1. What is the classic clinical presentation of these lesions?

2. What structure separates the internal auditory canal into superior and inferior portions?

3. Bilateral vestibular neuromas are seen with what syndrome?

4. Is cystic degeneration seen more commonly with meningiomas or schwannomas?

5-10).

Vestibular Schwannomas of the Internal Auditory Canal

1. Sensorineural hearing loss.

2. The crista falciformis.

3. Neurofibromatosis type 2.

4. Schwannomas.

Reference

Salzman KL, Davidson HC, Harnsberger HR, Glaston-
bury CM, Wiggin RH, Ellul S: Dumbbell schwannomas
of the internal auditory canal, *AJNR Am J Neuroradiol*
22:1368–1376, 2001.

Cross-Reference

Neuroradiology: THE REQUISITES, 2nd ed, pp 106–107.

Comment

Schwannomas arise most commonly along sensory nerves. In the intracranial compartment, cranial nerve VIII is most commonly involved, with neuromas of the superior vestibular nerve being slightly more common than those of the inferior vestibular nerve. Schwannomas of the cochlear nerve are less common. The vestibular branches run in the superior and inferior portions of the posterior internal auditory canal (IAC), whereas the cochlear division runs in the anteroinferior portion of the IAC. Cranial nerves V (trigeminal) and VII (facial) are the next most common sites for schwannomas. When masses involve the IAC or the cerebellopontine angle (CPA), the role of the radiologist is usually in distinguishing a schwannoma from a meningioma because this may affect management. Imaging findings favoring a schwannoma are masses that involve both the cerebellopontine angle and IAC, associated flaring or widening of the porus acousticus (the opening of the IAC), and the absence of dural enhancement. Meningiomas infrequently (5%) extend into the IAC, and when they do, the IAC is not expanded and the enhancement pattern is that of peripheral enhancement "tram-tracking," rather than centrally, as is seen with schwannomas. Meningiomas arising in the CPA may have an associated dural tail (although a dural tail is not diagnostic of a meningioma), and they are usually centered superior or inferior and anterior or posterior to the porus acousticus. In these cases, an enhancing mass involving both the IAC and the CPA (Case A), and a purely intracanalicular tumor with extension to the cochlear aperture (Case B) favor schwannomas.

Schwannomas account for more than 90% of purely intracanalicular lesions. However, only 5% to 15% are located exclusively within the IAC, whereas approximately 15% of vestibular schwannomas present only in the cerebellopontine angle cistern. Approximately 75% of these schwannomas involve both structures. On MR imaging, schwannomas have variable signal intensity, depending on their cellularity, water content, and the presence of necrosis or cystic degeneration. Small lesions (<2 cm) typically are isointense to white matter, and enhancement is often homogeneous, as in these cases. Lesions larger than 2 cm frequently undergo necrosis or cystic degeneration, resulting in heterogeneous enhancement.

Notes

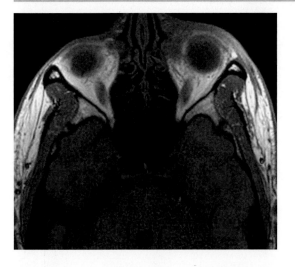

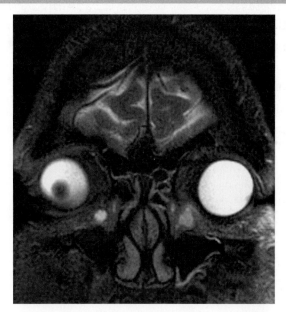

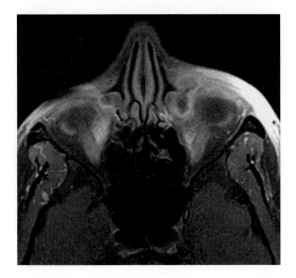

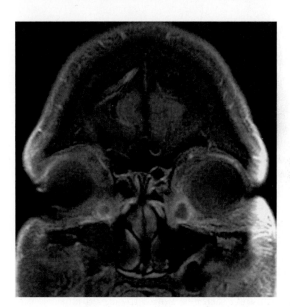

1. What are intracranial complications of this condition?

2. What is the typical clinical presentation of orbital pseudotumor?

3. What is the management of orbital pseudotumor?

4. What is the most common cause of orbital cellulitis?

Orbital Cellulitis and Abscess

1. Cavernous sinus thrombosis, meningitis, and brain abscess.

2. Pain, decreased ocular motility, and proptosis.

3. Steroid therapy.

4. Sinusitis. Dental infections and penetrating eyelid injury are also common predisposing conditions.

Reference

Caruso PA, Watkins LM, Suwansaard P, et al: Odonto-genic orbital inflammation: clinical and CT findings: initial observations, *Radiology* 239:187–194, 2006.

Cross-Reference

Neuroradiology: THE REQUISITES, 2nd ed, pp 504–505, 508–509.

Comment

It is important to distinguish orbital cellulitis that is a medical emergency from preseptal cellulitis. There are many superficial similarities between the two diseases, including lid edema and redness, and pronounced pain on palpation. However, orbital cellulitis manifests with proptosis and extraocular muscle restriction, whereas preseptal cellulitis does not. Also, patients with orbital cellulitis have fever and frequently have decreased vision. Proptosis develops due to intraorbital or postseptal abscess. Ophthalmoplegia results from toxic myopathy and soft tissue edema. Visual loss may occur due to increased intraorbital pressure from abscess and inflammation compressing the optic nerve. There typically will be a precipitating factor, such as sinusitis, penetrating lid trauma, odontogenic infection, or facial trauma. The patient may be systemically ill and have a fever. Orbital cellulitis results from microbial infection with subsequent inflammation of the postseptal orbital tissues. Common organisms include *Staphylococcus aureus*, *Streptococcus pyogenes*, *Streptococcus pneumoniae*, and *Haemophilus influenzae* in children. There is significant potential morbidity and even mortality as a postseptal lid infection can spread through a valveless venous system, leading to cavernous sinus thrombosis, meningitis, and brain abscess.

Often, the degree of proptosis in orbital cellulitis cannot be readily appreciated due to the extreme lid edema. For this reason, CT or MR imaging may be useful not only to identify orbital abscesses, but also to ascertain precipitating sinus involvement and to exclude intracranial extension. Management involves immediate hospitalization with inpatient parenteral antibiotic therapy.

Notes

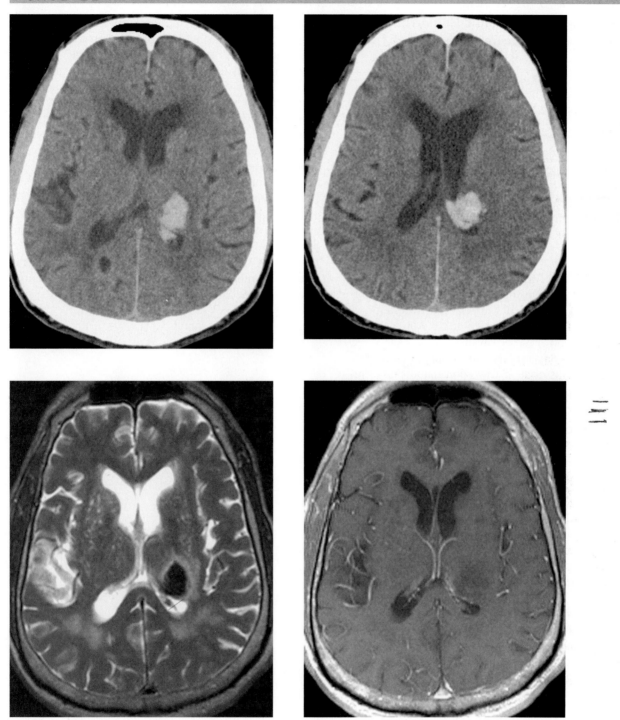

1. What was this patient's clinical presentation?

2. What is the most common cause of acute nontraumatic intracranial hemorrhage in adults?

3. What are the two common vascular causes of acute bilateral thalamic lesions?

4. What are the three most common locations of hypertensive bleeds?

Acute Hypertensive Thalamic Hemorrhage

1. Acute right-sided sensory deficit in the setting of elevated blood pressure (systolic/diastolic blood pressure of 190/110).

2. Hypertension.

3. Infarction of the artery of Percheron (a single perforating artery trunk that supplies the paramedian thalamic arteries) and deep venous thrombosis (internal cerebral veins).

4. The basal ganglia (especially the putamen), the thalamus, and the pons, in descending order of frequency.

References

Chan S, Kartha K, Yoon SS, Desmond DW, Hilal SK: Multifocal hypointense cerebral lesions on gradient-echo MR are associated with chronic hypertension, *AJNR Am J Neuroradiol* 17:1821–1827, 1996.

Tanaka A, Ueno Y, Nakayama Y, Takano K, Takebayashi S: Small chronic hemorrhages and ischemic lesions in association with spontaneous intracerebral hematomas, *Stroke* 30:1637–1642, 1999.

Cross-Reference

Neuroradiology: THE REQUISITES, 2nd ed, pp 216–219.

Comment

This case shows a typical acute left thalamic hypertensive hemorrhage with intraventricular extension. The hematoma is mildly hypointense to brain on T1W imaging and markedly hypointense on T2W imaging. Also noted are extensive sequelae of small vessel ischemic disease in the deep periventricular white matter and in the deep gray matter of the basal ganglia. In adults, the most common cause of intracerebral hemorrhage is hypertension, which accounts for approximately 80% of nontraumatic hemorrhages. Hemorrhages related to high blood pressure have a predilection to involve the deep gray matter (basal ganglia and thalamus) and brainstem, which are supplied by perforating vessels arising from the cerebral and basilar arteries. Rupture of microaneurysms (Charcot-Bouchard) arising from the deep perforating vessels may be the basis of hypertensive hemorrhages in a subset of patients. Approximately two thirds of hypertensive hemorrhages occur in the basal ganglia. Rupture into the ventricular system, as in this case, may be present in up to one half of these patients and is associated with a poorer prognosis.

The MR imaging evaluation of intracerebral hemorrhage is complex, and the imaging appearance is related to a multitude of factors. In hyperacute hemorrhage (within the first 6 hours and rarely captured on MR imaging), hemorrhage is hypointense to brain on T1W imaging and hyperintense on T2W imaging due to oxyhemoglobin in intact red blood cells. In the acute setting (hours to a few days), as in this case, hemorrhage may be isointense to hypointense to brain on T1W and is markedly hypointense on T2W images because of increasing deoxyhemoglobin. The microenvironment of the hematoma is such that oxyhemoglobin molecules rapidly deoxygenate to deoxyhemoglobin. In the early subacute phase (2 days to 1 week), hemorrhage is hyperintense on T1W imaging and hypointense on T2W imaging as a result of high protein concentrations and intracellular methemoglobin. In the late subacute phase (1 week to months), hemorrhage is hyperintense on both T1W and T2W imaging. Finally, in the chronic setting (months to years), hemorrhage is hypointense due to susceptibility effects of hemosiderin and ferritin.

Notes

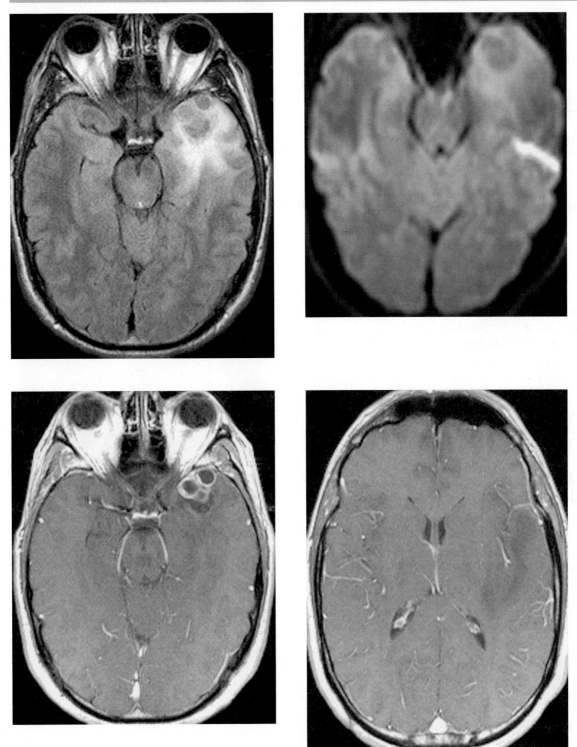

1. What is the differential diagnosis based on the first two images, the axial FLAIR and the corresponding enhanced axial T1W image? The patient's history is new-onset seizure.

2. The diffusion-weighted image makes what diagnosis less likely?

3. What finding on the enhanced images makes a glial neoplasm most likely?

4. What are the three subtypes of infiltrating astrocytic neoplasms?

CASE 23

Infiltrating Astrocytoma—Low Grade

1. Primary glial neoplasm, metastatic disease, and infection or abscess.

2. Brain abscess; however, it is important to recognize that not all abscesses have restricted diffusion.

3. On the enhanced image at the level of the left insula, the left insular gray matter is expanded and nonenhancing, consistent with infiltrating neoplasm.

4. According to the World Health Organization (WHO) classification, infiltrating astrocytic tumors may be divided into three subtypes: astrocytoma, anaplastic astrocytoma, and glioblastoma multiforme (GBM).

References

Bagley LJ, Grossman RI, Judy KD, et al: Gliomas: correlation of magnetic susceptibility artifact with histologic grade, *Radiology* 202:511–516, 1997.

Preul C, Kuhn B, Lang EW, Mehdorn HM, Heller M, Link J: Differentiation of cerebral tumors using multisection echo planar MR perfusion imaging, *Eur J Radiol* 48:244–251, 2003.

Cross-Reference

Neuroradiology: THE REQUISITES, 2nd ed, pp 128–129, 139, 142–143.

Comment

According to the WHO classification, infiltrating astrocytic tumors may be divided into three subtypes: astrocytoma, anaplastic astrocytoma, and GBM. The histologic criteria for these subdivisions depend on many factors, including cellular density, number of mitoses, presence of necrosis, nuclear or cytoplasmic pleomorphism, and vascular endothelial proliferation. GBM typically has all of these histologic features, whereas the lower-grade astrocytomas may only demonstrate minimal increased cellularity and cellular pleomorphism. The presence of necrosis and vascular endothelial proliferation in particular favor GBM, the most malignant of the glial neoplasms.

Astrocytomas are CNS neoplasms in which the predominant cell type is derived from an astrocyte. Two classes of astrocytic tumors are recognized: those with narrow zones of infiltration (pilocytic astrocytoma, subependymal giant cell astrocytoma, pleomorphic xanthoastrocytoma) and those with diffuse zones of infiltration (eg, low-grade astrocytoma, anaplastic astrocytoma, GBM). The latter group may diffusely infiltrate contiguous and distant CNS structures, regardless of histologic stage, and they have a tendency to progress to more advanced grades. Regions of a tumor demonstrating the greatest degree of anaplasia are used to determine the histologic grade of the tumor.

Low-grade infiltrating astrocytomas correspond to WHO grade II, and they grow slowly compared with their malignant counterparts, anaplastic astrocytomas. Several years can intervene between initial symptoms and establishment of the diagnosis of low-grade astrocytoma. Seizures, often generalized, are the initial presenting symptom in approximately one half of patients with low-grade astrocytoma.

Notes

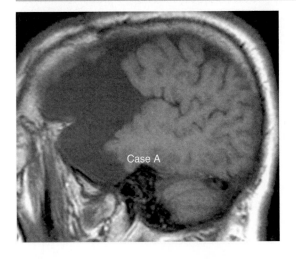

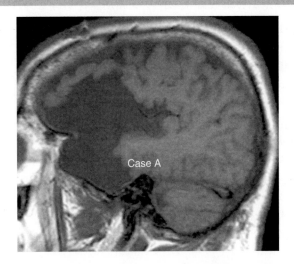

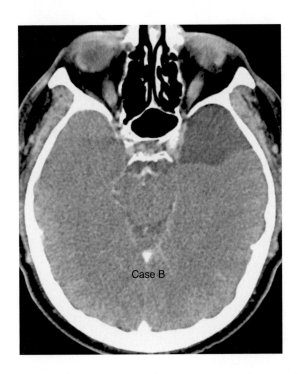

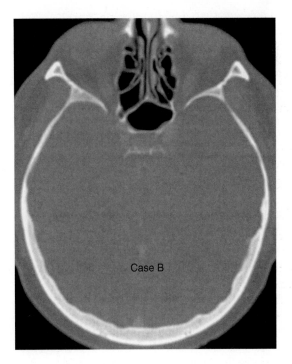

1. Are the masses in these two cases intra-axial or extra-axial?

2. What imaging findings differentiate an extra-axial mass from an intra-axial mass?

3. These lesions are derived from what structure?

4. Is this entity more commonly congenital or acquired?

Arachnoid Cyst

1. Extra-axial.

2. Buckling of the gray and white matter, as is seen of the anterior left frontal and temporal lobes in Case A; the cystic masses are broad-based up against the dural surface and inner table of the calvarium.

3. Meninx primitiva.

4. Congenital.

Reference

Sze G: Diseases of the intracranial meninges: MR imaging features, *AJR Am J Roentgenol* 160:727–733, 1993.

Cross-Reference

Neuroradiology: THE REQUISITES, 2nd ed, pp 413–417.

Comment

Most intracranial arachnoid cysts are congenital and are derived from the meninx primitiva, which envelops the developing CNS. As CSF fills the subarachnoid spaces, the meninx is resorbed. At the same time, a cleft may develop between layers of the arachnoid membrane and may behave as a one-way ball-valve mechanism. There is preferential flow of CSF into this cleft, resulting in formation of a cyst. Less commonly, arachnoid cysts may be acquired as a result of adhesions in the subarachnoid space related to a previous inflammatory process or hemorrhage.

The most common location for an arachnoid cyst is the middle cranial fossa. Other common locations include the cerebral convexities (most commonly, the frontal convexity, as in this case), the basal cisterns (suprasellar, cerebellopontine angle, and quadrigeminal), and the retrocerebellar region. On CT and MR imaging, arachnoid cysts usually follow the density or intensity of CSF, respectively. When large enough, cysts may cause smooth remodeling of the inner table of the bony calvarium and osseous expansion, as is seen of the greater wing of the sphenoid in Case B. There may also be hypogenesis of the underlying brain parenchyma (most commonly described in the temporal lobe with middle cranial fossa cysts). Calcification is unusual, and enhancement should not be present.

The major differential consideration is an epidermoid cyst. On unenhanced T1W images, an internal matrix, although subtle, is typically evident in epidermoid cysts. On FLAIR images, arachnoid cysts follow the signal intensity characteristics of CSF, whereas epidermoid cysts tend to be hyperintense relative to CSF. In addition, on diffusion-weighted images, arachnoid cysts are hypointense (similar to the CSF in the ventricles), resulting from an increased apparent diffusion constant, whereas epidermoid cysts do not have an increased apparent diffusion constant.

Notes

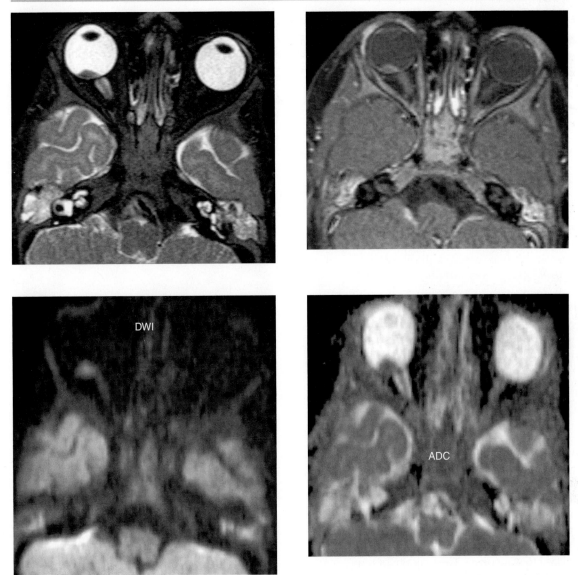

1. What are causes of intraocular calcification in children?

2. What is meant by the "third eye" in trilateral retinoblastoma?

3. How often are retinoblastomas bilateral?

4. What is the most common clinical presentation of retinoblastoma?

Retinoblastoma

1. Retinoblastoma, persistent hyperplastic primary vitreous, toxocaral endophthalmitis, Coats' disease (congenital retinal telangiectasia), and retrolental fibroplasia.

2. The third eye refers to a pineoblastoma of the pineal gland.

3. They are bilateral in 30% to 40% of patients.

4. Leukokoria.

References

Brisse HJ, Lumbroso L, Freneaux PC, et al: Sonographic, CT, and MR imaging findings in diffuse infiltrative retinoblastoma: report of two cases with histological comparison, *AJNR Am J Neuroradiol* 22:499–504, 2001.

Tateishi U, Hasegawa T, Miyakawa K, Sumi M, Moriyama N: CT and MRI features of recurrent tumors and second primary neoplasms in pediatric patients with retinoblastoma, *AJR Am J Roentgenol* 181:879–884, 2003.

Cross-Reference

Neuroradiology: THE REQUISITES, 2nd ed, pp 479–482.

Comment

Retinoblastoma represents the most common intraocular tumor in childhood. The typical clinical presentation is leukokoria, an abnormal pupillary reflex characterized by a "white" pupil. Other common clinical presentations include strabismus, decreased visual acuity, and eye pain (which may be related to glaucoma). The majority of retinoblastomas (98%) present before 3 years of age. Retinoblastomas most commonly represent isolated sporadic tumors; however, they may be heritable in an autosomal dominant pattern. Up to 30% to 40% of patients with retinoblastoma have bilateral tumors; familial disease should be considered in these cases.

Because the radiologic hallmark of retinoblastoma is the presence of intraocular calcification before the age of 3 years, CT remains the best imaging modality for the detection of retinoblastoma. CT is also important in assessing the other eye for small calcifications. MR imaging is not as sensitive in detecting calcification. This case shows a small retinoblastoma of the right eye with restricted diffusion. Not all retinoblastomas (particularly small ones) have calcification, so the absence of calcification does not exclude the possibility of retinoblastoma. MR imaging plays an important role in assessing these patients because retinoblastoma may spread along the nerves and vessels to the retrobulbar orbit, and there may be subarachnoid seeding. Both modes of transmission may result in intracranial dissemination of disease. Therefore, patients with retinoblastoma should be evaluated with MR imaging to determine the extent of disease. A small percentage (<5%) of patients with bilateral retinoblastomas may also have a pineoblastoma of the pineal gland ("third eye").

Notes

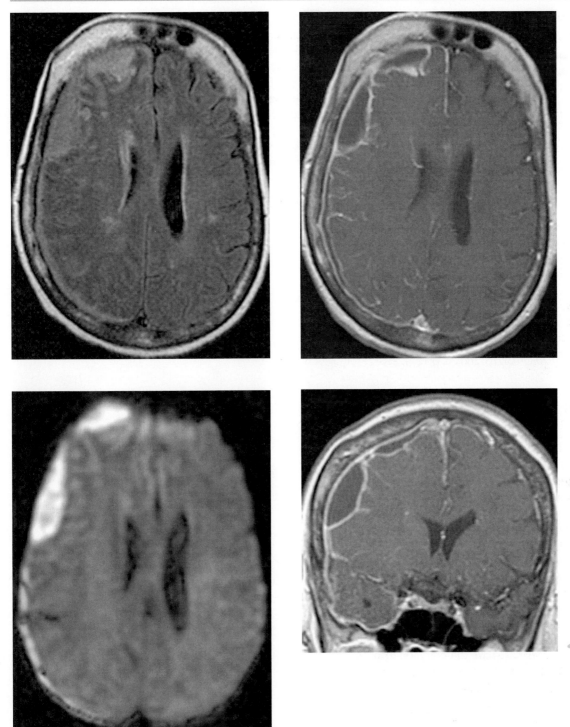

1. What is the diagnosis?

2. Cerebritis, brain abscess, and venous thrombosis are complications more commonly seen with epidural abscesses or subdural empyemas?

3. What type of subdural collection can mimic the MR image findings characteristic of a subdural empyema?

4. What is the standard treatment for subdural empyemas?

C A S E 2 6

Subdural Empyema—Complicated by Cerebritis

1. Subdural empyema complicated by cerebritis. There is meningitis as well, with prominent leptomeningeal enhancement along the right cerebrum.

2. Subdural empyemas.

3. Chronic subdural hematoma.

4. Craniotomy and surgical drainage and antibiotic therapy.

References

Fountas KN, Duwayri Y, Kapsalaki E, Dimopoulos VG, Johnston KW, Peppard SB: Epidural intracranial abscess as a complication of frontal sinusitis: case report and review of the literature, *South Med J* 97:279–282, 2004.

Cross-Reference

Neuroradiology: THE REQUISITES, 2nd ed, pp 274, 276–277.

Comment

Interruption of the arachnoid meningeal barrier by infection leads to the formation of subdural empyemas. Mechanisms by which subdural empyemas may develop include rupture of a distended arachnoid villus into the subdural compartment, thrombophlebitis of a bridging cortical vein, hematogenous spread, and direct spread of an extracranial infection (sinusitis, otomastoiditis, osteomyelitis). These serious infections may also occur as a complication after craniotomy or in patients with meningitis. Epidural abscesses are most frequently caused by direct extension of infection from the paranasal sinuses or mastoid air cells. Of conditions affecting the paranasal sinuses, frontal sinusitis is probably the most common cause of intracranial epidural abscesses and subdural empyemas.

On imaging, these lesions share the common appearance of other extracerebral collections. Epidural abscesses (like hematomas) are contained by the cranial sutures and may cross the midline. In contrast, subdural hematomas do not spread across the midline because they are confined by the falx, allowing differentiation from epidural collections. On MR imaging, these extracerebral infections are usually hypointense to isointense on T1W imaging (depending on the protein concentration and the cellular content) and hyperintense relative to the brain on FLAIR and T2W imaging. Empyemas typically are hyperintense on diffusion-weighted imaging (DWI) and have low apparent diffusion coefficients (ADCs), as in this case, whereas sterile subdural effusions are hypointense on DWI. There is usually prominent enhancement of thickened dura or a dural membrane. Epidural and subdural empyemas may be complicated by cerebritis (as in this case) and intraparenchymal abscess formation. In addition, dural venous or cortical vein thrombosis with venous infarction may occur. In the presence of suspected epidural abscess or subdural empyema, the radiologist (and the clinician!) should search for a site of origin of the infection, as well as its contiguous spread into the intracranial compartment.

Notes

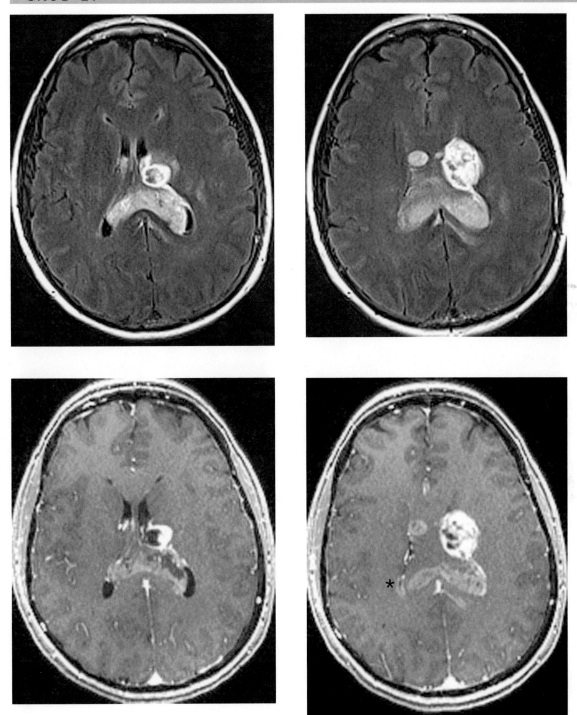

1. What mass lesions have a predilection for involving the corpus callosum?

2. Why is the corpus callosum relatively resistant to edema?

3. What white matter tracts are common conduits of spread of glial neoplasms from one cerebral hemisphere to the contralateral side?

4. What are the MR imaging findings of gliomatosis cerebri?

Glioblastoma Multiforme of the Corpus Callosum—"Butterfly Glioma"

1. Neoplasms (glioblastoma multiforme, lymphoma, and much less commonly, metastatic disease), demyelinating disease, and traumatic shear injury.

2. The corpus callosum is relatively resistant to edema because of the orientation and compact nature of the white matter fibers forming it.

3. The corpus callosum and the anterior and posterior commissures.

4. Gliomatosis cerebri is uncommon and refers to an extensive infiltrating glioma with imaging findings that are usually out of proportion to those on histologic evaluation and clinical examination. MR imaging shows extensive involvement of both the gray and white matter, with mild diffuse sulcal and ventricular effacement. There is often minimal or no enhancement of involved areas.

Reference

Rees JH, Smirniotopoulos JG, Jones RV, Wong K: Glioblastoma multiforme: radiologic-pathologic correlation, *RadioGraphics* 16:1413–1438, 1996.

Cross-Reference

Neuroradiology: THE REQUISITES, 2nd ed, pp 139, 142–143.

Comment

This case demonstrates findings characteristic of a butterfly glioma. There is a complex extensive mass with expansion of the splenium and body of the corpus callosum. Abnormal signal intensity and multiple more defined areas of necrotic mass are noted. Enhanced images better reveal the marked necrosis of certain portions of the tumor. Ventricular ependymal enhancement is shown (*).

Multicentric gliomas are uncommon, occurring in 1% to 5% of cases of GBM. They may represent true separate lesions; however, more often they represent contiguous spread of tumor (which is the case in this patient). Multicentric gliomas may be synchronous (multiple lesions detected at the time of presentation) or metachronous (occurring at different times and pathologically discontinuous). It may occasionally be difficult to distinguish such gliomas from metastases on imaging. When separate lesions are identified, it is important to evaluate for the presence of continuity between the separate lesions on the basis of abnormal T2W signal intensity. However, the connection may not be apparent on imaging and may be seen only on pathologic evaluation.

There is an increased association of multicentric gliomas in neurofibromatosis type I. In this case, a thin rind of ependymal enhancement is present along the body of the right lateral ventricles just medial to the (*). Of the infiltrative astrocytic tumors, GBM is most commonly associated with subependymal and ependymal spread.

Notes

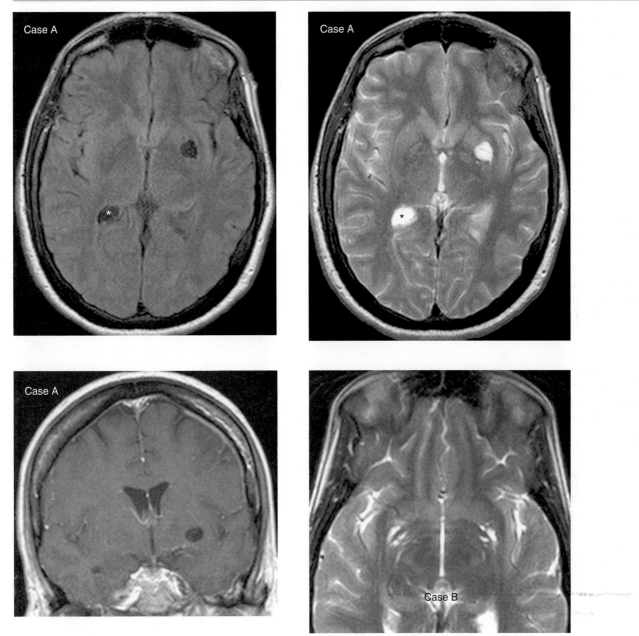

1. Do lacunar infarcts typically occur in the upper half or the bottom half of the putamen?

2. Virchow-Robin perivascular spaces classically occur along what structure?

3. Virchow-Robin spaces are extensions of what CSF space?

4. What CNS infection is associated with dilated Virchow-Robin spaces and pseudocysts within the basal ganglia?

Virchow-Robin Perivascular Spaces

1. The upper half of the putamen.

2. The anterior commissure.

3. The subarachnoid space.

4. *Cryptococcus* (especially in immunocompromised patients).

Reference

Song CJ, Kim JH, Kier EL, Bronen RA: MR imaging and histologic features of subinsular bright spots on T2-weighted MR images: Virchow-Robin spaces of the extreme capsule and insular cortex, *Radiology* 214:671–677, 2000.

Cross-Reference

Neuroradiology: THE REQUISITES, 2nd ed, pp 345–346.

Comment

This case illustrates the typical appearance of a Virchow-Robin perivascular space. Diagnostic considerations for deep basal ganglia lesions primarily include chronic lacunar infarcts; however, developmental cysts, cystic neoplasms, and occasionally chronic infections could potentially share many of the same imaging features. Dilated perivascular spaces can usually be distinguished from a lacunar infarct on the basis of typical imaging findings. Lacunar infarcts tend to occur in the upper half of the putamen, whereas perivascular spaces occur along the inferior half. In addition, whereas perivascular spaces are usually isointense to CSF on all pulse sequences, this is not the case with lacunar infarcts unless they have undergone cystic degeneration. Even when cystic, lacunar infarcts may have a thin surrounding hyperintense rim on T2-weighted and FLAIR images, representing gliosis. Dilated perivascular spaces are not associated with edema or enhancement, have a characteristic location along the anterior commissure, and are frequently bilateral and symmetric (as in Case B). In addition to the basal ganglia, they also frequently occur in the cerebral peduncles, in the subinsular white matter, and in the white matter lateral to and above the lateral ventricles. Frequently, a vessel can be seen coursing through these spaces, as in Case A.

Perivascular spaces are extensions of the subarachnoid space that follow the perforating vessels at the base of the brain into the basal ganglia. Virchow-Robin spaces may range from 1 to 15 mm in size, although occasionally they can be larger. They tend to enlarge with age and in the presence of hypertension. This makes sense because most vessels (including those along the perivascular spaces) become more ectatic under both of these circumstances. In addition, just as the subarachnoid spaces become more prominent with age in that the perivascular spaces are extensions of the subarachnoid space, it makes sense that they enlarge in a similar manner. Given the extension of the perivascular spaces from the subarachnoid space into the brain, they are a conduit for the spread of a variety of inflammatory and neoplastic processes (eg, *Cryptococcus*, sarcoid, carcinomatosis). Incidentally noted are cysts of the choriod plexus (*).

Notes

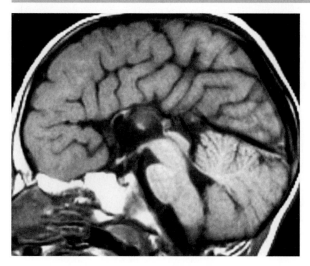
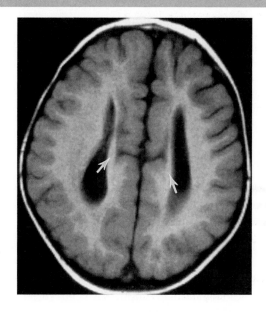

1. What are the names of these structures (*arrows*)?

2. The course of the mesial hemispheric sulci is uninterrupted in a radial manner all the way to the third ventricle because of the absence of what structure?

3. What congenital anomalies are associated with this entity?

4. In primary partial dysgenesis of the corpus callosum, which portions of the corpus callosum are typically spared?

Agenesis of the Corpus Callosum

1. The Probst bundles are the white matter tracts that were destined to cross the corpus callosum. The axons that would usually cross from right to left in the corpus callosum instead form tracts that run anterior to posterior along the medial walls of the lateral ventricles parallel to the interhemispheric fissure.

2. The cingulate gyrus.

3. Lipomas, migrational abnormalities, Dandy-Walker syndrome, Chiari malformations, and holoprosencephaly, to name just a few!

4. The anterior portions (except the rostrum).

References

Lee SK, Mori S, Kim DJ, Kim SY, Kim SY, Kim DI: Diffusion tensor MR imaging visualizes the altered hemispheric fiber connection in callosal dysgenesis, *AJNR Am J Neuroradiol* 25:25–28, 2004.

Quigley M, Cordes D, Turske P, Moritz C, Haughton V, Seth R: Role of the corpus callosum in functional connectivity, *AJNR Am J Neuroradiol* 24:208–212, 2003.

Cross-Reference

Neuroradiology: THE REQUISITES, 2nd ed, pp 424–425.

Comment

Axons arising from the right and left cerebral hemispheres grow into the lamina reuniens (the dorsal aspect of the lamina terminalis), giving rise to the corpus callosum (and the hippocampal commissures). The corpus callosum develops between the 11th and 20th gestational weeks in an organized manner, with formation of the anterior genu first followed in order by the anterior body, posterior body, splenium, and rostrum. Given this pattern of development, in partial dysgenesis of the corpus callosum, the anterior portion is formed and partial dysgenesis affects the posterior portions (posterior body, splenium) and rostrum. In cases in which the splenium is very small or is not visualized, partial dysgenesis of the corpus callosum can be readily distinguished from an insult to a previously fully developed splenium by checking for the presence of the rostrum. If the rostrum is absent, the splenial abnormality corresponds to partial dysgenesis. However, if the rostrum is present, given that it forms after the splenium, a splenial abnormality must have occurred on the basis of an insult resulting in secondary atrophy or volume loss.

Imaging findings in complete agenesis of the corpus callosum include lack of convergence of the lateral ventricles, which are displaced laterally and oriented in a vertical fashion; a high-riding third ventricle (which may form an interhemispheric cyst); and ex vacuo enlargement of the occipital and temporal horns (colpocephaly) related to deficient white matter. The Probst bundles are the white matter tracts that were destined to cross the corpus callosum. The axons that would usually cross from right to left in the corpus callosum instead form tracts that run anterior to posterior along the medial walls of the lateral ventricles parallel to the interhemispheric fissure.

Notes

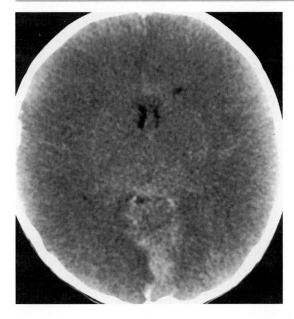

1. In the absence of known significant head trauma, the radiologist must be highly suspicious of what diagnosis in this case?

2. What other cranial manifestation is frequently present in child abuse?

3. What finding in the eyes is characteristic of this diagnosis?

4. What is the cause of a leptomeningeal cyst?

Nonaccidental Trauma—Child Abuse

1. Child abuse (nonaccidental trauma).

2. Skull fractures (particularly depressed or multiple).

3. Retinal hemorrhages.   *Gradient eche / EPI*

4. Skull fracture complicated by a dural tear.

Leptomeningial cyst

References

Demaerel P, Casteels I, Wilms G: Cranial imaging in child abuse, *Eur Radiol* 12:849–857, 2002.

Mogbo KI, Slovis TL, Canady AI, Allasio DJ, Arfken CL: Appropriate imaging in children with skull fractures and suspicion of abuse, *Radiology* 208:521–524, 1998.

Cross-Reference

Neuroradiology: THE REQUISITES, 2nd ed, pp 264–266.

Comment

The presence of skull fractures or intracranial hemorrhage, particularly in children younger than the age of 2 years, in the absence of known trauma to explain such injuries, should raise the suspicion of child abuse (nonaccidental trauma). There are more than 1 million reported cases of child abuse each year, and closed head injury is among the leading causes of morbidity and death in these children. Approximately 10% of neurologic developmental delays can be attributed to nonaccidental trauma. Brain injury may be the result of direct trauma, aggressive shaking, or strangulation or suffocation. There is often little or no evidence of external trauma.

The most common type of intracranial hemorrhage in the setting of child abuse is a subdural hematoma, although subarachnoid hemorrhage, epidural hematoma, intraventricular hemorrhage, hemorrhagic cortical contusion, and diffuse axonal injury are all manifestations of nonaccidental trauma. Bilateral retinal hemorrhages are highly suggestive of child abuse (shaken baby syndrome). In the absence of significant head trauma, the presence of skull fractures (especially bilateral, depressed, or occipital fractures), which are found in as many as 45% of nonaccidental trauma cases, should raise suspicion for child abuse. Because it is not fully developed, the infant skull is extremely pliable and relatively resistant to fracture. In the worse case, diffuse cerebral edema resulting in mass effect and herniation may occur in nonaccidental trauma. Cerebral infarction may occur as a result of strangulation or anoxic-hypoxic injury, and vascular compromise may be caused by intracranial mass effect. Infarctions in multiple vascular territories should be viewed with suspicion.

The radiologist plays an important role in identifying nonaccidental head trauma. The clinical presentation can be nonspecific. The radiologist is sometimes in a position to suggest the possibility of child abuse. It is therefore important to know the spectrum of sometimes subtle imaging findings that may be encountered. Skull x-ray and head CT are regularly used. Repeat or serial imaging may be necessary. Brain MR imaging may contribute to the diagnostic workup, particularly in the absence of characteristic CT findings.

Notes

high: Metaph #   post rib #
       sternal
       scapula
       spinus procen
medium:
       Multiple # of varying age
       depressed skull #

low: clavicle #
      long bone #
      linear skull

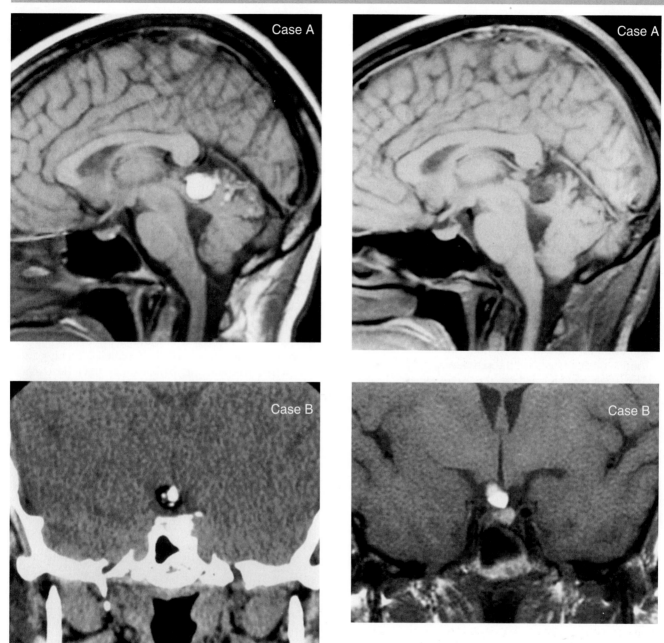

1. What substances are hyperintense on unenhanced T1W imaging?

2. On MR imaging, what artifact is indicative of the presence of fat?

3. What lesions on imaging may contain both fat and calcium?

4. What causes chemical shift artifact?

Dermoid Cysts

1. Fat, proteinaceous material, methemoglobin (hemorrhage), manganese, some calcium, liquid cholesterol, pantopaque contrast, and melanin.

2. Chemical shift artifact. Fat is hyperintense on fast spin echo T2W images. When there is a question, fat suppressed T1W imaging may confirm the presence of fat.

3. Dermoid cysts and teratomas. Lipomas may occasionally have calcification; however, this is less common than with teratomas and dermoid cysts. Calcification may be seen with "tumefactive" lipomas in the interhemispheric fissure that are usually associated with dysgenesis of the corpus callosum, allowing differentiation from dermoid cysts and teratomas.

4. Fat and water precess at slightly different Larmor frequencies (fat precesses more slowly). For correct spatial localization, the Larmor frequency must be uniform throughout the section. Chemical shift artifact results because the position of fat protons relative to water is altered during frequency encoding because its signal is assumed to originate from an incorrect location. Chemical shift artifact on long TR images is identified by the presence of a hyperintense rim and a hypointense rim at opposite margins of the lesion in the frequency encoding direction.

Reference

Calabro F, Capellini C, Jinkins JR: Rupture of spinal dermoid tumors with spread of fatty droplets in the cerebrospinal fluid pathways, *Neuroradiology* 42: 572–579, 2000.

Cross-Reference

Neuroradiology: THE REQUISITES, 2nd ed, pp 116, 543–544.

Comment

Epidermoid and dermoid lesions are developmental anomalies that may be considered congenital inclusions within the neural tube related to incomplete dysjunction of the neuroectoderm from the cutaneous ectoderm. Both lesions are of epidermal origin and may be associated with dermal sinuses or a bone defect. Dermoid cysts and teratomas are typically midline lesions, and both occur more commonly in men. In the intracranial compartment, they may be found in the parasellar or suprasellar region (as in Case B), frontal or basal surface of the brain, and in the posterior fossa. Within the posterior fossa, the superior cerebellar cistern (as in Case A) and fourth ventricular regions are the most common locations.

On CT, dermoids are decreased in attenuation (< -120 Hounsfield units) because of their fat content. Calcification may be seen in the periphery of the lesion. On MR imaging dermoids show the signal characteristics of fat, and chemical shift artifact is frequently present. When necessary, fat suppression can be applied to confirm the diagnosis. Compare the first image in Case A, which is an unenhanced T1W image, with the second image, which is an unenhanced T1W image with frequency selective fat saturation applied. Other common MR imaging findings in these relatively uncommon lesions include the presence of fat-fluid levels within dermoid cysts, and peripheral enhancement. On the other hand, teratomas often have areas of solid enhancement.

Dermoid cysts may contain dermal appendages, including sebaceous and sweat glands, as well as hair follicles. They are often asymptomatic but may enlarge over time due to recurrent glandular secretions and/or recurrent desquamation of the epithelial lining of the cyst. When symptomatic, patients may have headaches. A serious complication of dermoid cysts is their propensity to rupture into the subarachnoid space (as in Case A), which may result in an inflammatory chemical meningitis, vasospasm with ischemia, and even death. It is important on imaging to check for fat droplets within these locations.

Notes

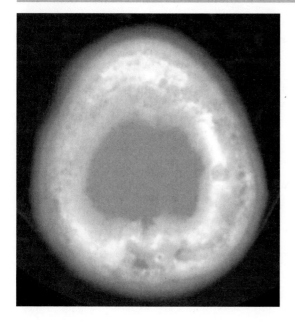
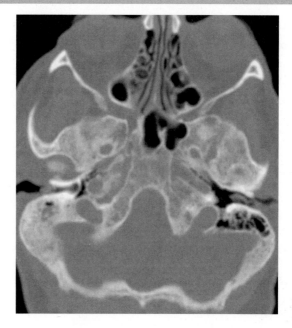

1. What is the differential diagnosis in this case?

2. What finding on the current examination is suggestive of an aggressive process as opposed to Paget's disease?

3. What are the most common causes of skull metastases in children?

4. What is the normal signal intensity on T1W imaging of the calvarial diploic space or marrow in adults?

Calvarial Metastases—Breast Carcinoma

1. Blastic metastases, Paget's disease.

2. Destruction of the cortex. In Paget's disease of the calvaria, there is typically cortical thickening rather than thinning.

3. Neuroblastoma and sarcoma.

4. The marrow normally is hyperintense due to the presence of fat.

References

Loevner LA, Tobey JD, Yousem DM, Sonners AI, Hsu WC: MR imaging characteristics of cranial bone marrow in adults with underlying systemic disorders compared with healthy controls, *Am J Neuroradiol* 23:248–254, 2002.

West MS, Russel EJ, Breit R, Sze G, Kim IKS: Calvarial and skull base metastases: comparison of nonenhanced and Gd-DTPA-enhanced MR images, *Radiology* 174: 85–91, 1990.

Cross-Reference

Neuroradiology: THE REQUISITES, 2nd ed, p 149.

Comment

This case shows mixed blastic and lytic metastases in a patient with breast carcinoma. Prostate carcinoma is the most common cause of blastic metastases in men. Other carcinomas that may present with blastic metastases include breast carcinoma (as shown here) and, less commonly, carcinoid, Hodgkin's lymphoma, and mucinous carcinomas of the lung, colon, and bladder. In older patients, blastic or mixed metastases (blastic and lytic) can be mistaken for the "cotton-wool" appearance of diffuse calvarial Paget's disease. On close examination of a CT scan, these can often be distinguished. In addition to having regions of sclerosis or lysis, Paget's disease is usually associated with thickening of the diploic space, as well as cortical thickening. In contrast, metastatic disease (as in this case) is typically not associated with significant bone expansion, and usually there is not cortical thickening. In this case, there are erosion and destruction of the outer cortical table in the right frontoparietal skull (not cortical thickening), suggesting a more aggressive process.

When there is a question about the diagnosis, particularly in a patient without a known systemic malignancy, a bone scan may be performed. In most instances, both pagetoid bone and metastatic disease will be "hot"; however, the reason to perform the bone scan is not to assess the skull, but rather to assess the remainder of the skeleton for evidence of additional foci of metastatic disease. Paget's disease is not infrequently polyostotic (involving multiple sites); however, plain radiographs of additional pagetoid lesions detected on bone scans usually have a characteristic appearance.

Notes

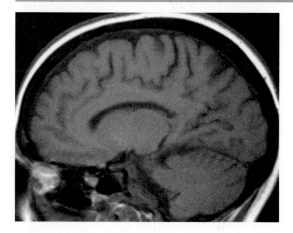

1. What factors determine the normal signal intensity of marrow?

2. What is the normal T1W signal intensity of marrow in children?

3. What is the cause of hypointense marrow on T1W imaging in chronic anemia?

4. What are infiltrative processes that may replace bone marrow?

C A S E   3 3

Chronic Anemia—Diffuse Replacement of Fat in the Calvarial Marrow

1. Ratio of marrow cellularity, fat, and water content.

2. In children, hematopoietic (red) marrow has a high cell:fat ratio and is hypointense.

3. Hematopoietic marrow in response to the chronic blood loss.

4. Primary hematologic malignancies, myelofibrosis, metastatic cancer, and granulomatous diseases, such as sarcoid.

References

Loevner LA, Tobey JD, Yousem DM, Sonners AI, Hsu WC: MR imaging characteristics of cranial bone marrow in adults with underlying systemic disorders compared with healthy controls, *Am J Neuroradiol* 23:248–254, 2002.

Ricci C, Cova M, Kang YS, et al: Normal age-related patterns of cellular and fatty bone marrow distribution in the axial skeleton: MR imaging study, *Radiology* 177:83–88, 1990.

Cross-Reference

Neuroradiology: THE REQUISITES, 2nd ed, p 806.

Comments

The normal signal intensity of marrow is dependent on the ratio of cells, fat, and water. In children, hematopoietic (red) marrow has a high cell:fat ratio and is hypointense. As we age, the amount of fat increases such that by early adulthood the marrow has undergone fatty conversion (yellow marrow), and on T1W images, it is isointense to hyperintense to white matter. Unenhanced T1W imaging is probably the best way to assess for marrow abnormalities, especially because it is part of all standard brain MR imaging protocols.

Hematopoietic (red) marrow is composed of approximately 40% fat, 40% water, and 20% protein; in contrast, inactive fatty (yellow) marrow contains approximately 80% fat, 10% to 15% water, and 5% protein. On unenhanced T1W images, yellow marrow has high signal intensity relative to that of muscle; it approaches the intensity of subcutaneous fat. Cellular red marrow has intermediate signal intensity and may be isointense or slightly hyperintense relative to muscle. Marrow conversion represents a normal process in which yellow marrow gradually replaces red marrow. At birth, marrow is predominantly red in both the appendicular and axial skeletons. In the appendicular skeleton, most of the marrow has undergone conversion by the time an individual is 21 years of age. Residual red marrow is found in the proximal metaphyses of the femurs and humeri. In the axial skeleton, in adults, a larger portion of the marrow remains hematopoietic compared with the appendicular skeleton.

The differential diagnosis of diffuse replacement of the fatty marrow with hypointense tissue (cells or water) includes hematologic malignancies (lymphoma, leukemia, and myeloma); granulomatous disease (sarcoid and tuberculosis); chronic anemias, such as thalassemia, sickle cell disease, or chronic blood loss; and AIDS (hypointense marrow has been attributed to several factors, including chronic anemia and low CD4 counts). Metastases may diffusely replace the marrow (most common with breast carcinoma in women and prostate carcinoma in men). More often, metastatic disease presents with multiple focal lesions.

Notes

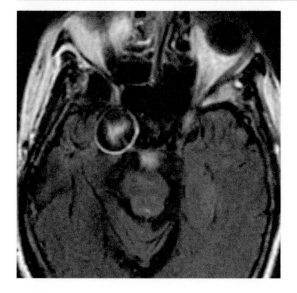 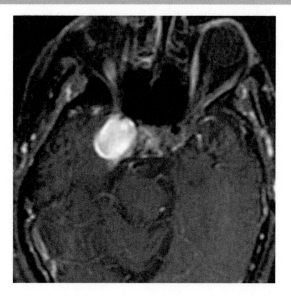

1. What is the clinical presentation of these lesions when they involve the cavernous internal carotid artery?

2. What is the definition of a giant aneurysm?

3. What are common vessels of origin of these lesions?

4. What is the shortcoming or pitfall of catheter angiography in the evaluation of giant aneurysms?

CASE 34

Giant Aneurysm—Middle Cerebral Artery

1. Painful ophthalmoplegia.

2. An aneurysm with a maximal diameter larger than 2.5 cm.

3. Middle cerebral artery, cavernous internal carotid artery, and tip of the basilar artery.

4. Although angiography will adequately assess the patent lumen, it cannot evaluate the true size of these aneurysms because the thrombosed portions are not visualized.

Reference

Jayaraman MV, Mayo-Smith WW, Tung GA, et al: Detection of intracranial aneurysms: multi-detector row CT angiography compares with DSA, *Radiology* 230: 510–518, 2004.

Cross-Reference

Neuroradiology: THE REQUISITES, 2nd ed, pp 224–230.

Comment

The middle cerebral artery bifurcation or trifurcation has a propensity for the development of giant aneurysms. Giant aneurysms may present with subarachnoid hemorrhage or symptoms caused by mass effect (nausea, vomiting, focal neurologic deficits) related to aneurysm size or intraparenchymal rupture or hematoma.

A thrombus may form within large aneurysms and may be a source of distal emboli. Unenhanced CT may show the giant aneurysm as a hyperdense mass. At its periphery there may be heterogeneous density related to the presence of thrombus. On MR imaging, giant aneurysms have a characteristic appearance, as in this case. Findings include signal void consistent with flow in the patent lumen; phase artifact related to flow, as is seen in this case; and heterogeneous signal intensity representing thrombi of varying ages.

Recent investigations with CT angiography in the setting of subarachnoid hemorrhage have shown detection rates for all aneurysms as high as 96%. False-negative findings may be related to CT angiography technique, aneurysm size (especially those < 3 mm), and aneurysm location. Aneurysms originating from the posterior communicating artery, the infraclinoid internal carotid artery, and the ophthalmic artery that are in close proximity to bone now are readily detected due to improved bone subtraction techniques. Advantages of CT angiography include its rapidity, noninvasiveness, ability to provide information about potential neuroangiographic intervention, and ability to provide preoperative information about the relationship of an aneurysm to adjacent bony landmarks. Catheter angiography is still the most commonly used technique and the accepted standard in the assessment of acute subarachnoid hemorrhage.

Notes

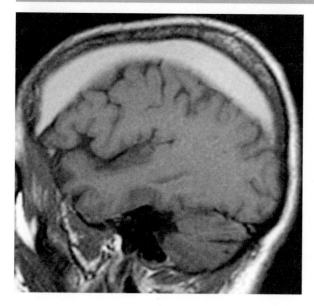
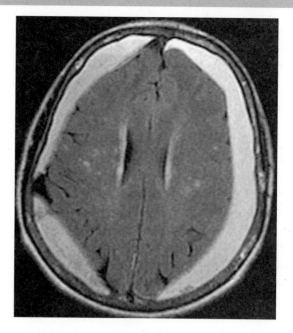

1. What factors contribute to the appearance of blood products on MR imaging?

2. How many unpaired electrons does methemoglobin have?

3. What patients are at increased risk for bilateral subdural hematomas?

4. What are the MR imaging signal characteristics of subacute (weeks to months old) hematomas?

CASE 35

Bilateral Subacute Subdural Hematomas

1. The structure of hemoglobin at the time of imaging is most important. Susceptibility effects, proton–electron dipole–dipole interactions, and other factors contribute to the variable signal characteristics of blood products.

2. Five unpaired electrons.

3. Elderly patients with atrophy and recurrent falls, patients who have undergone shunting for hydrocephalus, patients with central hypotension.

4. Hyperintense on T1W (methemoglobin) and T2W imaging.

References

Atkinson JL, Lane JI, Aksamit AJ: MRI depiction of chronic intradural (subdural) hematoma in evolution, *J Magn Reson Imaging* 17:484–486, 2003.

Pollo C, Meuli R, Porchet F: Spontaneous bilateral subdural haematomas in the posterior cranial fossa revealed by MRI, *Neuroradiology* 45:550–552, 2003.

Cross-Reference

Neuroradiology: THE REQUISITES, 2nd ed, pp 248–251.

Comment

The appearance of blood products on MR imaging is dependent on several factors, most importantly, the structure of hemoglobin at the time of imaging. Oxyhemoglobin (oxygen bound to the iron of hemoglobin) is diamagnetic because it effectively has no unpaired electrons. On giving up its oxygen, deoxyhemoglobin is formed and hemoglobin undergoes a small but significant structural change such that water molecules in the vicinity of deoxyhemoglobin are unable to bind to the iron. Deoxyhemoglobin has four unpaired electrons and may be oxidized to methemoglobin. Methemoglobin has five unpaired electrons, and water molecules are able to bind to the iron atom.

Susceptibility effects, proton–electron dipole–dipole interactions, and other factors contribute to the variable signal characteristics of blood products on MR imaging. When placed in a magnetic field, certain substances may induce an additional smaller magnetic field that may add to the externally applied field. This phenomenon may be seen with paramagnetic substances (deoxyhemoglobin and methemoglobin). Alternatively, other substances, when placed in a magnetic field, may induce magnetic fields that subtract from the externally applied field (seen with diamagnetic materials, such as oxyhemoglobin). Susceptibility effects of blood products depend on the proportionality constant between the strength of the applied magnetic field and the induced magnetic field.

Methemoglobin induces a local magnetic field significantly greater than that of a proton. Therefore, if a proton gets close enough to this field, a spin transition may occur. To have a proton–electron dipole–dipole interaction, water must bind to heme. Even though the number of heme molecules is small relative to that of water, the exchange rate of water molecules is quite rapid compared with the repetition time; hence, many water molecules are bound to heme during MR imaging. Proton–electron dipole–dipole interactions result in shortening of T1 and T2.

Notes

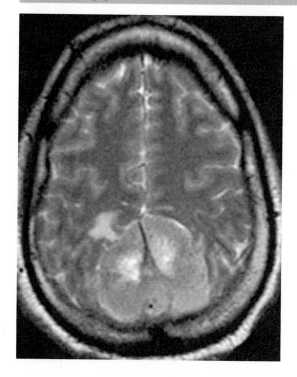 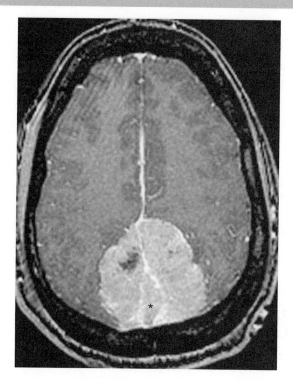

1. What are the clinical signs and symptoms of intracranial venous hypertension?

2. What is the differential diagnosis?

3. What vascular structure is involved (*)?

4. What findings on an imaging study suggest venous infarction?

Parafalcine Meningioma Invading the Superior Sagittal Sinus

1. Headaches, papilledema, and focal neurologic deficits if there is venous infarction.

2. Meningioma is most likely; however, other neoplastic processes must be considered, including dural metastases and hemangiopericytomas.

3. There is invasion of the superior sagittal sinus.

4. Imaging findings suggesting venous infarction include subcortical high signal intensity, bilateral parenchymal hemorrhages (particularly in cases of superior sagittal sinus thrombosis), and hemorrhagic infarctions that are not in arterial distributions. This patient does not have venous infarction.

References

Takeguchi T, Miki H, Shimizu T, et al: The dural tail of intracranial meningiomas on fluid-attenuated inversion-recovery images, *Neuroradiology* 46:130–135, 2004.

Tsuchiya K, Katase S, Yoshino A, Hachiay J: MR digital subtraction angiography in the diagnosis of meningiomas, *Eur J Radiol* 46:130–138, 2003.

Cross-Reference

Neuroradiology: THE REQUISITES, 2nd ed, pp 98–105, 217, 218–220.

Comment

This case shows a well-demarcated extra-axial mass (CSF cleft separating the mass from the brain on T2W image) in the posterior interhemispheric fissure along the falx cerebri. The mass is predominantly isointense to gray matter (because of its cellularity) and enhances avidly, with the exception of a few small areas of cystic degeneration (T2W hyperintense, nonenhancing regions). Enhancing tumor is noted obliterating the superior sagittal sinus (*).

In trying to determine the cause of this lesion, it is important to view the remainder of the brain as well as the calvaria for other abnormalities. This is because the vast majority of malignant extra-axial neoplasms are caused by bone metastases. Destructive or infiltrative lesions within the calvaria that may affect the inner and outer cortical tables should be sought. In addition, metastases may be associated with extraosseous soft tissue masses within the scalp. The finding of multiple lesions within the calvaria favors metastatic disease. Additional malignant extra-axial masses include metastases and lymphoma (which may involve the leptomeninges, dura, or bone). Finally, the absence of significant associated vasogenic edema in this case makes a malignant process unlikely. The opposite is not true, however; the presence of significant vasogenic edema would support meningioma or a more aggressive neoplasm (eg, metastases, lymphoma).

The most common cause of an extra-axial neoplasm in adults is meningioma. Although meningiomas may demonstrate changes along the inner table of the skull (hyperostosis and, less commonly, lysis), a dural-based mass in the absence of disease involving the diploic space or the outer table of the skull still favors meningioma (as do statistics!)

Notes

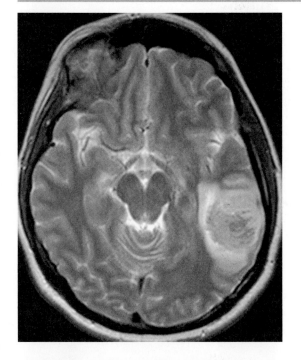

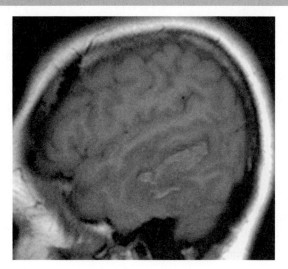

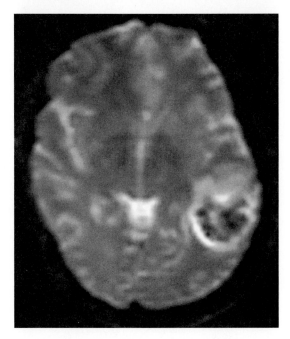

1. What are the two most common types of antiphospholipid antibodies?

2. In hypercoagulable states related to antiphospholipid antibodies, are cerebral arterial or venous infarcts more common?

3. What images in this case identify the presence of blood products?

4. What kidney disorder is associated with a hypercoagulable state?

Hemorrhagic Venous Infarction

1. Lupus anticoagulant and anticardiolipin. There is a high incidence of these circulating antibodies in patients with systemic lupus erythematosus.

2. Arterial infarcts.

3. The mass shows hyperintensity on the T1W image and mild hypointensity on the T2W image. The baseline images from the diffusion-weighted data set (T2W EPI) show more convincing decreased intensity because they are more sensitive to susceptibility effects than the relatively insensitive fast spin-echo T2W sequence. More optimal demonstration of susceptibility effects could be obtained with T2W gradient echo imaging (not acquired in this patient).

4. Nephrotic syndrome. The hypercoagulable state is multifactorial and includes the combined effects of endothelial injury, platelet hyperaggregability, and abnormalities in the coagulation cascade (such as protein S or C deficiency).

Reference

Tong KA, Ashwal S, Obenaus A, Nickerson JP, Kido D, Haacke EM: Susceptibility-weighted MR imaging: a review of clinical applications, *Am J Neuroradiol* 29:9–17, 2008.

Cross-Reference

Neuroradiology: THE REQUISITES, 2nd ed, pp 217, 219–220.

Comment

This case illustrates a hemorrhagic venous infarction in the left temporal lobe. Unlike arterial infarctions, the anatomic territories for venous occlusive disease are less consistent than with the territory supplied by arteries. Several findings should raise the suspicion of a venous infarct: (1) the presence of hemorrhage, especially in the white matter or at the gray–white matter interface; (2) the presence of an abnormality that is not in a single arterial distribution; and (3) an infarct in a young patient. This patient had acute thrombosis of the vein of Labbé and the distal left transverse sinus. The hemorrhagic infarct in the left temporal lobe is in the territory drained by the vein of Labbé.

Symptoms of venous occlusion are related to the rate at which collateral venous drainage is established, the location of the clot, and the rate of clot formation. Because of the network of venous collaterals in the brain, if the venous occlusive process is slow enough to allow time for collateral circulation to develop, the patient may remain asymptomatic. However, in the setting of acute occlusion of a large vein or dural venous sinus, venous congestion will result in back-pressure that extends to the capillary bed, where the flow will be diminished such that there is ischemia and, if extensive enough, infarction.

Before MR imaging and CT venography, the diagnosis of venous occlusive disease was more difficult, and a high index of suspicion was necessary. Many conventional CT findings have been described (including the delta sign, in which there is enhancement around the clot or filling defect in the sinus, and the cord sign, in which high density is seen in a venous sinus or vein); however, they are inconsistent.

Notes

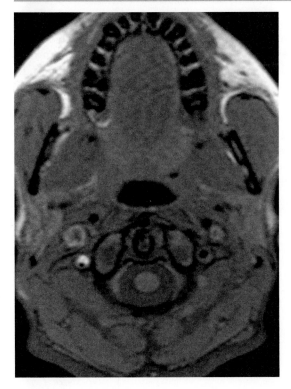 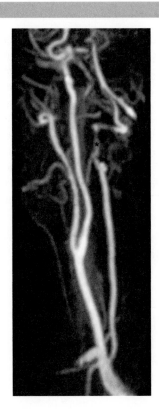

1. What are common injuries of the vertebral arteries?

2. Do traumatic dissections more commonly affect the extracranial or intracranial vasculature?

3. What are risk factors for intracranial dissections?

4. What are common complications of vascular dissections?

Vertebral Artery Dissection—Spontaneous

1. Vascular dissection, laceration or traumatic occlusion, and arteriovenous fistulization.

2. Extracranial.

3. Trauma associated with skull base fractures (particularly the sphenoid bone, carotid canal, and petrous apex) increases the risk of injury to the internal carotid arteries. Dissections also occur in patients with vascular dysplasia (eg, fibromuscular dysplasia, Marfan syndrome) and in patients with hypertension.

4. Transient ischemic attack and stroke related to embolic or thrombo-occlusive changes. Pseudoaneurysms may also occur.

References

Naggara O, Oppenheim C, Toussaint JF, et al: Asymptomatic spontaneous acute vertebral artery dissection: diagnosis by high-resolution magnetic resonance images with a dedicated surface coil, *Eur Radiol* 17:2434–2435, 2007.

Cross-Reference

Neuroradiology: THE REQUISITES, 2nd ed, pp 221–224, 263–264.

Comment

These MR images show narrowing of the lumen of the distal extracranial right vertebral artery (*) with surrounding mural hematoma that is hyperintense on the fat-suppressed unenhanced T1W image. Vascular dissections may be asymptomatic. When symptomatic, the symptoms may occur days to weeks after the actual injury. As a result, dissections often escape clinical detection. In addition, symptomatic lesions can be overlooked or masked by other injuries in patients with acute injuries. Therefore, the key to making the diagnosis is considering it in the appropriate clinical scenario. Although CT is not a sensitive study for detecting vascular injuries, it may identify patients at increased risk (those with skull base fractures or fractures of the vertebral bodies extending through the foramen transversarium, which houses the cervical vertebral artery). It is also important to recognize that vertebral artery dissections may be spontaneous (no clear etiology, minor trauma), and may occur in association with excessive vomiting, coughing, and excessive straining.

The combination of MR imaging and MR angiography is sensitive for detecting vascular injuries because these assess the vascular lumen, the vessel wall, and tissues around the vessel. MR imaging findings include intramural hematoma, which is typically hyperintense on unenhanced T1W images, as in this case, and narrowing and compromised flow in the arterial lumen (a narrowed but patent vessel can usually be distinguished from one that is occluded). Pseudoaneurysms may also be detected. The conventional angiographic appearance of a dissection may vary, and includes spasm, segmental tapering related to intramural hematoma (the hematoma is not visualized on angiography), aneurysmal dilation of the vessel, vascular occlusion, intimal flap, or retention of contrast material in the vessel wall.

Notes

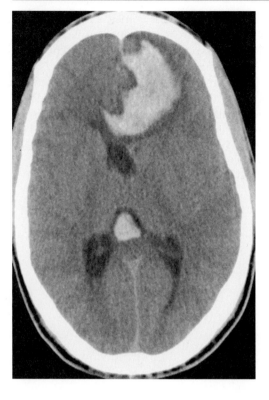

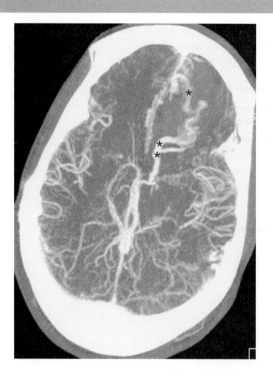

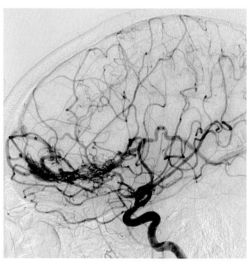

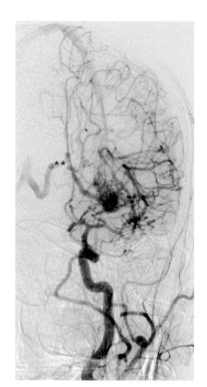

1. What is the differential diagnosis for a spontaneous, nontraumatic cerebral hematoma?

2. What entity would not be expected to be seen in patients younger than 60 years of age?

3. What is the cause of this young patient's spontaneous frontal lobe hematoma?

4. What are the anatomic structures marked with (*)?

Spontaneous Cerebral Hematoma—Ruptured Cerebral Arteriovenous Malformation

1. Hemorrhage into an underlying tumor, hemorrhage into an underlying vascular malformation (ruptured arteriovenous malformation [AVM], cavernoma), venous infarct, vasculitis, hemorrhagic arterial infarct, substance abuse (cocaine), amyloid angiopathy.

2. Amyloid angiopathy is usually seen in patients older than 60 years of age, and is a diagnosis of exclusion.

3. A ruptured AVM. The nidus is the tangle of blood vessels in the left frontal lobe on the conventional arteriogram.

4. Early draining veins to the superficial (*) and deep (**) venous systems.

References

Cloft HJ, Joseph GJ, Dion JE: Risk of cerebral angiography in patients with subarachnoid hemorrhage, cerebral aneurysm, and arteriovenous malformation, *Stroke* 30:317–320, 1999.

Spetzler RF, Martin NA: A proposed grading system for arteriovenous malformations, *J Neurosurg* 65:476–483, 1986.

Cross-Reference

Neuroradiology: THE REQUISITES, 2nd ed, pp 234–238.

Comment

This case shows a nontraumatic spontaneous hematoma in the left frontal lobe with surrounding hypodensity, consistent with edema and early clot retraction. There is local mass effect with sulcal effacement and mild posterior displacement of the frontal horn of the left lateral ventricle. There is blood in a persistent cavum vergae. In this case, the hematoma is due to a ruptured AVM. The vascular nidus is noted in the left frontal lobe. An AVM represents a vascular nidus made up of a core of entangled vessels fed by one or more enlarged feeding arteries. Blood is shunted from the nidus to enlarged draining veins that terminate in the deep or superficial venous system. In this case, there is superficial venous drainage (*) in the left frontal region that drains to the superior sagittal sinus, and there is deep venous drainage (**) to the internal cerebral veins.

On unenhanced CT, the vascular nidus of an AVM and enlarged draining veins are usually isodense or hyperdense to gray matter as a result of pooling of blood. Calcification may be present. AVMs enhance and have characteristic serpentine flow voids on MR imaging related to fast flow in dilated arteries. In lesions associated with an acute parenchymal hemorrhage, phase-contrast MR angiography best demonstrates the AVM (it subtracts out the signal intensity of the blood products in the hematoma, in contrast to time-of-flight MR angiography). Cerebral angiography shows enlarged feeding arteries, the vascular nidus, and early draining veins. In cases of very small AVMs, early venous filling should be sought on careful evaluation of the angiographic images.

Notes

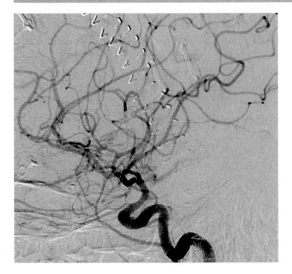

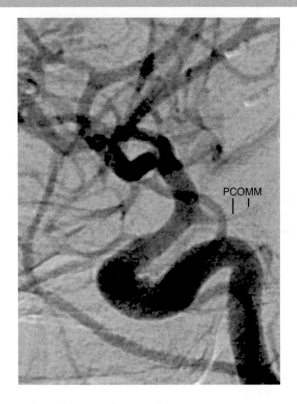

1. What is the first branch to arise from the supraclinoid internal carotid artery?

2. How does a clinician differentiate a posterior communicating artery aneurysm from an infundibulum?

3. What percentage of patients with nontraumatic subarachnoid hemorrhage will have unrevealing (negative) angiograms?

4. What are some causes of angiographically negative subarachnoid hemorrhage?

Vascular Infundibulum—Posterior Communicating Artery

1. The ophthalmic artery.

2. An infundibulum should meet the following criteria: (1) it measures 3 mm or smaller; (2) it is triangular or funnel-shaped; and (3) the posterior communicating artery arises from its apex.

3. Approximately 10% to 15%.

4. Aneurysms may not be detected because of vasospasm that inhibits filling of the aneurysm, spontaneous thrombosis of the aneurysm, or misinterpretation of the images. Other causes of angiogram-negative subarachnoid hemorrhage include perimesencephalic venous hemorrhages, vasculitis, venous thrombosis, and spinal vascular malformations.

References

Marshman LA, Ward PJ, Walter PH, Dossetor RS: The progression of an infundibulum to aneurysm formation and rupture: case report and literature review, *Neurosurgery* 43:1445–1448, 1998.

Ng SH, Wong HF, Ko SF, Lee CM, Yen PS, Wai YY: CT angiography of intracranial aneurysms: advantages and pitfalls, *Eur J Radiol* 25:14–19, 1997.

Cross-Reference

Neuroradiology: THE REQUISITES, 2nd ed, pp 226–227.

Comment

These angiographic images demonstrate the typical appearance of a posterior communicating artery infundibulum, showing its funnel shape as well as the origin of the posterior communicating artery from the apex of the infundibulum. Because the management is dramatically different, angiographic images in anteroposterior, lateral, and oblique projections should be obtained to accurately differentiate an aneurysm from an infundibulum.

Conventional catheter angiography and, increasingly, CT angiography are used in the diagnosis and evaluation of intracranial aneurysm. In the acute setting, there are several indications for prompt imaging evaluation, including nontraumatic subarachnoid hemorrhage; acute-onset third nerve palsy that involves the pupil (to exclude a posterior communicating or superior cerebellar artery aneurysm); and in the postoperative setting, to evaluate complications after placement of an aneurysm clip. In patients with angiogram-negative acute nontraumatic subarachnoid hemorrhage, follow-up angiography is usually indicated. It is important to remember that all potential sites of aneurysm formation must be assessed with conventional angiography. In the acute setting, postoperative angiography is often indicated in the evaluation of perioperative ischemic sequelae (which may be due to embolic phenomena, vasospasm, or vascular occlusion). Postoperative or intraoperative angiography on an elective basis may be performed to assess for residual aneurysm after aneurysm clipping.

Notes

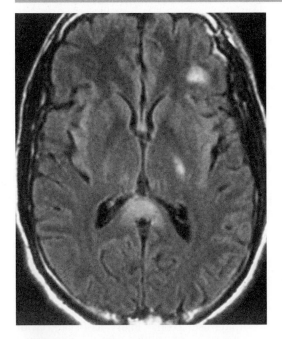
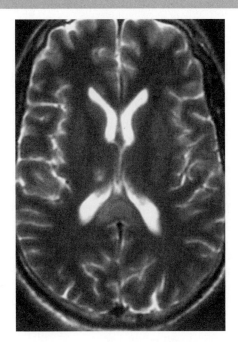

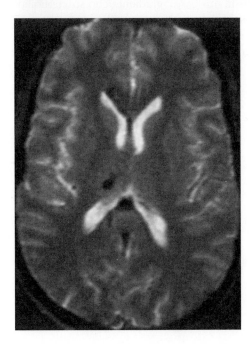

1. What are the most common locations for traumatic contusions?

2. What three anatomic locations are classically involved in diffuse axonal injury?

3. Why are the posterior and splenial regions of the corpus callosum more commonly affected by shear injury than the anterior portion?

4. In the absence of the gradient echo image, what other entities could result in similar imaging findings seen on the long TR images?

Closed Head Injury—Diffuse Axonal Injury

1. The frontal and temporal lobes. The anterior temporal lobes impact on the greater wing of the sphenoid bone, whereas the frontal lobes impact on the surfaces of the cribriform plate, orbits, and frontal bone.

2. The lobar white matter, the corpus callosum (most commonly the splenium, but also the undersurface of the posterior body), and the dorsolateral aspect of the upper brainstem (midbrain and pons).

3. With rotational acceleration of the head, shear forces develop across the corpus callosum. Anteriorly, there is less strain because the falx is shorter and allows transient displacement of the frontal lobes across the midline. Posteriorly, the falx is broader and more rigid, preventing motion of the cerebral hemispheres across the midline.

4. Demyelinating diseases (multiple sclerosis, acute disseminated encephalomyelitis) and neoplasm (primary glial and lymphoma).

References

Scheid R, Preul C, Gruber O, Wiggins C, von Cramon DY: Diffuse axonal injury associated with chronic traumatic brain injury: evidence from T2-weighted gradient-echo imaging at 3T, *AJNR Am J Neuroradiol* 24:1049–1056, 2003.

Tong KA, Ashwal S, Holshouser BA, et al: Hemorrhagic shearing lesions in children and adolescents with posttraumatic diffuse axonal injury: improved detection and initial results, *Radiology* 227:332–339, 2003.

Cross-Reference

Neuroradiology: THE REQUISITES, 2nd ed, pp 246, 256–258.

Comment

Diffuse axonal injury is the result of shear-strain forces induced by angular rotation or acceleration of the head that result in partial or complete disruption of involved axons. Patients have loss of consciousness and a spectrum of cognitive impairment and neurological dysfunction beginning at the moment of trauma. Symptoms may range from transient loss of consciousness at the time of injury to permanent coma (vegetative state) or death in the most severe diffuse forms. Diffuse axonal injury is most commonly seen in patients involved in high-velocity acceleration–deceleration motor vehicle accidents, but it can also be seen in more minor forms of trauma, such as a fall down stairs and occasionally falls from the standing position. It is characterized by multiple focal lesions in the lobar white matter at the gray–white matter interface, in the corpus callosum, and in cases of severe head trauma, in the dorsolateral brainstem. Shear injuries are typically elliptic in shape, with the long axis parallel to the direction of the involved axons.

Although MR imaging is the most sensitive imaging modality for the detection and evaluation of diffuse axonal injury, in the acute setting, the first radiologic study should be CT because the most critical issue is to detect potentially treatable acute intracranial hemorrhage (subdural and epidural hematomas, large parenchymal hematomas). If there is concern about shear injury, MR imaging should be performed when the patient is stable. Shear injuries, unless hemorrhagic or of substantial size, frequently go undetected on CT. The presence of intra-ventricular hemorrhage should raise suspicion of injury to the septum pellucidum or corpus callosum. On MR imaging, shear injuries are hyperintense on T2W images. Approximately 80% of shear injuries are non-hemorrhagic. In diffuse axonal injury associated with hemorrhage (as in this case), gradient echo susceptibility imaging shows blood products. In this case, the right thalamic and corpus callosal lesions are hypointense, consistent with the presence of blood products.

Notes

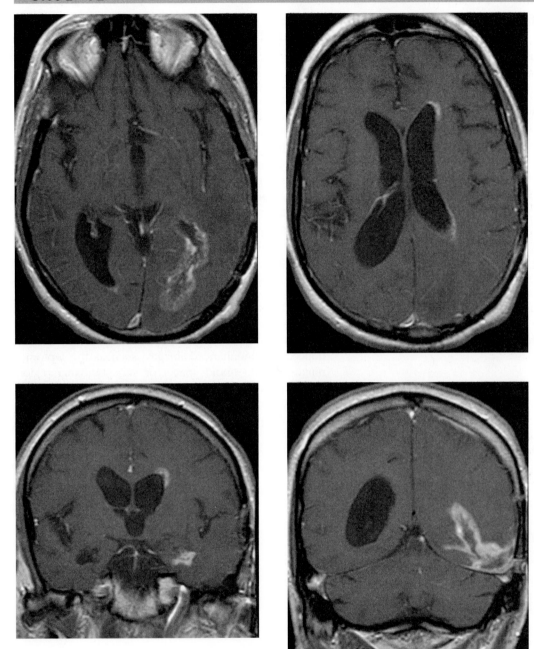

1. What is the primary imaging finding?

2. What is the differential diagnosis?

3. What is the best diagnosis in this case, and why?

4. In a patient with AIDS, what is the most likely cause of subependymal enhancement?

Glioblastoma Multiforme—Subependymal Spread

1. There is nodular enhancement along the subependyma of the left lateral ventricle (and a small amount along the right occipital horn).

2. Subependymal spread of neoplasm, including lymphoma, glioblastoma multiforme (GBM) [usually represents recurrent disease], and metastatic disease, such as breast and lung cancer. The inflammatory conditions that should be considered include sarcoid and tuberculosis. Although other infections can do this, the thick, nodular appearance in this case is more typical of neoplastic spread.

3. Recurrent subependymal GBM. The mild cerebral mass effect manifests as sulcal effacement in the left inferior frontal, temporal, and occipital lobes, consistent with infiltrating neoplasm. In addition, there is evidence of a previous craniotomy as well as an ill-defined parenchymal necrotic tumor extending to the left lateral ventricle seen on the second coronal image.

4. Lymphoma.

Reference

Christiforidis GA, Grecula JC, Newton HB, et al: Visualization of microvascularity in glioblastoma multiforme with 8-T high-spatial-resolution MR imaging, *AJNR Am J Neuroradiol* 23:1553–1556, 2002.

Cross-Reference

Neuroradiology: THE REQUISITES, 2nd ed, pp 128–129, 139, 142–143.

Comment

Glioblastoma multiforme classically presents with an ill-defined necrotic brain mass. The histologic grade of these aggressive neoplasms in adults progresses with age: the older the patient, the higher the histologic grade. Other imaging features that correlate with higher grades include enhancement, extensive mass effect, intratumoral necrosis, hemorrhage, vascularity and elevated relative cerebral blood volume, and elevated lactic acid on MR spectroscopy. Glioblastomas infiltrate the brain parenchyma, and this is manifest as T2W hyperintensity; however, there is little doubt that these neoplasms have also infiltrated into areas of the brain that appear normal on current diagnostic MR studies. Most GBMs enhance and usually demonstrate heterogeneity because of the presence of necrosis or hemorrhage. Enhancement may extend into the adjacent white matter. These tumors frequently cross the corpus callosum and the anterior or posterior commissures to spread to the contralateral cerebral hemisphere. Of the astrocytomas in adults, GBMs most commonly are associated with hemorrhage and subarachnoid seeding (2%–5%) of neoplasm. Occasionally, at presentation, GBMs will coat the subependyma or ependyma of the ventricles. However, it is important to recognize that although overall long-term survival rates in patients with GBM are still very poor, patients are living longer and in some instances with improved quality of life with changes in treatment protocols and in clinical trials looking at a spectrum of chemotherapeutic agents. Hence, in these patients, less typical patterns of disease progression on imaging, such as coating of the ventricles from subependymal tumor spread, will become more common, as in this case.

In a newly identified brain tumor in which biopsy is anticipated, regions of enhancement correlate with regions of solid tumor on pathology and have the best diagnostic yield. In addition, enhanced images may identify tumor spread to regions that otherwise would not be noticed on unenhanced images, such as the leptomeninges, subarachnoid space, or subependymal region along the ventricular margins, as in this case. In the postoperative setting, contrast may help to distinguish surgical change from residual tumor.

Notes

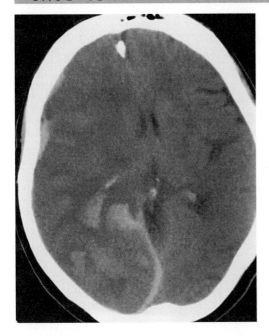 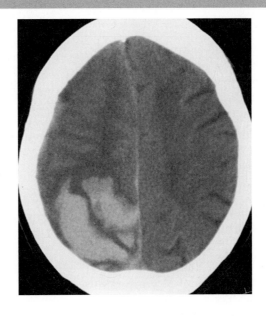

1. What are common causes of nontraumatic intracranial hemorrhage?

2. What is the most common cause of nontraumatic intracranial hemorrhage in adults?

3. What is the major risk factor for amyloid angiopathy?

4. What regions of the brain are typically spared in amyloid angiopathy?

Amyloid Angiopathy

1. The causes are numerous, and may be separated by age at presentation. Common etiologies include hypertension, underlying vascular malformations, hemorrhagic stroke, coagulopathies, blood dyscrasias, recreational drug use (cocaine), pregnancy (eclampsia), vasculitis, amyloid angiopathy, and infection (such as aspergillus).

2. Hypertension, which may account for more than 75% of nontraumatic intraparenchymal hemorrhages.

3. Age.

4. The basal ganglia, brainstem, deep white matter, and cerebellum.

Reference

Walker DA, Broderick DF, Kotsenas AL, Rubino FA: Routine use of gradient-echo MRI to screen for cerebral amyloid angiopathy in elderly patients, *Am J Roentgenol* 182:1547–1550, 2004.

Cross-Reference

Neuroradiology: THE REQUISITES, 2nd ed, p 220.

Comment

Central nervous system amyloid angiopathy results from deposition of β-pleated proteins within the media and adventitia of small- and medium-sized vessels of the superficial layers of the cortex and leptomeninges. Amyloid deposition increases with age and results in loss of elasticity of the walls of involved vessels. On pathologic examination, microaneurysms and fibrinoid degeneration are often present. Amyloid stains intensely with Congo red dye (previously referred to as congophilic angiopathy) and demonstrates yellow-green birefringence under polarized light.

On CT and MR imaging, hemorrhages are characteristically lobar in location, and they most commonly occur in the frontal and parietal lobes. Multiple hemorrhages of different ages, as well as multiple simultaneous hemorrhages, are often present. Subarachnoid and subdural blood may be present due to perforation of blood through the pia arachnoid or involvement of superficial blood vessels with amyloid deposition. MR imaging, including gradient echo images, may be especially useful for demonstrating the full extent of intracranial involvement (CT readily shows acute hemorrhage, as in this case; however, regions of old blood products are often occult). Patients may have numerous small subcortical regions of focal hypointensity (multiple hypointense foci may also be related to cavernomas or microhemorrhages, as is seen in hypertension). Importantly, there is no association of hypertension with the development of amyloid angiopathy.

Notes

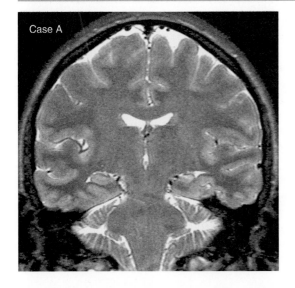

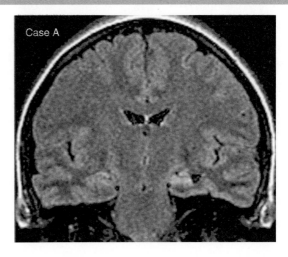

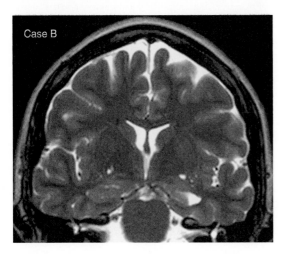

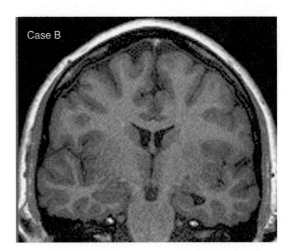

1. What is the "same" diagnosis in these two cases?

2. What is the patient's clinical presentation?

3. What imaging features help to differentiate mesial temporal sclerosis from a neoplasm?

4. What condition in infancy has been associated with mesial temporal sclerosis?

Mesial Temporal Sclerosis

1. Mesial temporal sclerosis.

2. Partial complex seizures.

3. Hippocampal sclerosis is characterized by volume loss of the hippocampus with associated ex vacuo dilation of the adjacent temporal horn. High signal intensity on T2W imaging in the hippocampus may (as in Case A) or may not (as in Case B) be present. Neoplasms are typically associated with hippocampal enlargement and local mass effect. Enhancement may or may not be present with neoplasms.

4. Complex infantile febrile seizures.

References

Briellman RS, Syngeniotis A, Fleming S, et al: Increased anterior temporal lobe T2 times in cases of hippocampal sclerosis: a multi-echo T2 relaxometry study at 3T, *Am J Neuroradiol* 25:389–394, 2004.

Hogan RE, Wang L, Bertrand ME, et al: MRI-based high dimensional hippocampal mapping in mesial temporal lobe epilepsy, *Brain* 127:1731–1740, 2004.

Cross-Reference

Neuroradiology: THE REQUISITES, 2nd ed, pp 447–449.

Comment

Temporal lobe epilepsy is the most common epilepsy syndrome in adults. Seizures usually begin in late childhood or adolescence. Virtually all patients have complex partial seizures. In most patients, the epileptogenic focus involves the structures of the mesial temporal lobe. These structures include the hippocampus, amygdala, and parahippocampal gyrus. The histologic substrate in approximately two thirds of cases is mesial temporal sclerosis. The hippocampal formation located in the mesial temporal lobe protrudes into the medial temporal horn and is roofed by the choroidal fissure. It is a complex structure composed of the hippocampus proper, subiculum, dentate gyrus, parahippocampal gyrus, fimbria, and fornix. The hippocampus proper (or cornu ammonis) can be subdivided into four subfields, CA1 though CA4, depending on the appearance of pyramidal neurons. Neuronal loss is accompanied by fibrillary gliosis, leading to hippocampal atrophy. In mesial temporal sclerosis, gliosis may also affect the amygdala, uncus, and parahippocampal gyrus.

The differential diagnosis for hippocampal sclerosis includes cortical dysplasias and primary brain neoplasm. Mesial temporal sclerosis is usually radiologically characteristic. MR imaging using high-resolution thin-section coronal FLAIR and T2W and T1W gradient volumetric sequences is the imaging modality of choice for evaluating patients with seizure disorders. These cases illustrate the classic MR imaging appearance of hippocampal sclerosis in which there is atrophy of the left hippocampus in both cases as well as mild ipsilateral dilation of the adjacent temporal horn. Case A also shows T2W hyperintensity in the abnormal hippocampus that is believed to reflect gliosis.

Whether mesial temporal sclerosis is the cause or the result of temporal lobe epilepsy is controversial. Some studies have shown a relationship between complex infantile febrile seizures and mesial temporal sclerosis. Patients with complex febrile seizures (duration > 15 minutes, convulsive activity, or > 3 seizures within 24 hours) have an increased incidence of mesial temporal sclerosis.

Notes

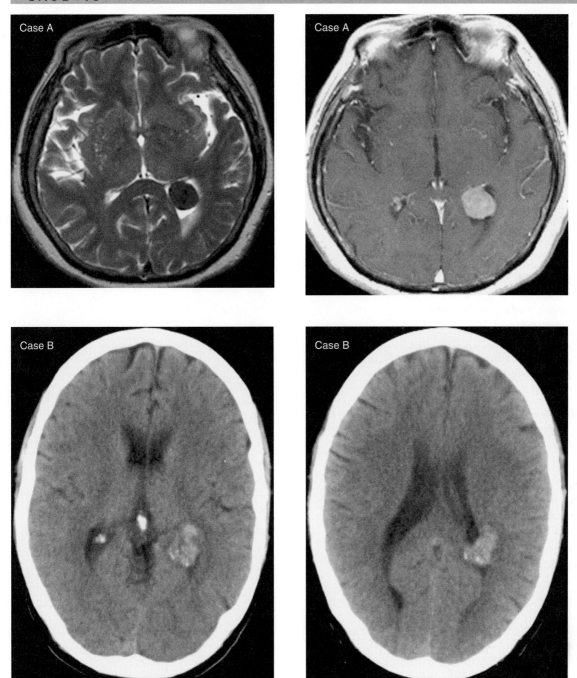

1. What factors significantly aid in limiting the differential diagnosis in these cases?

2. This particular tumor most often arises in what ventricle in adults?

3. What is the most common clinical presentation of these tumors?

4. In adults, choroid plexus papillomas most commonly occur in what ventricle? In children?

Intraventricular Meningioma

1. The age of the patient (child vs. adult) and the location of the mass (lateral, third ventricle, or fourth ventricle).

2. The lateral ventricle.

3. Asymptomatic. Many of these are incidental findings in patients being evaluated for unrelated reasons. Symptoms can include those of other intracranial mass lesions (eg, headaches, nausea).

4. The fourth ventricle. The trigone of the lateral ventricle.

References

Jelinek J, Smirniotopoulos JG, Parisi JE, Kanzer M: Lateral ventricular neoplasms of the brain: differential diagnosis based on clinical, CT, and MR findings, *AJR Am J Roentgenol* 155:365–372, 1990.

Majos C, Cucurella G, Aguilera C, Coll S, Pons LC: Intraventricular meningiomas: MR imaging and MR spectroscopic findings in two cases, *AJNR Am J Neuroradiol* 20:882–885, 1999.

Cross-Reference

Neuroradiology: THE REQUISITES, 2nd ed, p 101.

Comment

Cases A and B demonstrate well-demarcated mass lesions in the atria of the left lateral ventricle along the glomus of the choroid plexus, consistent with meningiomas. On T2W imaging, these tumors may range from mildly hyperintense to the brain parenchyma (however, markedly hypointense to CSF) to hypointense to brain tissue in cases of very cellular or calcified tumors. After contrast administration, there is homogeneous avid enhancement. In adults, this is the typical appearance of an intraventricular meningioma and the most common location for these neoplasms, which are speculated to arise from arachnoid rests within the choroid plexus. Like choroid plexus papillomas, intraventricular meningiomas occur slightly more often on the left, as illustrated in these cases. When large enough, intraventricular meningiomas may trap a particular segment of the lateral ventricle (usually the temporal or occipital horn), resulting in focal dilation and sometimes associated transependymal flow of CSF. When large enough, these tumors may compress the walls of the ventricles or grow through the ependyma, with resultant edema in the adjacent brain parenchyma. Their appearance on CT is similar to that of other intracranial meningiomas. On unenhanced CT images, these masses are often hyperdense with calcifications, as in Case B shown here. They avidly enhance after contrast administration.

The differential diagnosis of a mass in this location in adults includes glial neoplasms (astrocytomas, ependymomas), metastasis to the choroid plexus, and vascular lesions such as hemangiomas and cavernomas. Choroid plexus papillomas can usually be eliminated as a diagnostic consideration because they occur most commonly in children and because in adults they are usually located within the fourth ventricle.

Notes

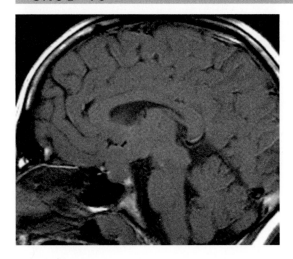 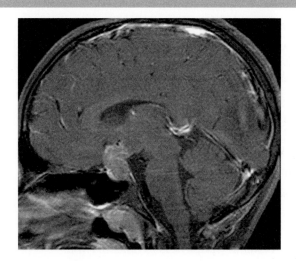

1. What is the clinical presentation of masses in this location?

2. Which category of pineal tumors does not have a sex predilection?

3. What is the most common germ cell tumor in the pineal region?

4. What is the typical imaging appearance of a germinoma on unenhanced CT?

Suprasellar Germinoma

1. Clinical presentation of suprasellar lesions is variable, but may include diabetes insipidus, hypopituitarism, or visual symptoms related to compression of the optic chiasm.

2. Those of pineal cell origin (pineoblastoma, pineocytoma).

3. Germinoma (also referred to as seminoma or dysgerminoma).

4. A hyperdense mass.

Reference

Mah E, Rahmat K: Neurohypophyseal germinoma with metastasis to the spine, *Eur J Radiol* 63:89–92, 2007.

Cross-Reference

Neuroradiology: THE REQUISITES, 2nd ed, pp 550–552.

Comment

This case demonstrates a solid, avidly enhancing suprasellar mass that represented a germinoma. Due to their marked cellularity and protein content, germinomas are typically hyperdense on unenhanced CT and isointense to brain on T2W MR imaging. Cystic change and calcification are uncommon, and these neoplasms typically show prominent enhancement. On diffusion-weighted imaging, these may restrict being hyperintense, with corresponding low signal on apparent diffusion coefficient maps. These tumors can metastasize by subarachnoid seeding, and screening MR imaging of the spine should be performed.

Germinomas are most common in children and young adults, and they arise from primitive germ cells. The pineal gland is the most common site, followed by the suprasellar region. Clinical presentation from suprasellar masses is variable, but may include diabetes insipidus, hypopituitarism, or visual symptoms related to compression of the optic chiasm. Germinoma is the most common pineal tumor, accounting for 65% of all pineal germ cell neoplasms and approximately 40% of all pineal region tumors. Other germ cell tumors include teratoma, embryonal carcinoma, and choriocarcinoma. Teratomas may be distinguished from other germ cell tumors due to the presence of fat, calcification, and cyst formation (the fat and calcification or bone may have characteristic appearances on imaging). Choriocarcinomas may be differentiated due to the high incidence of hemorrhage within these tumors. In addition, β-human chorionic gonadotropin is a good serum marker for choriocarcinoma. Less common germ cell tumors, including embryonal cell carcinoma, endodermal sinus (yolk sac) tumors, and teratomas, may have hormonal markers such as β-human chorionic-gonadotropin and α-fetoprotein.

Notes

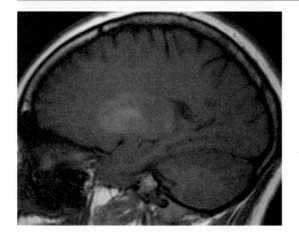
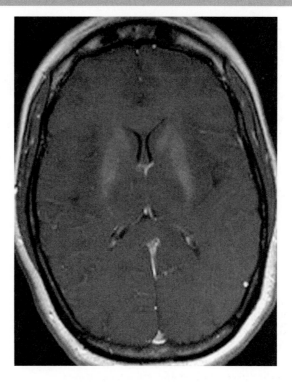

1. What is the pertinent finding?

2. What disorders of calcium and phosphate metabolism are associated with this finding?

3. What neurocutaneous syndrome is associated with high signal intensity foci in the brain on unenhanced T1W images?

4. What is the signal intensity of paramagnetic material on T2W images?

Mineral Deposition in the Basal Ganglia on T1W Imaging—Abnormal Calcium and Phosphate Metabolism

1. There is bilaterally symmetric hyperintensity in the basal ganglia on unenhanced T1W imaging.

2. Hyperparathyroidism and hypoparathyroidism (as well as every "pseudo" variety, including pseudohypoparathyroidism and pseudopseudo-hypoparathyroidism).

3. Neurofibromatosis type 1.

4. Low signal intensity.

References

Baba Y, Ohkubo K, Hamada K, Hokotate H, Nakajo M: Hyperintense basal ganglia lesions on T1-weighted images in hereditary hemorrhagic telangiectasia with hepatic involvement, *J Comput Assist Tomogr* 22:976–979, 1998.

Komiyama M, Nakajima H, Nishikawa M, Yasui T: Chronological changes in nonhaemorrhagic brain infarcts with short T1 in the cerebellum and basal ganglia, *Neuroradiology* 42:492–498, 2000.

Cross-Reference

Neuroradiology: THE REQUISITES, 2nd ed, p 395.

Comment

This case illustrates bilaterally symmetric high signal intensity in the basal ganglia on unenhanced T1W images in a patient with chronic abnormalities in calcium and phosphate metabolism. It is important to note that the axial image is a gadolinium-enhanced study, and the bilaterally symmetric high signal intensity in the basal ganglia should not be mistaken for enhancement. High signal intensity in the basal ganglia on unenhanced T1W images is also described in patients with chronic liver failure, patients receiving hyperalimentation, and those with portosystemic shunting. The high signal intensity is believed to be most likely related to deposition of paramagnetic ions, particularly manganese; however, other materials, such as copper, have been suggested. In the setting of liver failure, high signal intensity is frequently most pronounced in the globus pallidus; however, it may also be noted in the putamen, brainstem, and pituitary gland.

Neurofibromatosis type 1 is the most common neurocutaneous disorder. It is associated with a variety of intracranial lesions, the most common of which are foci of high signal intensity on long TR images within the brain parenchyma. The foci of high signal intensity are seen most commonly in the basal ganglia; however, they are frequently noted in the white matter tracts of the corpus striatum, in the brainstem, and in the cerebellum. The basal ganglia lesions may be hyperintense on unenhanced T1W images. It has been suggested that the pathologic basis of these foci in neurofibromatosis type 1 may be related to hypomyelination, migrational abnormalities, and nonneoplastic hamartomatous changes. A recent study in which pathologic correlation was obtained suggests that at least some of the foci of signal abnormality may be related to vacuolar or spongiotic change.

Notes

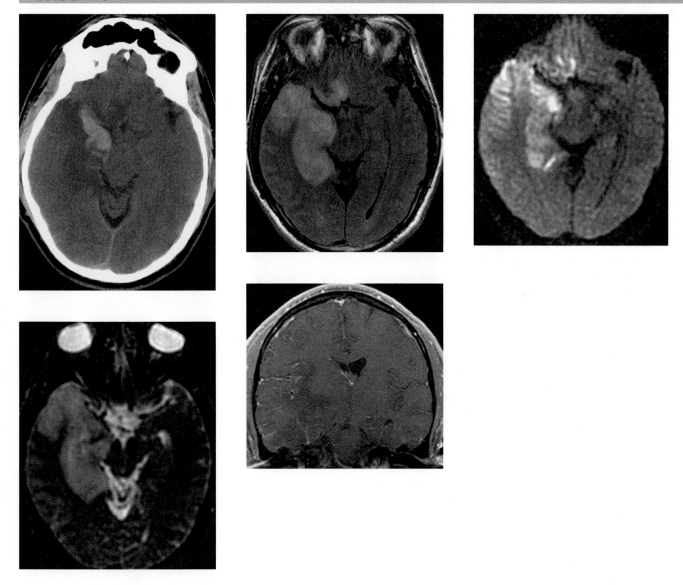

1. What is the differential diagnosis?

2. What imaging findings are typical for herpes simplex encephalitis?

3. What group of patients is at increased risk for herpes zoster infection?

4. Which herpes simplex virus is responsible for neonatal infection?

Herpes Simplex Encephalitis—Type 1

1. Encephalitis, primary neoplasm, and ischemia.

2. Medial bitemporal involvement and cortical gyriform enhancement.

3. Immunosuppressed patients.

4. Type II, acquired either transplacentally or through the birth canal of a mother with genital herpes.

Reference

Samann PG, Schlegel J, Muller G, Prantl F, Emminger C: Serial proton MR spectroscopy and diffusion imaging findings in HIV-related herpes simplex encephalitis, *Am J Neuroradiol* 24:2015–2019, 2003.

Cross-Reference

Neuroradiology: THE REQUISITES, 2nd ed, pp 288–290.

Comment

Type I herpes simplex virus produces necrotizing encephalitis in adults. The clinical presentation is varied, ranging from headache, fever, and seizures to coma. Radiologic evaluation frequently shows hypodensity with loss of gray–white matter differentiation in the temporal lobes and insular cortex on CT. Hemorrhage may also be present, as in this case. The CT appearance may simulate an infarct or a primary glial neoplasm. MR imaging findings in the acute stages of encephalitis show hyperintensity on long TR images within involved brain (usually the temporal lobes and inferomedial frontal lobes). There frequently is local mass effect, which is manifest by gyral expansion and sulcal effacement. Although bilateral disease is typical, herpes encephalitis usually involves the temporal lobes, insula, inferior frontal lobes, and cingulate gyrus in an asymmetric pattern. A proposed explanation for this pattern of involvement is the presence of the latent virus within the gasserian ganglion in Meckel's cave. Reactivated virus may spread along the trigeminal nerve fibers, with subsequent spread along the meninges around the temporal lobes and the undersurface of the frontal lobes. Meningoencephalitis commonly results. Diagnosis may depend on brain biopsy with a positive viral culture or identification of viral inclusion bodies. A positive result on herpes simplex virus polymerase chain reaction testing is diagnostic, and results of this test are available before those from cultures. Cortical gyriform enhancement is often present and may be associated with meningeal enhancement.

A good outcome from herpes simplex encephalitis relies on early diagnosis, which is of course dependent on considering herpes as a diagnosis! Delay in therapy (acyclovir) or untreated herpes is associated with a high mortality rate (50%–75%), with little chance of a full neurologic recovery.

Notes

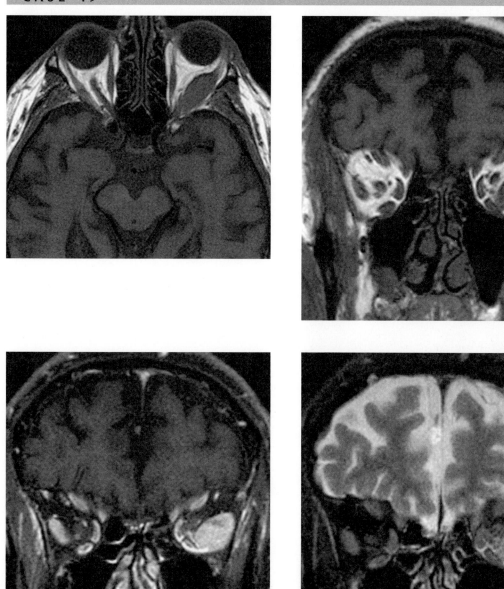

1. What is the most common location of orbital metastases?

2. What is the most common cause of orbital metastases in children?

3. What are the most common sites of primary orbital lymphoma?

4. What characteristic imaging finding, when present, is highly suggestive of metastatic breast carcinoma?

Primary Orbital Lymphoma

1. The globe (uveal tract).

2. Neuroblastoma.

3. Eyelid and extraocular muscles, as in this case when the left upper eyelid and lateral rectus muscle are involved.

4. Enophthalmos. Inward retraction of the globe (just like the skin of the involved breast) is characteristic of metastatic scirrhous breast carcinoma.

References

Holland D, Muane S, Kovacs G, Behrendt S: Metastatic tumors of the orbit: a retrospective study, *Orbit* 22:15–24, 2003.

Shields JA, Shields CL, Brotman HK, et al: Cancer metastatic to the orbit, *Ophthal Plast Reconstr Surg* 17:346–354, 2001.

Cross-Reference

Neuroradiology: THE REQUISITES, 2nd ed, pp 501, 503.

Comment

Clinical manifestations of ocular metastases and lymphoma are variable, depending on the site of involvement, ranging from asymptomatic to proptosis, diplopia, decreased vision, and less commonly, pain, red eye, and lid swelling. The symptoms of orbital metastasis may precede detection of the primary tumor in up to 25% of cases. In autopsy series, up to 7% of patients with known systemic carcinoma have metastases to the orbit. The presence of orbital metastases is an unfavorable prognostic sign, with an average mean survival time of less than 2 years. Management is palliative and may include radiation, chemotherapy, or surgery, and is intended to preserve vision, provide symptomatic relief, and improve quality of life.

The most common location of orbital metastases is to the globe. Ocular metastases characteristically involve the uveal region, resulting in thickening in this location on imaging. Intraconal retrobulbar disease is usually related to direct extension of an ocular metastasis. In most cases, metastasis occurs through hematogenous spread. The most common tumors to metastasize to the globe are breast, followed by prostate carcinoma in adults. Outside of the globe, orbital metastases most often are extraconal and are usually related to bone metastases (prostate carcinoma is most common). Extraosseous spread from a bone metastasis frequently invades the adjacent extraocular muscle.

Lymphoma of the orbit can be unilateral or bilateral and simultaneous and part of systemic disease, or can be isolated (primary) to the orbit. Primary orbital lymphomas histologically are usually low grade (60%) B-cell types. Primary lymphoma involves the eyelid and extraocular muscles in the majority of cases (up to 40%), the conjunctiva in 33% of cases, and the lacrimal apparatus in 25% of cases. These lesions are usually managed with radiation therapy, and some higher-grade lesions also receive chemotherapy. Distant recurrences are reported in approximately 15% of cases.

Notes

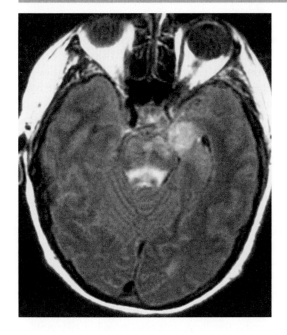 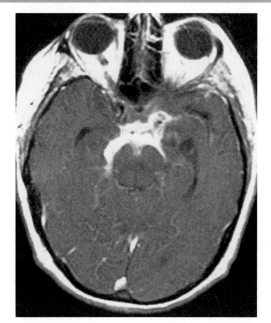

1. What are the imaging findings?

2. What disease processes affect the basilar meninges?

3. Is hydrocephalus associated with meningitis typically communicating or noncommunicating?

4. What primary CNS neoplasms have a predilection for subarachnoid seeding?

Basilar Meningitis and Encephalitis—Tuberculosis

1. Diffuse enhancement of the basal cisterns, T2W hyperintensity in the midbrain, and a ring-enhancing lesion in the medial left temporal lobe.

2. Infection (eg, tuberculosis, neurosyphilis, pyogenic infections, *Cryptococcus*), sarcoid, leptomeningeal seeding of tumor (carcinomatous from systemic malignancies or primary brain tumors), lymphoma, and chemical meningitides (eg, drugs, iodophenyl-undecylic acid [Pantopaque], fat from ruptured dermoids).

3. The hydrocephalus is usually communicating due to blockage of the basal cisterns and arachnoid villi with an inflammatory exudate. Hydrocephalus may also result from mass effect related to a parenchymal lesion, or from entrapment of a ventricle related to ependymitis.

4. Primitive neuroectodermal tumors (medulloblastoma, pineoblastoma), germinoma, glial neoplasms (glioblastoma multiforme, oligodendroglioma), and choroid plexus papilloma.

References

Bernaerts A, Vanhoenacker FM, Parizel PM, et al: Tuberculosis of the central nervous system: overview of neuroradiological findings, *Eur Radiol* 13:1876–1890, 2003.

Gupta RK, Vatsal DK, Husain N, Chawla S, Prasad KN, Roy R: Differentiation of tuberculous from pyogenic brain abscesses with in vivo proton MR spectroscopy and magnetization transfer MR imaging, *AJNR Am J Neuroradiol* 22:1503–1509, 2001.

Cross-Reference

Neuroradiology: THE REQUISITES, 2nd ed, pp 304–308.

Comment

There has been an increased incidence of tuberculosis in the United States. The cause of this is multifactorial and is related in part to AIDS and the emergence of drug-resistant strains of the bacillus. Approximately 5% to 10% of patients with tuberculosis go on to have CNS disease (approximately 5%–20% of patients with AIDS have CNS manifestations). Tuberculous infection in children is usually related to primary infection, whereas in adults it is usually caused by postprimary infection.

Central nervous system tuberculosis has a spectrum of clinical and radiologic presentations, including tuberculous meningitis, cerebritis or encephalitis, abscess formation, and tuberculoma. Intracranial tuberculosis has two related pathologic correlates—meningitis and the tuberculoma, which coexist in approximately 10% of cases. Tuberculomas are tubercles that form as a result of cell-mediated immunity. They are walled off by a fibrous capsule and are centrally necrotic, with surrounding lymphocytes and giant cells. Tuberculomas may be dormant for years. They may resolve, they may cause symptoms related to lesion location (seizure, mass effect), or they may rupture into the subarachnoid space, causing meningitis. FLAIR imaging is very sensitive in the detection of subarachnoid and leptomeningeal disease, which is manifest as hyperintensity in the affected areas. Avid enhancement of the involved areas is the rule. Arteritis may be seen in up to one third of patients with basilar meningitis. This is because the vessels coursing through this inflammatory exudate may become directly involved. Consequences of arteritis include vasospasm and infarction. CNS tuberculosis is usually related to hematogenous dissemination from a systemic source, most commonly, the lung, but also possibly the genitourinary system or gastrointestinal tract.

Notes

Fair Game

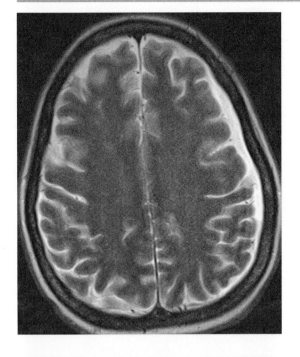
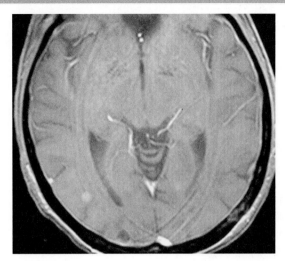
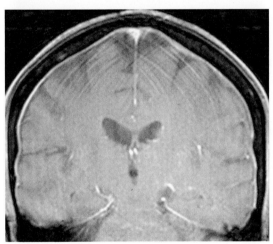
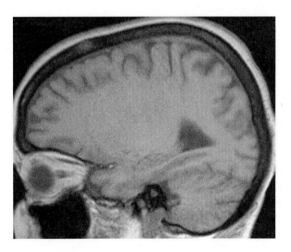

1. What is the most likely diagnosis?

2. What type (location) of metastases may be associated with minimal or no edema such that they are frequently missed on T2W imaging and necessitate the administration of intravenous contrast for their detection?

3. What is the most common neoplasm to be associated with purely dural metastases?

4. In children, dural metastases are most commonly associated with what extracranial tumors?

Dural Metastases—Breast Carcinoma

1. Metastatic disease.

2. Cortical metastases.

3. Breast carcinoma.

4. Adrenal neuroblastoma and leukemia.

References

Maki DD, Grossman RI: Patterns of disease spread in metastatic breast carcinoma: influence of estrogen and progesterone receptor status, *AJNR Am J Neuroradiol* 21:1064–1066, 2000.

Walker R, Kessar P, Blanchard R, et al: Turbo STIR magnetic resonance imaging as a whole-body screening tool for metastases in patients with breast carcinoma: preliminary clinical experience, *J Magn Reson Imaging* 11:343–350, 2000.

Cross-Reference

Neuroradiology: THE REQUISITES, 2nd ed, pp 109–113, 148–152.

Comment

This case of metastatic breast carcinoma illustrates several findings and imaging patterns of metastatic disease. There is a small left subdural effusion that follows the signal characteristics of CSF on all pulse sequences (including FLAIR and diffusion-weighted images, not shown). Note on the axial T2W image that the cortical veins seen as small black flow voids are closely up against the surface of the left cerebrum, consistent with a subdural effusion (in contrast to dilated subarachnoid spaces, as are seen in cerebral atrophy, in which the bridging cortical veins are noted to course through the CSF spaces). There is diffuse thin enhancement of the dura over the cerebral convexities. Axial images also demonstrate two cortical enhancing metastases. Lastly, best appreciated on the sagittal unenhanced T1W image is diffuse decreased signal intensity of the calvarial marrow, with superimposed areas of signal abnormality, consistent with diffuse marrow infiltration or metastases.

Dural metastases usually are secondary to hematogenous dissemination of tumor from extracranial systemic tumors. Dural metastases may also result from direct extension of adjacent calvarial or skull base bone metastases. Breast, lung, and prostate carcinoma as well as melanoma and lymphoma not uncommonly are associated with dural metastases in adults. In children, adrenal neuroblastoma and leukemia are most commonly associated with dural metastases. These malignant neoplasms may also metastasize to the cranial sutures. In infancy, this may present as widened sutures. Inflammatory processes that may mimic dural metastases include granulomatous infections (tuberculosis, syphilis, and fungal), sarcoid, Langerhans' cell histiocytosis, and Erdheim-Chester disease.

Notes

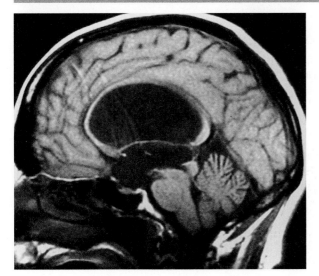
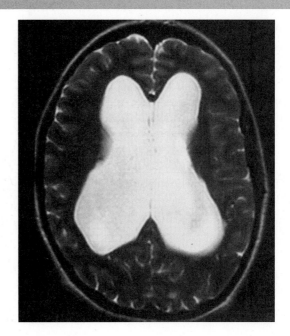

1. What is the level of ventricular obstruction in this case?

2. What can cause obstruction of the aqueduct of Sylvius?

3. In communicating hydrocephalus, where is the obstruction of CSF circulation?

4. What is the inheritance pattern in congenital aqueductal stenosis?

Aqueductal Stenosis

1. The aqueduct of Sylvius.

2. Obstruction may be congenital (webs or diaphragms within the aqueduct or gliosis). Acquired aqueductal stenosis may be intrinsic, related to clot or adhesions from previous subarachnoid hemorrhage or infection (meningitis or ventriculitis), or extrinsic on the basis of compression of the aqueduct related to tumors in this region (tectal gliomas, pineal tumors, cerebellar neoplasms), or cerebellar stroke.

3. Most commonly, in the arachnoid villi. Lesions at the level of the foramen magnum may also result in obstructive communicating hydrocephalus.

4. Congenital aqueductal stenosis may be seen as an inherited X-linked recessive disorder in boys.

Reference

Yoshimoto Y, Ochiai C, Kawamata K, Endo M, Nagai M: Aqueductal blood clot as a cause of acute hydrocephalus in subarachnoid hemorrhage, *AJNR Am J Neuroradiol* 17:1183–1186, 1996.

Cross-Reference

Neuroradiology: THE REQUISITES, 2nd ed, pp 372–373.

Comment

This case demonstrates the characteristic findings in congenital aqueductal stenosis. There is prominent dilation of the lateral and third ventricles, with a relatively normal-sized fourth ventricle. There is upward convexity or bowing of the corpus callosum related to the lateral ventricular dilation, and there is inferior bowing of the anterior recesses of the third ventricle, with depression of the optic chiasm. Congenital aqueductal stenosis may be seen as an inherited X-linked recessive disorder in boys. Children may present with an enlarging head circumference. Blockage of the aqueduct may be caused by webs, septae, or gliosis.

Aqueductal stenosis is often acquired in relation to previous subarachnoid hemorrhage, meningitis or ventriculitis, or extrinsic compression from a mass or tumor. MR imaging is the modality of choice in evaluating affected patients; sagittal MR imaging is particularly useful in distinguishing intrinsic aqueductal abnormalities from extrinsic mass compression. The presence of aqueductal CSF flow may be evaluated using spin-echo and gradient echo flow scans with gradient moment nulling. On spin-echo images, hypointensity within the aqueduct (signal void) is consistent with flow, whereas on gradient echo imaging. the presence of high signal intensity within the aqueduct is consistent with flow.

Notes

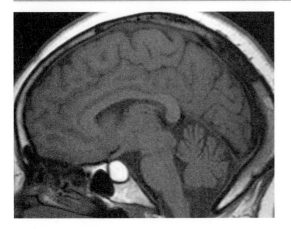
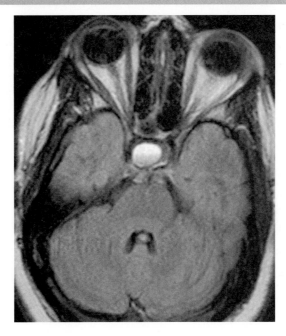

1. What is the differential diagnosis?

2. What radiologic findings would favor the diagnosis of craniopharyngioma?

3. Most Rathke's cleft cysts are localized in what part of the pituitary gland?

4. When large enough, this lesion may cause visual symptoms or hormonal dysfunction as a result of compression of what structures?

Rathke's Cleft Cyst

1. Rathke's cleft cyst, hemorrhagic pituitary adenoma, craniopharyngioma, choristoma.

2. The presence of calcification, an associated soft tissue mass, or areas of solid enhancement.

3. Unlike pituitary adenomas, which are more frequently localized in the lateral portion of the gland, large autopsy series have shown that the vast majority of Rathke's cleft cysts are localized in the center of the gland (pars intermedia).

4. The optic chiasm and the anterior lobe of the pituitary gland or stalk, respectively.

Reference

Byun WM, Kim OL, Kim D: MR imaging findings of Rathke's cleft cysts: significance of intracystic nodules, *Am J Neuroradiol* 2000:485–488, 2000.

Cross-Reference

Neuroradiology: THE REQUISITES, 2nd ed, pp 417, 542.

Comment

Rathke's cleft cysts are embryologic remnants of Rathke's pouch, the neuroectoderm that ascends from the oral cavity to the sella to form the anterior pituitary lobe and pars intermedia. In the majority of cases, Rathke's cleft cysts are incidental findings noted at autopsy or identified on imaging studies performed for other reasons. In a recent series of 1000 autopsy specimens, 11% of the pituitary glands had an incidental Rathke's cleft cyst. These lesions are typically localized within the pituitary sella, although they may also extend into the suprasellar region. In addition, Rathke's cleft cysts may be centered in the suprasellar cistern anterior to the hypothalamic stalk. A single layer of cuboidal or columnar epithelium, which may contain goblet cells, typically lines these cysts.

The contents within the cysts are mucoid, resulting in their typical MR imaging appearance. Most Rathke's cleft cysts are circumscribed and hyperintense on both unenhanced T1W and T2W images. Although this is the most common pattern, cysts may also be hypointense or isointense on either T1W or T2W images, depending on their protein concentration and viscosity. In this case, the cyst is hyperintense on unenhanced T1W imaging and hyperintense on T2W imaging, with a fluid–debris level (did you catch that?). These cysts do not enhance (although there may be mild peripheral enhancement). More recently, intracystic nodules have been described that are hyperintense on unenhanced T1W images and hypointense on T2W images. At surgery, these appear as yellow, waxy solid masses, and the pathologic correlate shows a mucin clump.

Although most Rathke's cleft cysts are incidental findings, symptoms may occur with larger lesions that compress the optic chiasm (resulting in headache and visual disturbances) or pituitary gland (patients may present with diabetes insipidus or hypopituitarism).

Notes

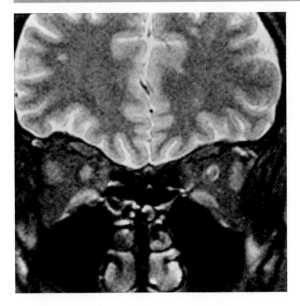 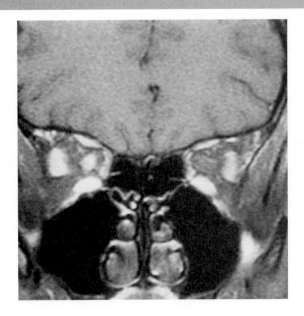

1. What are the imaging findings?

2. What is the differential diagnosis of this finding? What is the best diagnosis?

3. What is optic neuritis?

4. What are causes of optic neuritis?

Optic Neuritis (Demyelinating Disease)

1. High signal intensity within the right optic nerve associated with avid solid enhancement of the optic nerve sheath complex.

2. Optic neuritis (demyelinating disease), sarcoid, infection, primary tumor (glioma and meningioma), and metastatic disease. Multiple sclerosis is the best diagnosis.

3. Optic neuritis is inflammation of the optic nerve associated with decreased vision, abnormal color vision, and afferent papillary defect.

4. Demyelinating disease is most common. Less common etiologies include ischemia, vasculitis, sarcoid, systemic lupus erythematosus, infection (viral, Lyme, toxoplasmosis), and radiation therapy.

References

Al-Shafai, Mikulis DJ: Diffusion MR imaging in a case of acute ischemic optic neuropathy, *Am J Neuroradiol* 27:255–257, 2006.

Beck RW, Cleary PA, Trobe JD, et al: The effect of corticosteroids for acute optic neuritis on the subsequent development of multiple sclerosis, *N Engl J Med* 329:1764–1769, 1993.

Cross-Reference

Neuroradiology: THE REQUISITES, 2nd ed, pp 492–493.

Comment

A wide spectrum of disease processes may be associated with optic neuritis, most commonly, demyelinating disease followed by idiopathic disease. Approximately 50% of patients with optic neuritis have multiple sclerosis, and approximately 15% of patients with multiple sclerosis have optic neuritis as their initial clinical presentation. Devic's disease (neuromyelitis optica) represents a specific syndrome of multiple sclerosis in which patients have isolated transverse myelitis and optic neuritis. These two may present simultaneously or on separate occasions. In older patients, vasculopathies and ischemia are more common causes of optic neuritis.

Patients presenting with optic neuritis can be assessed using high-resolution, fat-suppressed, fast spin-echo T2W and enhanced T1W images, as in this case. Imaging in the coronal plane is particularly useful. Imaging may demonstrate increased T2W signal intensity within the nerve itself, and postcontrast images may demonstrate enhancement of the nerve as well as the nerve sheath due to perivenous inflammation (as in this case). In cases of clinically diagnosed optic neuritis, MR imaging of the brain is especially useful and is recommended because it may help to establish the diagnosis of demyelinating disease. In patients with their first episode of optic neuritis, up to 65% have asymptomatic cerebral white matter lesions on brain MR study. In addition, studies have shown that the presence of brain lesions on MR imaging in patients with optic neuritis may be important in determining prognosis and outcome.

Notes

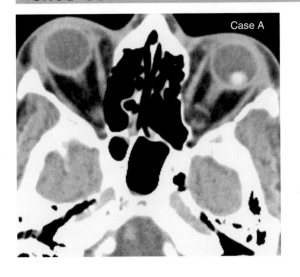

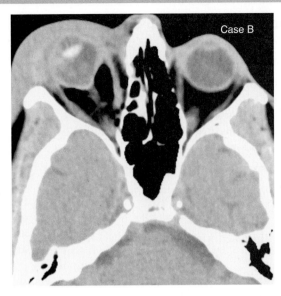

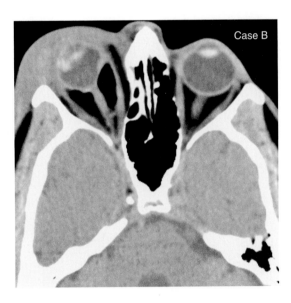

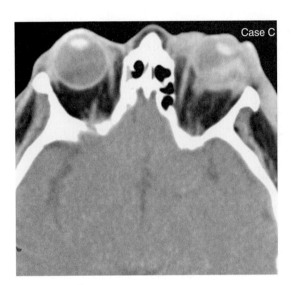

1. What is the diagnosis for Case A?

2. Regarding ocular foreign bodies, what are the CT and MR imaging appearances of wood?

3. What is the diagnosis for Cases B and C?

4. What connective tissue disorders (mesodermal abnormalities) are associated with dislocation or subluxation of the lens?

Ocular Trauma—Lens Dislocation and Globe Rupture

1. Traumatic lens dislocation.

2. Wood is hypodense on CT and hypointense on MR imaging. On CT, the orbits should be viewed on wide (bone) windows to distinguish wood from orbital emphysema, because wood can resemble air on soft tissue windows.

3. Globe rupture.

4. Marfan syndrome, Ehlers-Danlos syndrome, and homocystinuria.

References

Maguire AM, Enger C, Eliott D, Zinreich SJ: Computerized tomography in the evaluation of penetrating ocular injuries, *Retina* 11:405–411, 1991.

Weissman JL, Beatty RL, Hirsch WL, Curtin HD: Enlarged anterior chamber: CT finding of a ruptured globe, *Am J Neuroradiol* 16(Suppl):936–938, 1995.

Cross-Reference

Neuroradiology: THE REQUISITES, 2nd ed, pp 266–268, 469–470, 475–477.

Comment

On CT imaging, lens dislocation (Case A) may be differentiated from other intraocular foreign bodies by identifying that the intraocular density has the configuration of a lens and, importantly, observing that the lens in that eye is not located in its normal position. Lens dislocation may be confirmed on physical examination. CT is the imaging modality of choice in the initial assessment of patients with orbital trauma due to its availability as well as the ease and rapidity with which the examination can be performed. In addition, CT readily establishes the presence of orbital foreign bodies, delineates orbital fractures, and assesses for retrobulbar complications of trauma.

Subluxation or dislocation of the lens may be unrelated to trauma. It may be spontaneous or related to infection. There are also hereditary disorders that affect the connective (mesodermal) tissues that may be associated with lens dislocation, such as Marfan syndrome, Ehlers-Danlos syndrome, and homocystinuria. In Marfan syndrome, lens subluxation or dislocation is superior and at the periphery of the globe (and usually bilateral), whereas in homocystinuria, subluxations are inferior ("down and out").

Globe rupture indicates that the integrity of the outer membranes of the eye is disrupted. Globe rupture may occur when a blunt object impacts the orbit, causing anterior–posterior compression of the globe and raising intraocular pressure such that the sclera tears. Ruptures from blunt trauma usually occur at the sites where the sclera is thinnest, at the insertions of the extraocular muscles, at the limbus, and around the optic nerve. Sharp objects or those traveling at high velocity may perforate the globe directly. Globe rupture represents an ophthalmologic emergency and requires surgical intervention. Damage to the posterior segment of the eye is associated with a very high frequency of permanent visual loss. Early recognition and ophthalmologic intervention are critical to maximizing functional outcome. On CT imaging, the presence of vitreous hemorrhage suggests an associated globe rupture. An enlarged anterior chamber and retraction of the lens are indicative of rupture of the posterior sclera. Other findings of globe rupture are a small, misshapen globe that contains blood or air (as in Cases B and C).

Notes

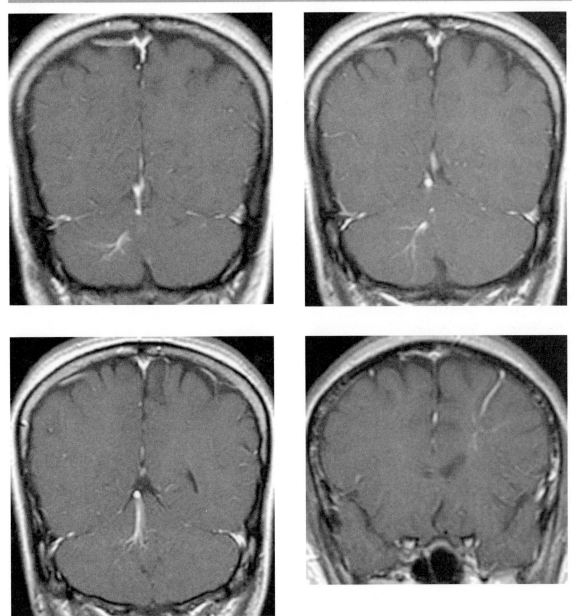

1. What is the diagnosis?

2. What is the most common infratentorial location of these lesions?

3. What neurocutaneous syndrome is associated with a diffuse venous malformation?

4. What would the arterial and venous phases of a conventional cerebral angiogram show?

CASE 56

Developmental Venous Anomaly

1. Developmental venous anomalies in the cerebellum and the left frontal lobe.

2. The cerebellum.

3. Sturge-Weber syndrome. This represents a more extensive venous malformation that results from failure of development of the normal venous system, often covering a large portion of a cerebral hemisphere. Large cerebral malformations may also be seen in Klippel-Trénaunay-Weber syndrome.

4. A normal arterial phase. The venous phase shows a pathognomonic collection of dilated medullary veins converging in an enlarged "draining" vein.

Reference

Lee C, Pennington MA, Kennedy CM III: MR evaluation of developmental venous anomalies: medullary venous anatomy of venous angiomas, *AJNR Am J Neuroradiol* 17:61–70, 1996.

Cross-Reference

Neuroradiology: THE REQUISITES, 2nd ed, pp 231, 234.

Comment

Developmental venous anomalies, also referred to as venous malformations or venous angiomas, likely occur late in the first trimester and early in the second trimester of gestation, when the medullary veins are developing. Insults leading to failure in the development of the normal draining venous structures are believed to be the cause of these anatomic variants. Instead of the normal parallel appearance of the medullary veins as they drain into subependymal or superficial cortical veins, a disorganized network of dilated medullary veins converges in a "caput medusa" appearance and drains into an enlarged venous channel that subsequently drains superficially to cortical veins or sinuses, or deeply to subependymal veins of the lateral ventricle and then into the galenic system. Normal cerebral tissue intervenes between the dilated veins. The brain parenchyma surrounding a venous angioma is typically normal, although occasional gliosis, seen as mild T2W hyperintensity, may be present. Developmental venous anomalies are found most commonly in the frontal lobes, followed by the parietal and temporal lobes. Infratentorial developmental venous anomalies occur most commonly in the cerebellum. These can drain to the fourth ventricle and then to the pontomesencephalic vein, or to the precentral cerebellar vein and into the galenic system.

More than 99% of developmental venous malformations are asymptomatic; however, rarely, these lesions may hemorrhage. Hemorrhagic complications are usually secondary to coexisting cavernous malformations. Rare hemorrhage related specifically to the venous angioma is most common with cerebellar lesions. Patients may present with headache, seizure, or focal neurologic symptoms. Asymptomatic (essentially all) developmental venous anomalies are not treated because they represent a compensatory venous drainage route for normal brain. Sacrifice of these lesions could result in venous infarction of the normal brain that they drain.

Notes

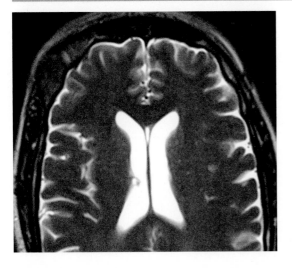

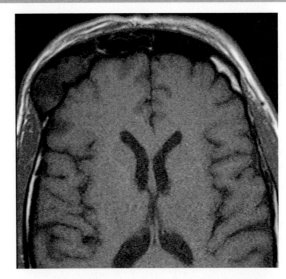

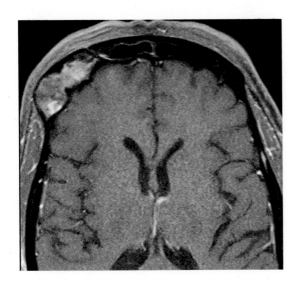

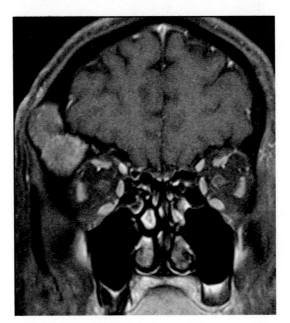

1. What is the differential diagnosis?

2. What imaging study could be done next to make the diagnosis?

3. How often is fibrous dysplasia polyostotic?

4. Which bones are most commonly affected in polyostotic fibrous dysplasia?

Fibrous Dysplasia of the Calvaria

1. Fibrous dysplasia and Paget's disease. Metastatic disease and lymphoma are less likely, given the imaging appearance (an expansile mass with preservation of the inner and outer cortical tables).

2. CT to identify the characteristic appearance of fibrous dysplasia.

3. Fibrous dysplasia is polyostic in approximately 25% of cases.

4. The skull and facial bones.

Reference

Jee WH, Choi KH, Choe BY, Park JM, Shinn KS: Fibrous dysplasia: MR imaging characteristics with radiopathologic correlation, *AJR Am J Roentgenol* 167:1523–1527, 1996.

Cross-Reference

Neuroradiology: THE REQUISITES, 2nd ed, pp 513, 662, 864.

Comment

Fibrous dysplasia is a developmental bone disorder in which osteoblasts do not undergo normal differentiation and maturation. The cause is unknown. Fibrous dysplasia may be monostotic (a solitary lesion) or polyostotic (multiple bones involved or multiple lesions in one bone). Approximately 75% of cases of fibrous dysplasia are monostotic (25% polyostotic). Polyostotic fibrous dysplasia involves the skull and facial bones more frequently than does monostotic disease. Common areas of calvarial involvement include the ethmoid, maxillary, frontal, and sphenoid bones. Involvement of these bones may result in orbital abnormalities such as exophthalmos, visual disturbances, and displacement of the globe. Involvement of the temporal bone may result in hearing loss or vestibular dysfunction.

Fibrous dysplasia of the skull or facial bones on plain radiography may present as radiolucent or sclerotic lesions. Sclerotic lesions are more common in the calvaria, skull base, and sphenoid bones. Although Paget's disease may occur in these same locations of the calvaria, unlike fibrous dysplasia, concomitant involvement of the facial bones is less common. In this case, there is a mass in the right frontal bone, with associated focal expansion of the diploic space. There is preservation of the inner and outer cortical tables without destruction or significant thickening of the cortex. These features are typical of fibrous dysplasia. In contrast, although there may be expansion of the diploic space in patients with Paget's disease, there is normally thickening of the cortex (which may be extensively involved).

Notes

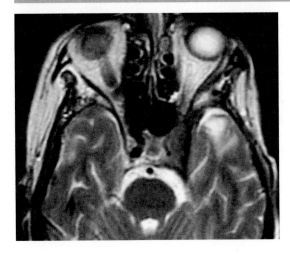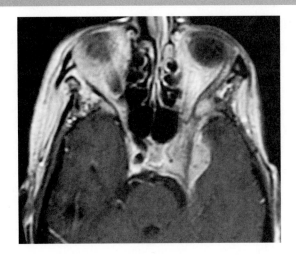

1. What is the anatomic location of the mass in this case?

2. What cranial nerves course through this anatomic space?

3. Which cranial nerve passes through the foramen ovale?

4. Given the presence of narrowing of the left cavernous internal carotid artery, what is the best diagnosis?

Cavernous Sinus Mass—Meningioma

1. The left cavernous sinus.

2. Cranial nerves III, IV, V (first and second divisions), and VI.

3. The third division of cranial nerve V.

4. Meningioma of the cavernous sinus.

References

Hirsch WL Jr, Hryshko FG, Sekhar LN, et al: Comparison of MR imaging, CT, and angiography in the evaluation of the enlarged cavernous sinus, *AJNR Am J Neuroradiol* 9:907–915, 1988.

Hudgins PA: Imaging of the cavernous sinus: management of cavernous sinus pathology, *Techniques in Neurosurgery* 8:211–219, 2003.

Cross-Reference

Neuroradiology: THE REQUISITES, 2nd ed, pp 522–525, 527, 551–558.

Comment

A variety of lesions can affect the cavernous sinus, including neoplasms primarily arising from bone (chondrosarcoma, chondroma, and chordoma) and bone metastases. Metastases and lymphoma primarily affecting the cavernous sinus and perineural spread of tumor are also common. Benign neoplasms include meningioma, schwannoma, and extension of a pituitary adenoma. A variety of vascular and inflammatory lesions may also involve the cavernous sinus.

Infectious processes include bacterial and fungal (actinomycosis, aspergillus, and mucormycosis) agents. In addition, the cavernous sinus may be affected indirectly by complications of infectious processes (eg, cavernous sinus thrombosis). Tolosa-Hunt syndrome represents an idiopathic granulomatous inflammatory disorder that may affect the orbital apex and cavernous sinus. Histologically, Tolosa-Hunt syndrome is identical to orbital pseudotumor (differing only in location). It may present with painful ophthalmoplegia, deficits of the cranial nerves coursing through the cavernous sinus, and retro-orbital pain. Symptoms may last for days to weeks, and may be recurrent. Like orbital pseudotumor, it responds rapidly to steroid treatment. MR imaging may show abnormal signal intensity or an enhancing mass within the cavernous sinus. There may be extension into the orbital apex. Thrombosis of the cavernous sinus or superior ophthalmic vein may occur.

These images demonstrate a mass within the left cavernous sinus that is hypointense to CSF (isointense to brain parenchyma) on T2W imaging. Neoplastic processes that may be hypointense on T2W imaging include lymphoma, meningioma, and less commonly, plasmacytoma and schwannoma. Sarcoid may also be hypointense on T2W imaging. Enhancement extends along the lateral dural margin, as well as posteriorly along the tentorial margin (an appearance that may be seen with meningiomas, lymphoma, and sarcoid). The marked narrowing of the left cavernous internal carotid artery with preserved antegrade flow makes meningioma the best diagnosis. Biopsy through a left temporal craniotomy revealed a meningioma.

Notes

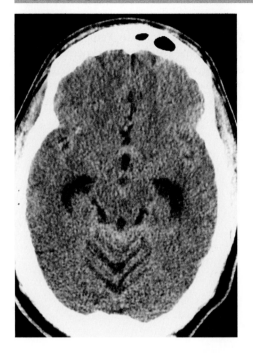 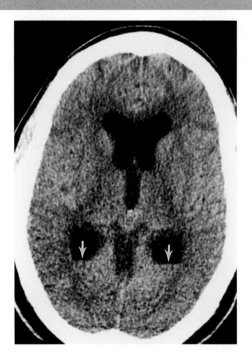

1. What are the pertinent imaging findings?

2. What are common secondary complications related to ventricloperitoneal shunts?

3. What infectious agents have a propensity to cause choroid plexitis?

4. What are common complications of meningitis?

C A S E 5 9

Pyogenic Ventriculitis with Acute Hydrocephalus

1. Acute hydrocephalus and pus levels layering in the lateral ventricles (*arrows*).

2. In addition to ventriculitis, other complications include overdrainage resulting in slit ventricle syndrome, subdural hematomas (which are frequently bilateral), and shunt malfunction.

3. *Cryptococcus* and *Nocardia*. choroid plexusitis

4. Subdural empyema, encephalitis, brain abscess, and ventriculitis with acute hydrocephalus, as in this case.

References

Kanamulla US, Ibarra RA, Jinkins JR: Imaging of cranial meningitis and ventriculitis, *Neuroimaging Clin N Am* 10:309–331, 2000.

Pezzullo JA, Tung GA, Mudigonda S, Rogg JM: Diffusion weighted MR imaging of pyogenic ventriculitis, *Am J Roentgenol* 180:71–75, 2003.

Cross-Reference

Neuroradiology: THE REQUISITES, 2nd ed, pp 284–286.

Comment

This case demonstrates acute hydrocephalus and fluid–fluid levels (*arrows*) within the occipital horns of the lateral ventricles, consistent with ventriculitis complicating pyogenic meningitis. Lumbar puncture yielded pus. Ventriculitis is due to the introduction of infectious organisms into the ependyma or ventricles, and may be secondary to bacteremia, extension of an intraparenchymal abscess, trauma, or surgical instrumentation (especially placement of ventricular shunts). In addition to ventriculitis, other complications of ventriculoperitoneal shunts include overdrainage resulting in slit ventricle syndrome, subdural hematomas (which are frequently bilateral), shunt malfunction, surgery-related complications, and metastases in the setting of neoplasm (such as primitive neuroectodermal tumor).

Approximately 20% of patients with pyogenic bacterial meningitis will have complications necessitating neurosurgical intervention (surgery or a ventriculostomy), even after antibiotic therapy. Such complications include subdural empyema; parenchymal brain abscess; ventriculitis with hydrocephalus, as in this case; and encephalitis. The development of such complications may correlate with inadequate treatment or with the duration of meningitis before the initiation of therapy.

Cytomegalovirus (CMV) ventriculitis is unusual, but may occur in patients with HIV infection. Most HIV-infected patients with CMV ventriculitis have already been diagnosed with an AIDS-defining condition. Pathologic findings include inflammation of the ependyma and periventricular structures, as well as ependymal necrosis with CMV intranuclear inclusion bodies. The differential diagnosis in this patient population includes non-Hodgkin's lymphoma.

Notes

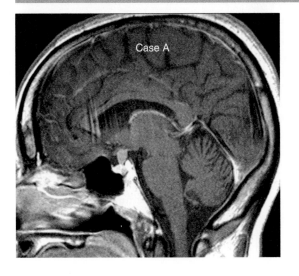

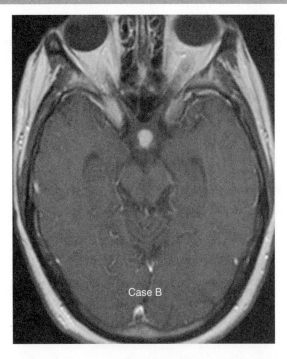

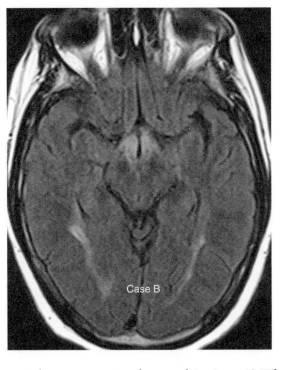

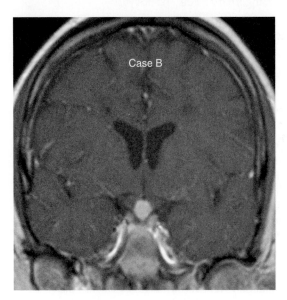

1. What structure is abnormal in Case A? Where is the lesion centered in Case B?

2. What was the clinical presentation in both of these cases?

3. What is the differential diagnosis of a mass in this location in adults?

4. Is the infundibular stalk normally wider at the median eminence or inferiorly along its insertion with the pituitary gland?

Lesions of the Pituitary Stalk and Hypothalamus: Case A—Sarcoidosis; Case B—Langerhans' Cell Histiocytosis

1. The pituitary stalk. In Case B, the mass is centered in the hypothalamus at the location of the upper pituitary stalk.

2. Diabetes insipidus.

3. The differential diagnosis of an infundibular lesion in adults includes granulomatous disease (sarcoid or tuberculosis), metastasis (especially lung and breast), and germinoma. Less commonly, lymphoma or a hypothalamic glioma may present in this way.

4. The pituitary stalk is normally widest at the median eminence and should taper as it extends inferiorly to its insertion at the pituitary gland.

Reference

Prayer D, Grois N, Prosch H, Gadner H, Barkovich AJ: MR imaging presentation of intracranial disease associated with Langerhans cell histiocytosis, *Am J Neuroradiol* 25:880–891, 2004.

Cross-Reference

Neuroradiology: THE REQUISITES, 2nd ed, pp 320, 541–542.

Comment

In Case A, the midline sagittal enhanced T1W MR image shows abnormal thickening and enhancement along the pituitary stalk that lacks normal tapering as it extends inferiorly toward the pituitary gland. This represented sarcoid, and responded well to steroid treatment. This patient had a history of sarcoid with pulmonary involvement. Involvement of the CNS by sarcoid occurs in approximately 5% to 15% of patients, with isolated involvement of the pituitary gland or stalk in fewer than 1% to 2% of all patients with sarcoid. When CNS sarcoid presents with leptomeningeal involvement, the pituitary stalk in these cases is commonly involved.

Case B shows an enhancing mass in the hypothalamic region at the level of the upper pituitary stalk, and this represented Langerhans' cell histiocytosis. The differential diagnosis of an infundibular mass in children includes germinoma, infection (meningitis or tuberculosis) and, less commonly, lymphoma or leukemia and glioma involving the hypothalamic region. In patients with Langerhans' cell histiocytosis, there may be absence of the normal "bright spot" of the posterior pituitary gland in the sella on unenhanced T1W images. Langerhans' cell histiocytosis uncommonly affects the CNS. It is a disorder of the reticuloendothelial system. The most common

cranial bone abnormality is a lytic, circumscribed, enhancing mass of the calvaria or skull base. In the cranium, it most commonly involves the temporal bone along the mastoid segment. It also may involve the frontal bone along the orbit.

The differential diagnosis of an infundibular lesion in adults includes granulomatous disease (sarcoid or tuberculosis) and metastasis (especially lung and breast). Less commonly, lymphoma or a hypothalamic glioma may present in this way. Lymphocytic adenohypophysitis is a unique condition that almost always affects women. It is most common in the postpartum period or in the late stages (third trimester) of pregnancy. It is characterized by lymphocytic infiltration of the adenohypophysis and is usually self-limited.

Notes

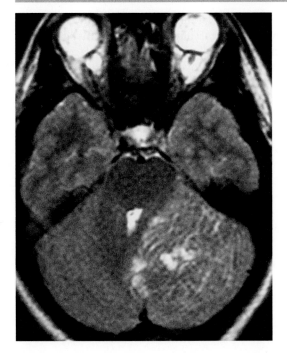
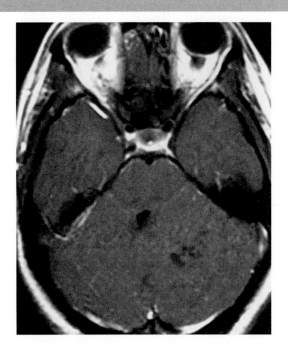

1. What are the MR imaging findings in this case that are characteristic for this disease?

2. With what uncommon neurocutaneous syndrome are dysplastic gangliocytomas associated?

3. In what part of the cerebellum do PNETs (primitive neural ectodermal tumors) occur in adults?

4. Following intravenous gadolinium administration, what would you expect to see with this patient's mass?

Lhermitte-Duclos Disease (Dysplastic Gangliocytoma of the Cerebellum)

1. There is T2W hyperintensity and thickening of involved cerebellar folia giving a laminated or corduroy appearance. These lesions typically do not demonstrate avid enhancement, but they often exert mass effect, as is noted in this patient.

2. Cowden disease (multiple hamartoma syndrome).

3. Lateral cerebellar hemisphere.

4. No significant enhancement.

References

Moonis G, Ibrahim M, Melhem ER: Diffusion-weighted MRI in Lhermitte-Duclos disease: report of two cases, *Neuroradiology* 46:351–354, 2004.

Nagaraja S, Powell T, Griffiths PD, Wilkinson ID: MR imaging and spectroscopy in Lhermitte-Duclos disease, *Neuroradiology* 46:355–358, 2004.

Cross-Reference

Neuroradiology: THE REQUISITES, 2nd ed, pp 137–138, 162–163.

Comment

Lhermitte-Duclos disease is also known as dysplastic gangliocytoma of the cerebellum. When symptomatic, patient typically presents with complaints related to mass effect in the second and third decades of life. Lhermitte-Duclos disease has been associated with Cowden disease (multiple hamartoma syndrome), an autosomal dominant disorder associated with an increased incidence of neoplasms in the pelvis, breast, colon, and thyroid. Intracranial meningiomas have also been noted with this syndrome.

Although controversial, Lhermitte-Duclos disease is considered to represent a complex hamartomatous malformation, not a true neoplasm. Dysplastic gangliocytomas often occur in the cerebellar hemispheres. These lesions tend to be poorly demarcated, presenting on CT as a mildly hypodense mass. Calcification has been reported. On MR imaging, these lesions have a more characteristic appearance in which the gray and white matter of the cerebellar hemisphere are both involved and are thickened and hyperintense on T2W imaging, showing a somewhat characteristic laminated or "corduroy" appearance. They may exert mass effect. Hydrocephalus may be present. Dysplastic gangliocytomas do not demonstrate significant enhancement. On pathologic evaluation they usually appear as dysplasia with cellular disorganization of the normal laminar structure of the cerebellum, and hypertrophied granular cell neurons. Histologically there is hypermyelination of axons, and pleomorphic ganglion cells replace the granular and Purkinje cell layers.

Notes

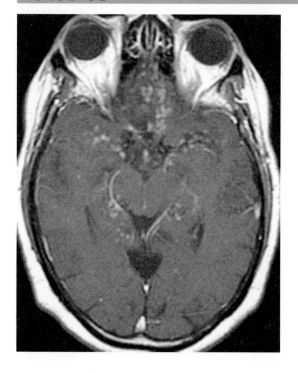 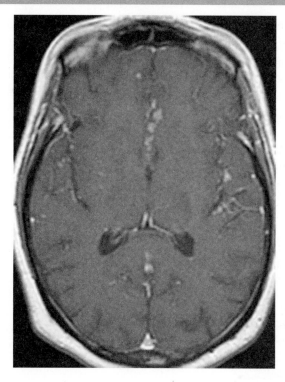

1. What is the major imaging finding?

2. What disease processes affect the basilar leptomeninges?

3. In cases of meningitis with associated hydrocephalus, is the hydrocephalus typically communicating or noncommunicating?

4. What primary CNS neoplasms have a predilection for subarachnoid seeding?

Basilar Meningitis—Sarcoidosis

1. Nodular enhancement of the basal cisterns or leptomeninges and subarachnoid spaces. Enhancement is noted around the optic chiasm and infundibular stalk.

2. Infection (eg, tuberculosis, neurosyphilis, pyogenic infections, *Cryptococcus*), sarcoidosis, leptomeningeal seeding of tumor (eg, carcinomatous from systemic malignancies or primary brain tumors), lymphoma, and chemical meningitis (eg, drugs, iodophenylundecylic acid [Pantopaque], fat from ruptured dermoids).

3. Communicating because of blockage of the cisterns from an inflammatory exudate. Occasionally, hydrocephalus may be secondary to mass effect from a parenchymal lesion or from entrapment of a ventricle related to ependymitis.

4. Primitive neuroectodermal tumors (medulloblastoma, pineoblastoma), germinoma, glial neoplasms (glioblastoma multiforme, oligodendroglioma), and choroid plexus papilloma.

Reference

Singer MB, Atlas SW, Drayer BP: Subarachnoid space disease: diagnosis with fluid-attenuated inversion-recovery MR imaging and comparison with gadolinium-enhanced spin-echo MR imaging—blinded reader study, *Radiology* 208:417–422, 1998.

Cross-Reference

Neuroradiology: THE REQUISITES, 2nd ed, pp 198, 277–281, 320–322, 541.

Comment

Sarcoidosis is a systemic disorder characterized pathologically by noncaseating granulomas. Typical presentation is in the third and fourth decades of life, and it is slightly more common in women than in men. CNS involvement has been reported in 5% to 15% of cases, and isolated CNS involvement occurs in fewer than 2% to 4% of cases. Multiple patterns of CNS involvement may occur. The most common is chronic meningitis with a predilection for the leptomeninges of the basal cisterns, as in this case. These patients may present with chronic meningeal symptoms, cranial neuropathies (especially involving the facial and optic nerves), or symptoms related to involvement of the hypothalamus and pituitary stalk. Imaging findings are best demonstrated with MR imaging and include nodular enhancement of the leptomeninges that tends to be most pronounced in the basal cisterns (but may be seen in any of the subarachnoid spaces, as in this case). Another common pattern of CNS sarcoid is brain involvement, with multiple regions of abnormality that may occur as a result of direct extension from leptomeningeal disease; white matter lesions mimicking multiple sclerosis may be present because of disease extension along the perivascular spaces or related to sarcoid-induced small vessel vasculitis. There may also be granulomas in the brain. Less commonly, dural-based disease may be the predominant imaging finding and may be mistaken for a meningioma.

Central nervous system tuberculosis may have a variety of clinical and radiologic presentations, including nodular tuberculous meningitis similar to sarcoid, cerebritis, abscess formation, tuberculoma, or a combination of these. CNS tuberculosis is normally related to hematogenous dissemination from a systemic source, such as the lung, genitourinary system, or gastrointestinal tract. Arteritis may be seen in up to one third of patients with basilar meningitis. This is because the vessels coursing through this inflammatory exudate may become directly involved. Consequences of arteritis include vasospasm and infarction.

Notes

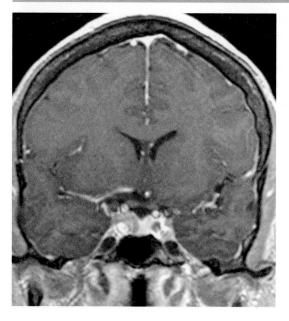 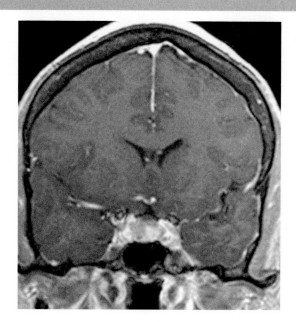

1. What was the clinical presentation in this patient?

2. What is the abnormality on imaging?

3. What is pituitary apoplexy?

4. What treatment is associated with an increased incidence of hemorrhage within an adenoma?

Pituitary Microadenoma

1. Irregular menses and galactorrhea.

2. Subcentimeter mass in the right lateral pituitary with differential enhancement (less enhancement) relative to the normal pituitary gland seen on the left.

3. A clinical syndrome manifested by the acute onset of headache, nausea and vomiting, visual disturbance, cranial neuropathies, or a change in mental status. It is most commonly associated with hemorrhage within an adenoma, although it has been described with infarction. Most pituitary hemorrhages are asymptomatic.

4. Bromocriptine treatment (a dopamine agonist) used to treat prolactinomas.

Reference

Indrajit IK, Chidambaranathan N, Sundar K, Ahmed I: Value of dynamic MRI imaging in pituitary adenomas, *Indian J Radiol Imaging,* 11:185–190, 2001.

Cross-Reference

Neuroradiology: THE REQUISITES, 2nd ed, pp 532–524.

Comment

Pituitary adenomas are slow-growing, benign epithelial neoplasms arising from the anterior lobe of the gland. They are typically demarcated with a "pseudocapsule" that separates them from the normal gland. Pituitary adenomas larger than 10 mm are referred to as macroadenomas, and those less than 10 mm in diameter are referred to as microadenomas. Many adenomas are incidental findings (asymptomatic).

The clinical presentation of pituitary adenomas depends on their size, the presence of hormone secretion resulting in endocrine hyperfunction, and the presence of extension beyond the sella (leading to visual symptoms or cranial nerve palsies related to compression). In vivo, approximately 75% of pituitary adenomas are hormonally active (however, in autopsy series, nonsecreting adenomas are much more common).

The most common clinically significant secreting adenoma is the prolactinoma (which arises from the prolactin-secreting cells [lactotrophs]). In women, the most common clinical presentation is irregular menses, galactorrhea, and infertility. In men, impotence may be present. Hormonally active pituitary adenomas arising from somatotrophs, the growth hormone-secreting cells, cause acromegaly in adults and gigantism in children. In acromegaly, endochondral and periosteal bone formation is stimulated, as is proliferation of connective tissue. These changes result in bone overgrowth and increased soft tissue thickness, especially in the "acral" regions (feet, hands, mandible). There is enlargement of the mandible, thickening of the cranial vault, and frontal bossing (the result of enlargement of the frontal sinuses and prominence of the supraorbital ridges).

Notes

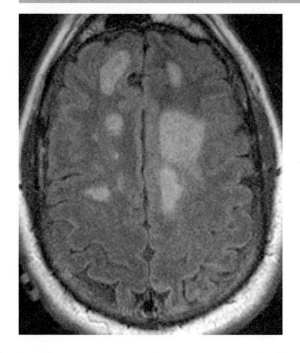
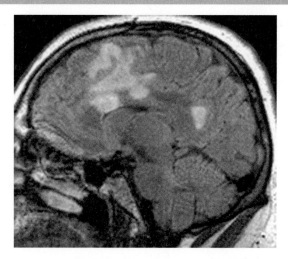

1. What percentage of patients with multiple sclerosis present in childhood and adolescence?

2. What clinical and imaging factors might help differentiate demyelinating disease from a glioma?

3. What percentage of patients with multiple sclerosis present after 50 years of age?

4. What findings may be present in the CSF in patients with multiple sclerosis?

Multiple Sclerosis—Marburg Type

1. Approximately 3% to 5%.

2. Young age, the presence of additional lesions separate from the mass, and neurologic symptoms spaced over time and location favor demyelinating disease.

3. Approximately 10%.

4. Elevated oligoclonal bands (≥90% of cases) and elevated IgG (approximately 75% of patients).

Reference

Cianfoni A, Niku S, Imbesi SG: Metabolite findings in tumefactive demyelinating lesions utilizing short echo time proton magnetic resonance spectroscopy, *Am J Neuroradiol* 28:272–277, 2007.

Cross-Reference

Neuroradiology: THE REQUISITES, 2nd ed, pp 332–336, 341.

Comment

Although the etiology of multiple sclerosis is unknown, several causative factors have been implicated. These include autoimmune disease, infection (viral agent), and genetic factors. The prevalence of multiple sclerosis varies with geographic location.

Variants of multiple sclerosis may be present on a clinical or imaging basis. A handful of rare borderline types of multiple sclerosis occur, including Marburg type (also known as acute, fulminant, or malignant multiple sclerosis), a form of acute multiple sclerosis usually seen in younger patients that may be preceded by fevers, is typically rapidly progressive, and can result in death. In such cases, there is extensive demyelination and there may be defined rings within or surrounding plaques of acute demyelination. Enhancement is typically seen in the region of these rings. Concentric sclerosis or Balo-type sclerosis is characterized histologically by alternating rings of demyelination and myelination (normal brain or areas of remyelination) and has a characteristic MR imaging appearance. Schilder's disease is a rare progressive demyelinating disorder that usually begins in childhood. Symptoms may include dementia, aphasia, seizures, personality changes, tremors, balance instability, incontinence, muscle weakness, headache, and visual impairment.

A type of multiple sclerosis that is usually limited to the optic nerves and spinal cord (either simultaneously or separately) is Devic's disease or neuromyelitis optica. The main symptoms of Devic's disease are loss of vision and spinal cord dysfunction. The visual impairment can consist of reduced visual fields, diminished light sensitivity, or loss of color vision. Spinal cord dysfunction includes muscle weakness and lack of coordination, reduced sensation, and incontinence. The brain is usually spared.

"Tumefactive" multiple sclerosis on imaging may be mistaken for a neoplasm or occasionally an abscess, particularly in the absence of a clinical history. The age of the patient may be helpful (multiple sclerosis typically occurs in younger patients). In addition, on close questioning, patients often have neurologic symptoms that are spaced in both time and location. MR imaging may show white matter lesions separate from the mass, suggesting multiple sclerosis. Unlike neoplasms, tumefactive multiple sclerosis often has relatively little mass effect for the amount of signal abnormality present.

Notes

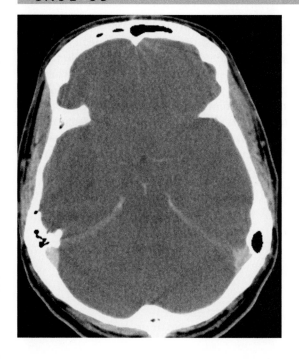

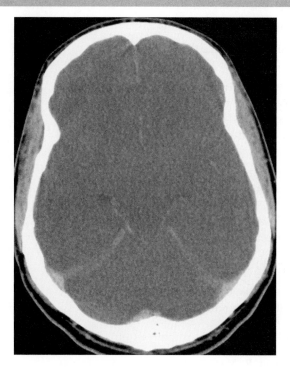

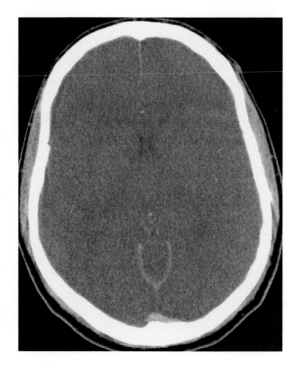

1. What type of CT scan is this?

2. What are the imaging findings? What is the diagnosis?

3. What are the imaging findings in subfalcine herniation?

4. What are causes of upward herniation (superior vermian herniation)?

Transtentorial Herniation

1. It is important to recognize that the study is an unenhanced head CT to correctly interpret the images.

2. Effacement of the cerebral sulci, basilar cisterns, and ventricles; loss of gray–white matter differentiation; pseudosubarachnoid hemorrhage; and pseudovenous sinus thrombosis. Transtentorial herniation.

3. Herniation of the cingulate gyrus beneath the anterior free edge of the falx, best seen on coronal MR imaging. Secondary changes include ischemia in the anterior cerebral artery territory related to vascular compression.

4. Rapid reduction of supratentorial increased intracranial pressure (as with decompression of large extra-axial hematomas) or posterior fossa lesions, resulting in cerebellar mass effect.

Reference

Leistner S, Boegner F, Marx P, Koennecke HC: Transtentorial herniation after unilateral infarction of the anterior cerebral artery, *Stroke* 32:649–651, 2001.

Cross-Reference

Neuroradiology: THE REQUISITES, 2nd ed, pp 261–262.

Comment

This case illustrates global cerebral swelling after resuscitation from a cardiac arrest resulting in transtentorial herniation. The brain is confined by the cranial vault and an inelastic dura. CSF surrounding the brain serves as a shock absorber. With increased intracranial pressure, herniation of brain from one compartment to another may occur. There are multiple patterns of herniation. In the posterior fossa, there may be inferior tonsillar and cerebellar herniation, with displacement of these structures into the foramen magnum, or there may be upward herniation (superior vermian herniation) in which cerebellar tissue obliterates the quadrigeminal and superior vermian cisterns. Herniation syndromes in the supratentorial compartment include subfalcine, temporal lobe, and central transtentorial herniation.

Transtentorial herniation is typically caused by supratentorial mass lesions or global cerebral swelling, resulting in vector forces that are directed medially and inferiorly. There is resultant effacement of the basilar cisterns and ventricles, as well as caudal displacement of the upper brainstem. The temporal lobe shifts over the tentorium. Caudal displacement of the brainstem and effacement of the ambient cisterns may result in compression of the oculomotor nerve (resulting in ipsilateral pupillary dilation) and compression of the posterior cerebral arteries, resulting in ischemic changes in the occipital lobes and brainstem or diencephalon. There may be secondary small hemorrhages (Duret), which are typically centrally located within the rostral pons and midbrain. Other findings include pseudosubarachnoid hemorrhage and pseudovenous sinus thrombosis, in which the subarachnoid spaces and venous sinuses appear hyperdense on unenhanced imaging relative to the diffuse hypodensity of the edematous cerebrum, as in this case.

Notes

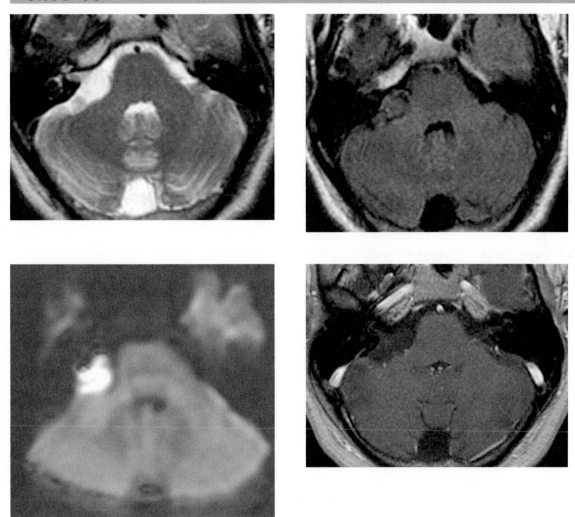

1. Is the entity shown in this case more often extradural or intradural?

2. What are the characteristic MR imaging findings of an arachnoid cyst?

3. What are common locations for intradural epidermoid cysts?

4. Which entity is considered a true neoplasm: epidermoid cyst, dermoid cyst, or teratoma?

C A S E 6 6

Epidermoid Cyst—Cerebellopontine Cistern

1. Intradural. For every extradural epidermoid cyst, the clinician will see 10 intradural epidermoid cysts. Extradural epidermoid cysts arise in the diploic space of the calvarium and in the temporal bone and petrous apex.

2. They are circumscribed lesions that follow the signal characteristics of CSF on all pulse sequences (T1W, FLAIR, T2W) and do not restrict on diffusion-weighted images.

3. The cerebellopontine angle cistern, prepontine cistern, suprasellar cistern, cisterna magna, and the pineal region.

4. Teratoma. Epidermoid cysts and dermoid cysts are of ectodermal origin. The epidermoid cyst has desquamated skin, whereas dermoid cysts also have skin appendages, such as hair follicles. Teratomas are true neoplasms of multipotential germ cells.

References

Kallmes DF, Provenzale JM, Cloft HJ, McClendon RE: Typical and atypical MR imaging features of intracranial epidermoid tumors, *AJR Am J Roentgenol* 169:883–887, 1997.

Tien RD, Felsberg GJ, Lirng JF: Variable bandwidth steady-state free-precession MR imaging: a technique for improving characterization of epidermoid tumor and arachnoid cyst, *AJR Am J Roentgenol* 164:689–692, 1995.

Cross-Reference

Neuroradiology: THE REQUISITES, 2nd ed, pp 114–116.

Comment

Epidermoid cysts are congenital lesions that result from incomplete separation of the neural and cutaneous ectoderm at the time of closure of the neural tube. These cysts are lined by a single layer of stratified squamous epithelium, and they contain desquamated epithelium, keratin, and cholesterol crystals. Many of these cysts are incidental findings, but when symptomatic, epidermoid cysts typically present in the third or fourth decade of life. Men and women are equally affected. These are frequently asymptomatic, but in the cerebellopontine cistern, they may present with dizziness, trigeminal neuralgia, and facial nerve weakness.

This case illustrates the typical appearance of an epidermoid cyst. There is a mass in the right cerebellopontine angle cistern that exerts mild mass effect on the adjacent brainstem. On the unenhanced T1W images (not shown), this mass is mildly hyperintense to CSF, with a fine internal architecture. On T2W image, the lesion is isointense to CSF. Unlike arachnoid cysts, which are typically isointense to CSF on proton density and FLAIR images, epidermoid cysts are hyperintense relative to CSF on these pulse sequences. Furthermore, this case illustrates hyperintensity on DW images, consistent with restricted diffusion, characteristic of these lesions. After contrast, there is no enhancement, as in this case. Other characteristic features of epidermoid cysts that distinguish them from arachnoid cysts (the major differential consideration here) are also presented in this case, including the lobulated and scalloped borders of this lesion and its insinuating nature, which fills and conforms to the shape of the space that it occupies.

Notes

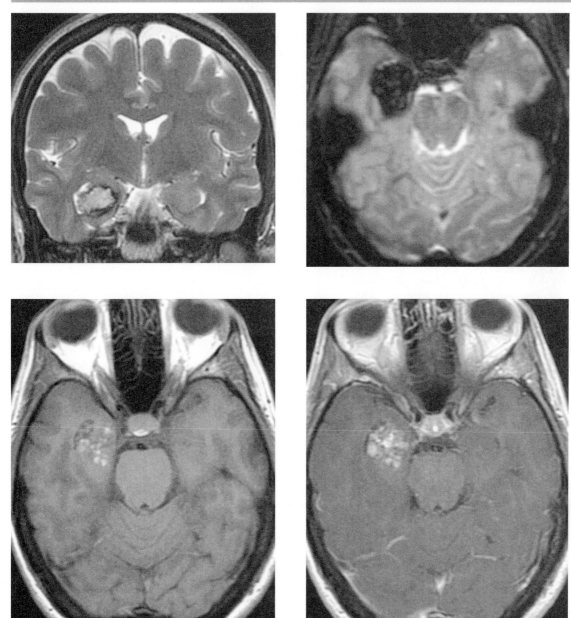

1. What do the central regions of T1W and T2W hyperintensity represent?

2. What findings on T2W and gradient echo susceptibility images help to distinguish this entity from other lesions?

3. In what percentage of cases is this entity multiple?

4. De novo development of these lesions has been reported in what subsets of patients?

CASE 67

Cavernous Malformation (Cavernous Hemangioma, Occult Cerebrovascular Malformation)

1. Methemoglobin.

2. The presence of a complete circumferential hemosiderin ring and the absence of edema are typical of uncomplicated cavernous malformations.

3. Approximately 25% of patients have multiple lesions.

4. Patients with a family history of cavernous malformations (CMs) or a history of radiation therapy to the brain.

Reference

Porter RW, Detwiler PW, Spetzler RF, et al: Cavernous malformations of the brainstem: experience with 100 patients, *J Neurosurgery* 90:50–58, 1999.

Cross-Reference

Neuroradiology: THE REQUISITES, 2nd ed. pp 231–234, 551.

Comment

Cavernous malformations, also referred to as cavernomas, cavernous hemangiomas, and angiographically occult cerebrovascular malformations, represent a sinusoidal network of blood vessels without intervening normal brain parenchyma. Frequently, gliosis is also present. On unenhanced CT, CMs may be mildly hyperdense as a result of pooling of blood in the sinusoids. They may also be associated with focal calcification. On MR imaging, CMs are recognized by their characteristic appearance, representing blood products of different ages. Typically, cavernomas have a central region of high signal intensity on unenhanced T1W and T2W images, representing methemoglobin, surrounded by a complete rim of hemosiderin that is hypointense on T2W and gradient echo susceptibility images (as in this case). In the absence of recent hemorrhage, there should be no associated T2W signal abnormality (edema) within the surrounding brain parenchyma.

Angiographically, CMs are usually occult. Unlike other occult vascular malformations, such as capillary telangiectasias and venous angiomas, these patients may present clinically with seizures or symptoms related to mass effect in cases in which there has been recent hemorrhage.

Cavernous malformations may be present in as much as 5% of the population. The majority of CMs are located superficially in the cerebrum and are often closely associated with the adjacent subarachnoid space. They may occur deep within the cerebral hemispheres, although this is less common. CMs occur less frequently in the infratentorial compartment. The most common brainstem location is the pons. Symptoms may be related to lesion location or acute hemorrhage. In the cerebrum, the most common presentation is seizures. In the infratentorial compartment, neurologic deficits may occur on the basis of acute hemorrhage, thrombosis, or progressive enlargement of a CM related to recurrent hemorrhage.

Notes

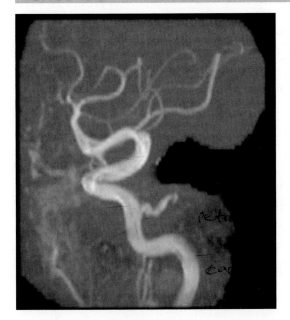
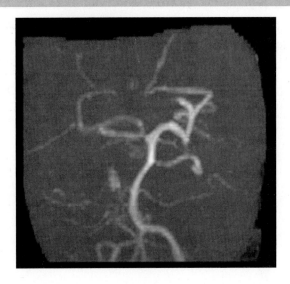

1. What is the anatomic variant in this case?

2. What are the three intracranial embryologic anastomoses between the carotid (anterior) and vertebrobasilar (posterior) circulations?

3. What other intracranial vascular abnormalities have been associated with persistent trigeminal arteries?

4. What percentage of cerebral arteriograms reveal a persistent trigeminal artery?

C A S E   6 8

Persistent Trigeminal Artery

1. Persistent trigeminal artery.

2. The trigeminal, otic, and hypoglossal arteries.

3. Aneurysms and arteriovenous malformations.

4. Approximately 0.1% to 0.5%.

References

Boyko OB, Curnes JT, Blatter DD, Parker DL: MRI of basilar artery hypoplasia associated with persistent primitive trigeminal artery, *Neuroradiology* 38:11–14, 1996.

Piotin M, Miralbes S, Cattin F, et al: MRI and MR angiography of persistent trigeminal artery, *Neuroradiology* 38:730–733, 1996.

Cross-Reference

Neuroradiology: THE REQUISITES, 2nd ed, pp 82–83.

Comment

The trigeminal, otic, and hypoglossal arteries (named after the cranial nerves with which they course) are the three embryologic anastomoses between the anterior internal carotid artery and the posterior vertebrobasilar circulations. The persistent trigeminal artery is the most common embryonic carotid–vertebrobasilar anastomosis to persist into adulthood, reported in as many as 0.1% to 0.5% of cerebral arteriograms. Persistence of a trigeminal artery may be associated with hypoplasia or absence of the ipsilateral posterior communicating artery, or with hypoplasia of both posterior communicating arteries. In addition, the proximal basilar artery and the distal vertebral arteries are often hypoplastic.

A persistent trigeminal artery usually arises from the precavernous internal carotid artery; however, origin from the intracavernous internal carotid artery has been reported. In some cases, trigeminal arteries may course through the sella turcica before joining the basilar artery (knowledge of this variant is critical in patients before transsphenoidal surgery). Persistent trigeminal arteries are associated with a variety of intracranial vascular abnormalities, including aneurysms and arteriovenous malformations, as well as a spectrum of clinical syndromes, such as tic douloureux (cranial nerve V), other cranial neuropathies, and vertebrobasilar insufficiency. Aneurysms arising from the trigeminal artery itself have been reported. Correct identification and an understanding of this anatomic variation are important because interventional neuroradiologic and neurosurgical procedures (often performed to treat an associated vascular abnormality) may need to be modified appropriately.

Notes

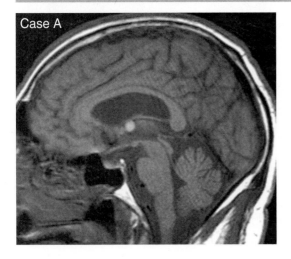

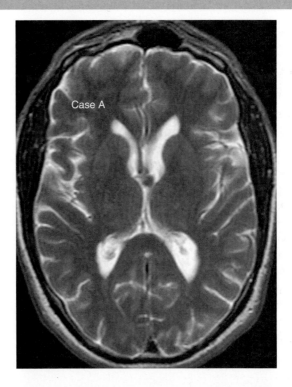

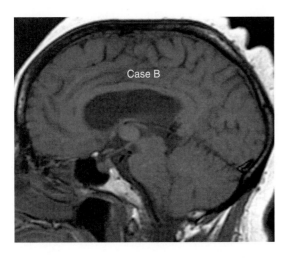

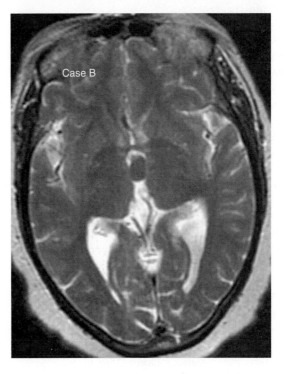

1. What is the radiologic diagnosis?

2. What is responsible for the variable density (CT) or intensity (MR) seen on imaging?

3. What is the precise anatomic location of these lesions?

4. When patients are symptomatic, what is the typical clinical presentation?

Colloid Cyst

1. Colloid cyst.

2. Protein concentration, water content, viscosity, and presence of paramagnetic ions.

3. Between the columns of the fornices.

4. Symptoms of acute hydrocephalus, including "positional" nausea, vomiting, and headache.

References

Armao D, Castillo M, Chen H, Kwock L: Colloid cyst of the third ventricle: imaging-pathologic correlation, *AJNR Am J Neuroradiol* 21:1470–1477, 2000.

El Khoury C, Brugieres P, Decq P, et al: Colloid cysts of the third ventricle: are MR imaging patterns predictive of difficulty with percutaneous treatment? *AJNR Am J Neuroradiol* 21:489–492, 2000.

Cross-Reference

Neuroradiology: THE REQUISITES, 2nd ed, p 162.

Comment

Colloid cysts are benign masses typically located in the superior aspect of the anterior third ventricle between the columns of the fornices. They are lined by a single layer of epithelium and represent the most common type of neuroepithelial cyst (the origin of these cysts has been debated). Many of these lesions are incidental findings in patients being evaluated for other reasons. Alternatively, signs and symptoms of hydrocephalus (headache, nausea, vomiting) that may be positional in nature may occur intermittently due to obstruction of the foramen of Monro. These benign masses, even if an incidental finding, are usually treated because their mobility with changes in head position put the patient at risk for acute obstructive hydrocephalus. Management options include stereotactic aspiration, surgical resection, and shunting, or a combination of these treatments.

These cystic masses usually are radiologically characteristic, allowing them to be distinguished from other mass lesions in this location that are typically more solid, including those related to the choroid plexus (the occasional choroid plexus papilloma), craniopharyngiomas, gliomas, and occasionally meningiomas. Within colloid cysts is found thick, mucoid material, as well as a variety of other products, including old blood, CSF, other proteins, and paramagnetic ions, such as magnesium. The location of these cysts and their contents give them a characteristic radiologic appearance, including variable density and intensity characteristics on CT and MR imaging, respectively. Depending on the specific contents within an individual cyst, on unenhanced CT, these lesions may range from isodense (low protein concentration) to extremely hyperdense (high protein concentration) to the CSF and brain tissue. Colloid cysts also vary extensively in their signal characteristics on T1W and T2W MR imaging, ranging from very hyperintense (Case A) to isointense or hypointense (Case B) on unenhanced T1W images. The signal characteristics will depend on protein concentration, viscosity, water content, and cross-linking of glycoproteins. A thin wall is usually seen that commonly enhances after contrast administration. With the exception of this mild, thin, peripheral enhancement of the epithelial lining, these lesions should not demonstrate solid or central enhancement.

Notes

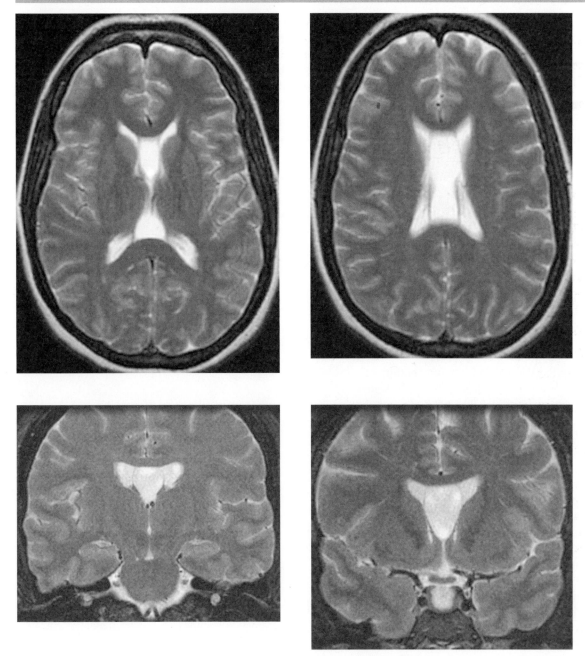

1. Above what ventricle does the cistern of the velum interpositum lie?

2. Development of the corpus callosum is intimately associated with development of what other structure?

3. What structures traverse the cistern of the velum interpositum?

4. What is the normal volume of CSF in the entire CNS?

Cavum Septum Pellucidum and Cavum Vergae

1. The third ventricle.

2. The septum pellucidum.

3. The internal cerebral veins and the vein of Galen traverse it.

4. Approximately 150 mL. Approximately 75 mL is distributed around the spinal cord, 25 ml is in the ventricular system, and 50 ml is in the subarachnoid spaces around the brain.

References

Cowley AR, Moody DM, Alexander E Jr, Ball MR, Laster DW: Distinctive CT appearance of cyst of the cavum septi pellucidi, *AJR Am J Roentgenol* 133:548–550, 1979.

Nakano S, Hojo H, Kataoka K, Yamasaki S: Age related incidence of cavum septi pellucidi and cavum vergae on CT scans of pediatric patients, *J Comput Assist Tomogr* 5:348–349, 1982.

Silbert PL, Gubbay SS, Vaughan RJ: Cavum septum pellucidum and obstructive hydrocephalus, *J Neurol Neurosurg Psychiatry* 56:820–822, 1993.

Cross-Reference

Neuroradiology: THE REQUISITES, 2nd ed, pp 53, 56, 261.

Comment

The cavum pellucidum is bordered superiorly by the corpus callosum and posteriorly by the body of the fornix. The cavum extending posterior to the columns of the fornix and the foramen of Monro is called the cavum vergae. The cavum septum pellucidum and cavum vergae are potential cavities that lie between the membranes of the septum pellucidum. They most commonly represent a normal anatomic variant. On obstetric ultrasound, the cavum septum pellucidum is present in essentially all normal fetuses between 18 and 37 weeks' gestation. During the latter half of gestation, the cavum septum pellucidum decreases in size. At birth, approximately 50% to 80% of term infants have a small residual cavum septum pellucidum that continues to decrease in size with age. Review of the literature shows considerable variation in the reported prevalence of a cavum septum pellucidum and cavum vergae in normal adults. Autopsy studies have also shown significant variability (range, 3%–30%). When a cavum septum pellucidum and cavum vergae are present concomitantly, as in this case, they usually communicate with one another; however, they do not typically communicate with the ventricular system. They are usually asymptomatic. Cysts may arise in this location and exert mass effect. In addition, enlargement of the cavum septum pellucidum, with intermittent obstruction of the foramen of Monro, resulting in hydrocephalus, has rarely been reported. Cysts may be treated with surgical resection, shunting, or fenestration.

Notes

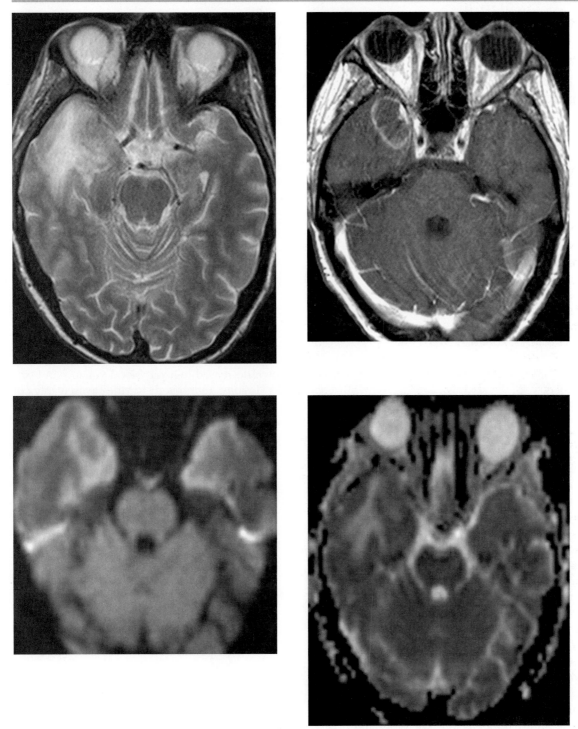

1. In differentiating a necrotic brain neoplasm from infection or abscess, which is typically associated with restricted diffusion?

2. How is *Toxoplasma gondii* infection transmitted?

3. In infants congenitally infected with toxoplasmosis, what are the typical neuroimaging findings?

4. In differentiating toxoplasmosis from primary CNS lymphoma, which demonstrates increased uptake on thallium-201 scintigraphy?

Toxoplasmosis Infection in Acquired Immunodeficiency Syndrome

1. Pyogenic brain abscess.

2. *Toxoplasma* can be transmitted through raw meat, milk, blood products, and cat feces, and by in utero exposure.

3. There are multiple calcifications in the basal ganglia and cortex as well as in the hydrocephalus. In severe cases, there may be microcephaly.

4. Lymphoma.

References

Camacho DL, Smith JK, Castillo M: Differentiation of toxoplasmosis and lymphoma in AIDS patients by using apparent diffusion coefficients, *AJNR Am J Neuroradiol* 24:633–637, 2003.

Ernst TM, Chang L, Witt MD, et al: Cerebral toxoplasmosis and lymphoma in AIDS: perfusion MR imaging experience in 13 patients, *Radiology* 208:663–669, 1998.

Cross-Reference

Neuroradiology: THE REQUISITES, 2nd ed, p 297.

Comment

Central nervous system toxoplasmosis is caused by the intracellular protozoan *Toxoplasma gondii*. *Toxoplasma* encephalitis is most commonly seen in immunocompromised patients with impaired cellular immunity, especially in the setting of AIDS. Other immunodeficient conditions associated with increased infection include following organ transplantation, long-term steroid therapy or chemotherapy, and impaired immunity from an underlying malignancy. In the setting of AIDS, radiologic differentiation between toxoplasmosis and lymphoma can be difficult. Both entities may have multiple lesions, and both may have solid or ring enhancement. Toxoplasmosis has a predilection for the basal ganglia and the corticomedullary junction. Lesions are often hyperintense on T2W imaging, but vary widely in their signal characteristics. Lesions may be hemorrhagic. Findings favoring lymphoma are hyperdense masses on unenhanced CT, ependymal spread on enhanced MR imaging (rare in toxoplasmosis), and a periventricular distribution.

Distinguishing these two disease processes is important because they are treated differently. Primary lymphoma responds to radiation therapy; however, the benefit of radiation therapy is diminished when treatment is delayed, as may happen in patients first treated empirically for toxoplasmosis. Thallium-201 SPECT can be effective (sensitive and specific) in distinguishing lymphoma (takes up thallium) from toxoplasmosis (normally does not take up thallium). Positron emission tomography has been shown to be useful in the accurate differentiation of hypometabolic toxoplasmosis lesions versus metabolically active lymphoma.

Diffusion-weighted imaging with apparent diffusion coefficient (ADC) maps has been used to distinguish these two lesions. Toxoplasmosis lesions have demonstrated significantly greater diffusion than lymphoma, with increased diffusion relative to that in normal white matter, in contrast to the restricted diffusion seen within pyogenic abscesses. Increased diffusion in toxoplasmosis lesions has been postulated to reflect relatively decreased viscosity within the central cores of the lesions, perhaps due to an impaired cellular immune response related to the immunocompromised state of these patients. Although considerable overlap of ADC ratios between 1.0 and 1.6 has been reported, ADC ratios greater than 1.6 have been associated solely with toxoplasmosis. The core of the lesion in this case demonstrates increased diffusion relative to white matter: the ADC value was 1.3. Recent investigations with perfusion MR imaging have shown decreased regional blood volumes in toxoplasmosis lesions (attributed to the avascularity of abscesses) compared with increased blood volumes in lymphoma (attributed to increased vascularity in regions of metabolically active tumor).

Notes

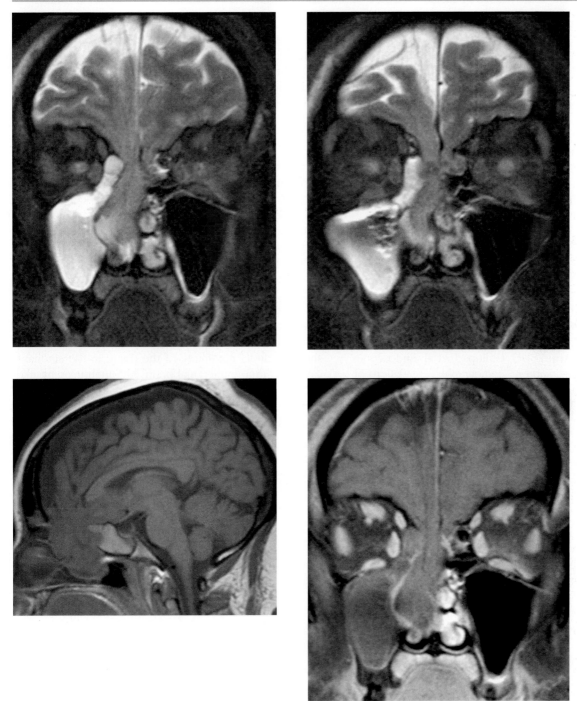

1. What are the most common causes of acquired meningocele (encephalocele)?

2. What finding in this case suggests that this abnormality is developmental rather than acquired?

3. What is a nasal glioma?

4. In the postoperative setting, what is the most common presentation of an encephalocele?

Encephalocele—Developmental

1. Trauma and iatrogenic (postoperative) causes.

2. There is also cortical dysplasia of the bilateral frontal lobes.

3. A misnomer in that the benign mass is composed of heterotopic glial tissue and is not a true tumor. Unlike meningoceles (encephaloceles), nasal gliomas do not have CSF spaces that communicate with the intracranial subarachnoid spaces or ventricles. In 15% of cases, nasal gliomas are connected with the intracranial compartment via fibrous or glial bands. They are more commonly extranasal than intranasal too!

4. Rhinorrhea—CSF leak.

References

Allbery SM, Chaljub G, Cho NL, Rassekh CH, John SD, Guinto FC: MR imaging of nasal masses, *RadioGraphics* 15:1311–1327, 1995.

Hudgins PA, Browning DG, Gallups J, et al: Endoscopic paranasal sinus surgery: radiographic evaluation of severe complications, *AJNR Am J Neuroradiol* 13: 1161–1167, 1992.

Cross-Reference

Neuroradiology: THE REQUISITES, 2nd ed, pp 418–419, 616–617, 623, 628–629.

Comment

This case illustrates a large congenital basal encephalocele associated with bilateral frontal lobe cortical dysplasia. Meningocele (encephalocele) refers to herniation of the meninges, CSF, or brain through an osseous defect in the cranium. Meningoencephaloceles are more common than meningoceles. Congenital encephaloceles are due to an abnormality in the process of invagination of the neural plate. During embryogenesis, the dura around the brain contacts the dermis in the facial or nasion region as the neural plate regresses. When there is failure of dermal regression, an encephalocele, dermoid cyst, sinus tract, or nasal glioma may develop. Dermoid sinus tracts may have an intracranial connection in up to 25% of cases, and may be complicated by infection (osteomyelitis, meningitis, and abscesses). Vietnamese and southeastern Asian women have a higher incidence of congenital nasofrontal and sphenoethmoidal meningoencephaloceles. Nasofrontal and sphenoethmoidal encephaloceles are frequently clinically occult, and the differential diagnosis is broad when this entity is seen through the nasoscope on office examination. Anterior basal encephaloceles have an association with other developmental anomalies, as in this case, including migrational abnormalities, agenesis of the corpus callosum, and cleft lip and palate.

In the setting of trauma or surgery, most meningoencephaloceles involve the nasal cavity and paranasal sinuses or the temporal bone. Patients may present with rhinorrhea.

A combination of imaging modalities, including nuclear scintigraphy, CT, and MR imaging, can be used to assess CSF leaks and meningoencephaloceles. It is important to determine whether the CSF leak is due to a dural laceration or a meningocele (encephalocele). After the placement of pledgets in the nares, intrathecal instillation of indium diethylene triamine pentaacetic acid may be used to confirm and localize the CSF leak. Once a leak is established, coronal CT may be performed for anatomic localization. In the hands of skilled ear, nose, and throat surgeons and radiologists, iodinated contrast CT cisternography is rarely necessary. If an encephalocele is suspected, MR imaging in the sagittal and coronal planes is most useful in establishing this diagnosis by showing direct continuity of the tissue in the sinonasal cavity with the intracranial brain. Although imaging may be useful in detecting CSF leaks, fluorescein injected intrathecally, followed by endoscopic evaluation, may allow direct visualization of an active leak.

Notes

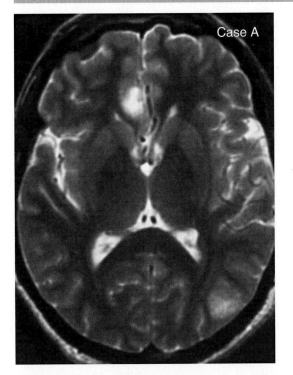

Case A

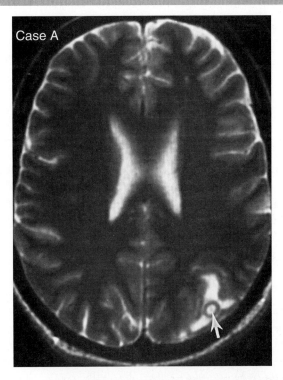

Case A

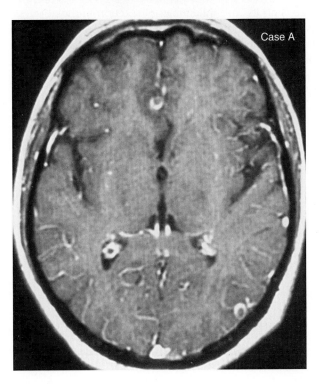

Case A

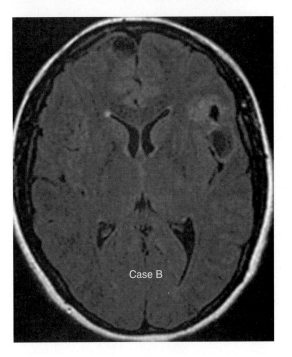

Case B

1. What is the differential diagnosis in these cases?

2. What is the most likely diagnosis in these cases?

3. What is the most common clinical presentation of patients with this entity?

4. What is the most common location of intraventricular neurocysticercosis?

Cysticercosis of the Central Nervous System

1. The differential diagnosis of multiple superficial (cortical and gray–white matter junction) lesions includes a spectrum of infectious and inflammatory processes (eg, septic emboli, bacterial abscesses, cysticercosis) and metastatic disease.

2. Cysticercosis.

3. Seizures, seen in 30% to 90% of symptomatic patients. Symptoms are dependent on the stage of infestation, as well as the sites of parasitic CNS involvement. Initial cerebral infection and the mature cystic phase of infection, when the larvae are alive, are frequently asymptomatic. Patients may be most symptomatic as the larvae die because the larvae incite a significant inflammatory reaction.

4. The fourth ventricle.

References

Arriada-Mendicoa N, Celis-Lopez MA, Higuera-Calleja J, Corona-Vazquez T: Imaging features of sellar cysticercosis, *AJNR Am J Neuroradiol* 24:1386–1389, 2003.

Braga F, Rocha AJ, Gomes HR, Filho GH, Silva CF, Fonseca RB: Noninvasive MR cisternography with fluid-attenuated inversion recovery and 100% supplemental O$_2$ in the evaluation of neurocysticercosis, *AJNR Am J Neuroradiol* 25:295–297, 2004.

Cross-Reference

Neuroradiology: THE REQUISITES, 2nd ed, pp 316–319.

Comment

Cysticercosis is the most common parasitic infection of the CNS. It usually involves the intracranial compartment, and it may very, very, very rarely involve the spinal contents. Cysticercosis is endemic to Central and South America, parts of Asia, Mexico, Africa, and India. The pork tapeworm (*Taenia solium*) is the causative agent. Humans may become the definitive host (the parasite sexually reproduces) by eating inadequately cooked pork that harbors the larvae of the pork tapeworm (cysticerci). These larvae develop into tapeworms in the small intestine that release eggs that pass into the stool. If humans ingest food or water contaminated by these ova, they may serve as an intermediate host. In the stomach, the ova release oncospheres (primary larvae), which enter the bloodstream through the gastrointestinal mucosa. These primary larvae may deposit within muscle and subcutaneous tissue, although they have a propensity to infect the CNS. There are multiple patterns of neurocysticercosis, including the parenchymal pattern (the larvae penetrate directly into the brain), the intraventricular pattern (involves the ependyma or choroid plexus), and the subarachnoid pattern (involves the meninges). In mixed neurocysticercosis, there is involvement of the parenchyma, ventricles, or subarachnoid spaces. Patients with parenchymal involvement may present with seizures and neurologic signs (confusion, dementia, paresis, paraesthesias, visual disturbances). Intraventricular involvement may be symptomatic if there is obstructive hydrocephalus, and meningeal involvement may result in communicating hydrocephalus.

There is a spectrum of radiologic appearances, depending on the stage of disease; however, imaging findings are frequently characteristic. In the initial stage of cerebral infection, the larvae result in small, edematous lesions that are hypodense on CT and hyperintense on T2W images. The cysticerci then develop into cysts that range in size from millimeters to centimeters and contain a scolex. There may be mild surrounding edema in the brain, as in Case B. On the more cephalad T2W image in Case A, the left parietal lobe lesion has a characteristic appearance, with a defined capsule that has a hypointense rim and a small (1 mm), hypointense focus (*arrow*), representing the scolex. As the cysts die, there is an intense inflammatory reaction in the adjacent brain parenchyma that may result in prominent edema and mass effect. It is at this time that patients may be most symptomatic, presenting with seizures or focal neurologic signs. After years of infestation, the cysts finally collapse and often calcify. Rim enhancement has been described in as many as 38% of calcified lesions.

Notes

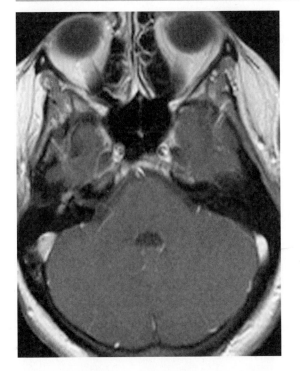

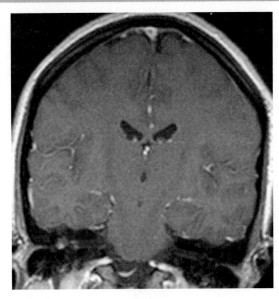

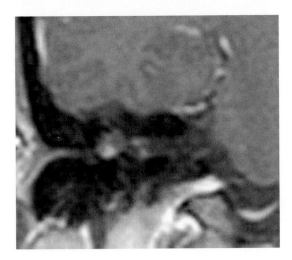

1. What is the differential diagnosis?

2. What portions of the facial nerve normally enhance?

3. What structure separates the internal auditory canal into superior and inferior components?

4. What cranial nerve runs in the anteroinferior portion of the internal auditory canal?

Facial Nerve—Inflammation (Viral)

1. Inflammatory conditions, including viral infection, Lyme disease, and sarcoidosis. Neoplasm is less likely, but metastatic disease can appear like this. Schwannoma is unlikely given that multiple cranial nerves are involved.

2. The portions within the temporal bone (descending, tympanic, and geniculate ganglia) because they have a rich circumneural venous plexus. The labyrinthine portion, the portion within the internal auditory canal, and the cisternal portions do not normally enhance, and the presence of enhancement implies pathology.

3. The crista falciformis.

4. The cochlear division of the vestibulocochlear nerve.

Reference

Gebarski SS, Telian SA, Niparko JK: Enhancement along the normal facial nerve in the facial canal: MR imaging and anatomic correlation, *Radiology* 183:391–394, 1992.

Cross-Reference

Neuroradiology: THE REQUISITES, 2nd ed, pp 79–80, 591, 603–604.

Comment

This case shows enlargement and thickening of the right facial nerve (cranial nerve VII) along the tympanic portion, as well as enhancement of the facial nerve in the fundus of the internal auditory canal. Enhancement of the right cochlear nerve below the facial nerve in the anteroinferior internal auditory canal is also seen. The patient presented with Bell's palsy. Statistically speaking, inflammatory processes (ie, viral) are most likely. Other infectious etiologies associated with cranial nerve VII involvement, in addition to viral causes, include Lyme disease. In immunocompromised patients, especially those with HIV infection, cytomegalovirus can affect the nerves in the internal auditory canal. Other inflammatory processes that affect the cranial nerves here include sarcoidosis.

Neoplasms that may involve cranial nerve VII include schwannoma (unlikely in this case because there are multiple cranial nerves involved and this patient's clinical presentation was acute in onset). Subarachnoid seeding of tumor may involve the internal auditory canals and can be seen in lymphoma and carcinomatosis (lung, breast, or seeding of primary brain tumors). Perineural spread of malignancies along the facial nerve is often associated with destructive changes in the temporal bone. Perineural spread of temporal bone squamous cell carcinoma, primary parotid malignancies, and skin cancers of the ear and cheek are probably most common.

Frequently, imaging is not necessary in the workup of Bell's palsy. However, when Bell's palsy is bilateral, is recurrent, or does not show significant improvement in 6 to 8 weeks, imaging is indicated to assess for causes other than viral disease.

Notes

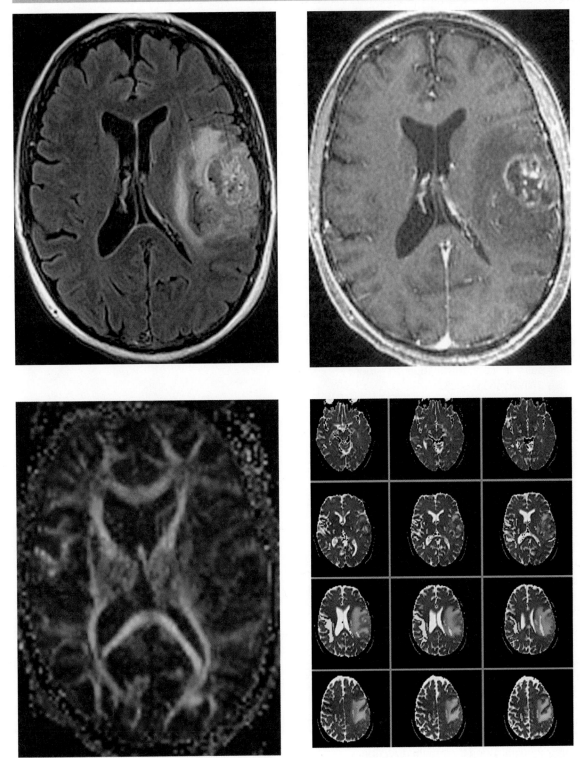

1. What is the best diagnosis for the brain lesion?

2. What MR technique has been performed in addition to conventional MR imaging?

3. What structures are denoted in *green*?

4. In diffusion tensor imaging, diffusion gradients are applied in at least how many directions?

Magnetic Resonance Tractography— Preoperative Mapping of the Corticospinal Tracts for Glioblastoma Multiforme Resection

1. A high-grade primary glial neoplasm or glioblastoma multiforme.

2. MR tractography from diffusion tensor imaging. The imaging of this property is an extension of diffusion MR imaging.

3. The corticospinal tracts.

4. In at least six directions. This allows calculation of a tensor for each voxel that describes the three-dimensional shape of diffusion. The fiber direction is indicated by the tensor's main eigenvector that can be color-coded, yielding a cartography of the position and direction of the tracts.

Reference

Holodny AI, Gor DM, Watts R, Gutin PH, Ulug AM: Diffusion-tensor MR tractography of somatic organization of corticospinal tracts in the internal capsule: initial anatomic results in contradistinction to prior reports, *Radiology* 234:649–653, 2005.

Cross-Reference

Neuroradiology: THE REQUISITES, 2nd ed, pp 16–17, 189–191.

Comments

White matter tractography based on diffusion tensor imaging is an MR technique that can depict white matter tracts in the brain in vivo. Diffusion tensor sequences may be analyzed with combined volume analysis and tractography extraction software, giving indirect visualization of white matter connections. Rapid data processing allows imaging of the normal and diseased fiber pathways to be part of a routine MR imaging examination.

Diffusion tensor imaging enables the measurement of the restricted diffusion of water in tissue. The principal application currently is in the imaging of white matter, where the location, orientation, and anistrophy of the tracts can be measured. The architecture of the axons and their myelin sheaths facilitates the diffusion of water molecules preferentially along their main direction, referred to as anisotropic diffusion.

The corticospinal tract (CST) is the main white matter connection between the motor cortex and the spinal cord, serving as the main conduit of information between the higher cortical structures and voluntary muscular motion. The location and internal organization of the CST, as it passes through the corona radiata and the posterior limb of the internal capsule, have important clinical applications. Precise localization of the CST is useful for planning functional neurosurgery in patients with Parkinson disease and in the management of stroke, and importantly, preoperative localization of the CST may avoid inadvertent iatrogenic injury of these structures in patients with brain tumors, as in this case. Accurate depiction of the relationship of the CST and other main white matter tracts relative to a tumor preoperatively may improve neurosurgical planning. The superior longitudinal fasciculus (SLF) is a pair of long, bidirectional bundles of neurons connecting the front and the back of the cerebrum. Each association fiber bundle is lateral to the centrum semiovale and connects the frontal, occipital, parietal, and temporal lobes. Note the left SLF (*yellow*) passing through the tumorigenic edema in this case.

Notes

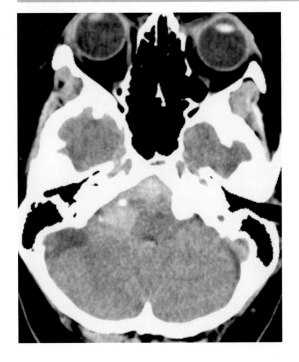 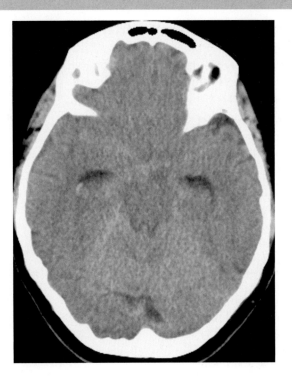

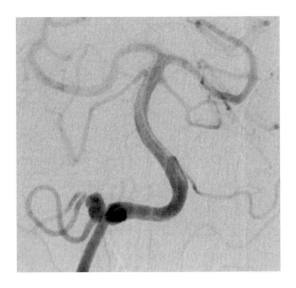

1. What are the CT imaging findings?

2. What is the differential diagnosis?

3. What does the conventional catheter angiogram show?

4. What is the most common site of origin for aneurysms in the posterior circulation?

Right Posterior Inferior Cerebellar Artery Aneurysm Rupture

1. Acute subarachnoid hemorrhage, predominantly in the posterior fossa, and early hydrocephalus, with dilation of the temporal horns.

2. Given the predominance of subarachnoid blood in the right prepontine and premedullary cisterns, rupture of a right posterior inferior cerebellar artery (PICA) aneurysm and intradural right vertebral artery dissection are the primary considerations.

3. A multilobed right PICA aneurysm.

4. The tip of the basilar artery.

Reference

Jayaraman MV, Mayo-Smith WW, Tung GA, et al: Detection of intracranial aneurysms: multi-detector row CT angiography compared with DSA, *Radiology* 230:510–518, 2004.

Cross-Reference

Neuroradiology: THE REQUISITES, 2nd ed, pp 224–227.

Comment

The majority of intracranial aneurysms arise from the supraclinoid segment of the internal carotid artery and its branches. More than 80% of saccular aneurysms arise from the anterior communicating artery, the distal internal carotid artery at the origin of the posterior communicating artery, the bifurcation of the supraclinoid internal carotid artery, and the middle cerebral artery bifurcation. Intracranial aneurysms are multiple in approximately 20% of cases. Aneurysms arising from the distal internal carotid artery at the origin of the ophthalmic artery account for 5% of intracranial aneurysms and have interesting features, including a preponderance in women, multiplicity in 10% to 20% of cases, and bilaterality in up to 20% of cases.

Aneurysms arising from the posterior circulation are not uncommon; however, they occur much less frequently than do their anterior counterparts. Most originate from the tip of the basilar artery. Basilar tip aneurysms may become quite large, and not uncommonly, the origins of one or both posterior cerebral arteries may be incorporated into the aneurysm. The next most common site for aneurysms in the posterior circulation is the origin of the posterior inferior cerebellar artery. Rarely, aneurysms may arise from the superior cerebellar artery or the anteroinferior cerebellar artery.

Aneurysms arising from distal arterial branches are usually acquired rather than congenital. They are frequently secondary to infection of the arterial wall (mycotic) or to trauma (aneurysms arising from the posterior circulation may be related to compression along the tentorium), and occasionally, they may be related to tumor.

Notes

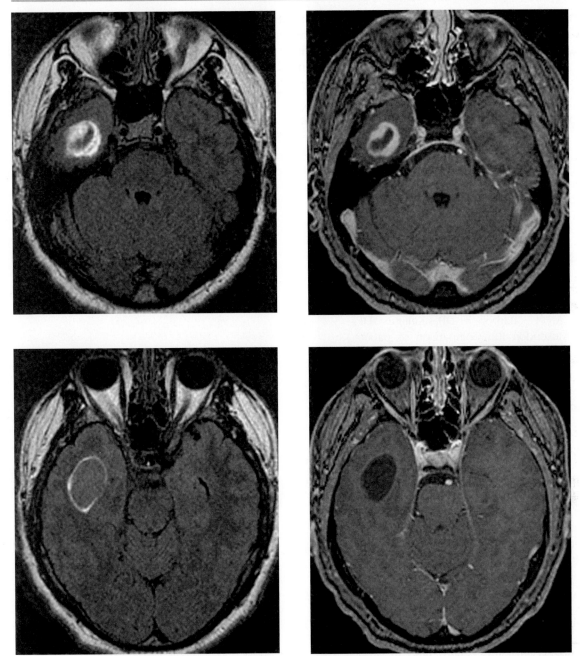

1. What is the differential diagnosis in this 17-year-old patient?

2. What are the classic MR imaging findings in mesial temporal sclerosis?

3. Gangliogliomas most commonly arise in what part of the cerebrum?

4. What is the cell of origin of pleomorphic xanthoastrocytomas?

CASE 77

Ganglioglioma

1. Astrocytoma, ganglioglioma, dysembryoplastic neuro-epithelial tumor, and pleomorphic xanthoastrocytoma.

2. Mesial temporal sclerosis is usually associated with hippocampal volume loss with ex vacuo dilation of the temporal horn. T2W signal abnormality may or may not be present.

3. The temporal lobe, followed by the frontal lobe.

4. The astrocyte. Histology shows pleomorphic cells ranging from fibrillary to giant multinucleated cells with intracellular lipid vacuoles ("xanthoma" cells).

References

Koeller KK, Henry JM: From the archives of the AFIP: superficial gliomas. Radiologic-pathologic correlation, *RadioGraphics* 21:1533–1556, 2001.

Provenzale JM, Ali U, Barboriak DP, Kallmes DF, Delong DM, McLendon RE: Comparison of patient age with MR imaging features of gangliogliomas, *AJR Am J Roentgenol* 174:859–862, 2000.

Cross-Reference

Neuroradiology: THE REQUISITES, 2nd ed, pp 136–137.

Comment

Gangliogliomas and ganglioneuromas are slow-growing, benign tumors that most commonly affect children and young adults. Gangliogliomas have a predominance of glial tissue and typically occur in the cerebrum, most commonly arising in the temporal lobe, followed by the frontal lobe, parietal lobe, occipital lobe, and region of the hypothalamus and third ventricle. They may also be infratentorial, arising within the cerebellum or brainstem. Gangliogliomas are typically circumscribed tumors that occur superficially in the brain parenchyma, with little or no surrounding edema. They are usually cystic (purely cystic or cystic with solid components), although solid tumors without cyst formation may occur. Calcification is frequently present, and these neoplasms may demonstrate variable contrast enhancement, ranging from mild to marked. However, contrast enhancement need not be present.

Because gangliogliomas are composed of both glial (usually astrocytes) and neural elements, they may undergo malignant degeneration. When neuronal elements make up the majority of the mass, the neoplasm is referred to as a ganglioneuroma. Gangliocytomas are composed of mature ganglion cells. They rarely have glial elements and therefore have no potential for malignant change.

In children and young adults, the main differential considerations for ganglioglioma on imaging studies include low-grade astrocytoma, juvenile pilocytic astrocytoma, dysembryoplastic neuroepithelial tumor, and pleomorphic xanthoastrocytoma.

Notes

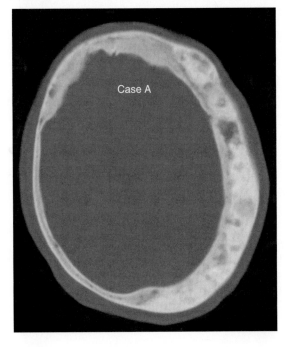

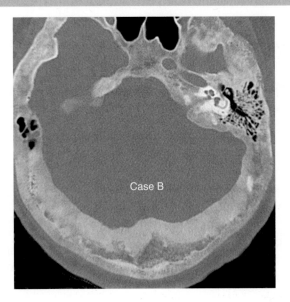

1. What is the name of the characteristic radiologic appearance that typifies the osteolytic phase of this disease in the calvaria?

2. What systemic conditions may result from this disorder?

3. How can Paget's disease be distinguished from fibrous dysplasia?

4. Why is bone affected with this disease more prone to metastatic deposits?

CASE 78

Paget's Disease—Osteitis Deformans

1. Osteoporosis circumscripta. Osteolysis is most commonly seen in the frontal or occipital region.

2. Heart disease and kidney stones.

3. Paget's disease is a disease of middle-aged and elderly persons, whereas fibrous dysplasia is typically seen in children and young adults. In contrast to fibrous dysplasia, extensive involvement of the facial bones is uncommon in Paget's disease. Paget's disease causes cortical thickening, compared with fibrous dysplasia, in which the cortex is relatively spared.

4. Increased blood flow within pagetoid bone may make it more susceptible to deposition of metastases.

References

Richards PS, Bargiota A, Corrall RJ: Paget's disease causing an Arnold-Chiari type 1 malformation: radiographic findings, *AJR Am J Roentgenol* 176:816–817, 2001.

Tehranzadeh J, Fung Y, Donohue M, Anavim A, Pribram HW: Computed tomography of Paget's disease of the skull versus fibrous dysplasia, *Skeletal Radiol* 27:664–672, 1998.

Cross-Reference

Neuroradiology: THE REQUISITES, 2nd ed, p 599.

Comment

In Paget's disease, there is malfunction in the normal process of bone remodeling. When an area of bone is destroyed, the new bone replacing it is soft and porous. Bone affected with Paget's disease also has increased vascularity. The cause of Paget's disease is unknown; however, a viral etiology is favored. Paget's disease is more common in men than in women, and it usually presents after the age of 40 years. It is often an incidental finding detected on radiographs obtained for other reasons. Patients may be symptomatic, depending on the distribution of disease. Involvement of the calvarium (Case A) may present with enlarging head size. Involvement of the skull base, resulting in platybasia, may lead to neurologic symptoms (weakness and paralysis). Conductive hearing loss may result if there is involvement of the ossicles. Compression of the eight cranial nerves due to overgrowth of bone may cause sensorineural hearing loss. There is usually relative sparing of the otic capsule (Case B). Paget's disease has multiple stages, including an initial osteolytic phase characterized by osteoclastic activity with resorption of normal bone. This phase is followed by excessive and sporadic new bone formation as a result of osteoblastic activity. Eventually, Paget's disease enters its inactive stage.

Neoplastic involvement within pagetoid bone is not uncommon and includes sarcomatous degeneration, giant cell tumors, superimposed hematologic neoplasms (myeloma, lymphoma), and metastatic disease. Giant cell tumors are typically confined to the skull and less often to the facial bones. It is speculated that the increased blood flow within pagetoid bone may make it more susceptible to deposition of metastases. Clinically, the development of neoplastic disease in pagetoid bone should be suspected if there is increased pain or an associated soft tissue mass.

The differential diagnosis of Paget's disease of the skull includes other sclerotic bone lesions, hyperostosis frontalis, fibrous dysplasia, and metastatic disease. In the elderly, metastatic disease may have the cotton-wool appearance of Paget's disease (prostate cancer in men and breast cancer in women).

Notes

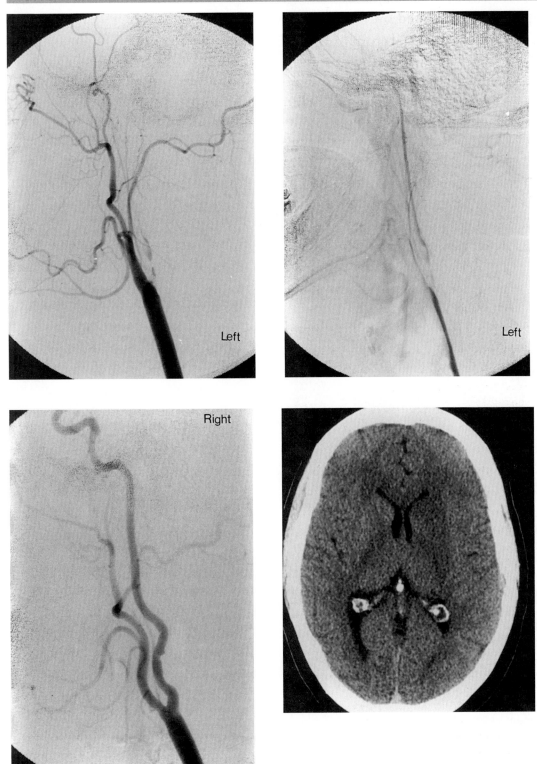

1. What is the cause of this patient's acute stroke?

2. Which layer of the arterial wall is most commonly affected in fibromuscular dysplasia?

3. What systemic vessels are most commonly involved with fibromuscular dysplasia?

4. What is the most common location for an intracranial arterial dissection?

Fibromuscular Dysplasia—Complicated by Acute Stroke

1. There is a dissection of the left cervical internal carotid artery complicating fibromuscular dysplasia, resulting in a distal embolus with stroke.

2. Involvement of the media with hyperplasia or dysplasia is most common.

3. The renal arteries.

4. The supraclinoid internal carotid artery.

Reference

Manninen HI, Koivisto T, Saari T, et al: Dissecting aneurysms of all four cervicocranial arteries in fibromuscular dysplasia: treatment with self-expanding endovascular stents, coil embolization, and surgical ligation, *AJNR Am J Neuroradiol* 18:1216–1220, 1997.

Cross-Reference

Neuroradiology: THE REQUISITES, 2nd ed, p 202.

Comment

Conventional catheter angiography demonstrates findings consistent with an extracranial dissection of the proximal left internal carotid artery, distal to the carotid bifurcation. There is marked narrowing and irregularity of the proximal internal carotid artery, with poor distal filling and very slow antegrade flow seen on the delayed image. An extracranial dissection may result from major or minor trauma, including chiropractic manipulation. Alternatively, extracranial dissection may result from an underlying vascular abnormality or dysplasia. In this case, injection of the right internal carotid artery demonstrates a normal appearance of the proximal internal carotid artery distal to the carotid bifurcation; however, there is irregularity, with regions of narrowing alternating with dilation, producing a "string of beads" appearance that is commonly described in fibromuscular dysplasia. There are many subtypes (medial, intimal, and adventitial) of fibromuscular dysplasia in which one or all of the layers of the arterial wall may be involved; however, involvement of the media with hyperplasia or dysplasia is most common, seen in up to 90% of cases. Thinning of the media is associated with abnormalities in the internal elastic lamina, resulting in the dilations seen in this condition. The cervical internal carotid artery is most commonly affected, and the proximal 2 cm of this vessel is usually spared due to architectural differences in this part of the vessel's wall. The extracranial vertebral artery and external carotid arteries may be involved; however, intracranial fibromuscular dysplasia is relatively uncommon. The incidence of intracranial aneurysms is increased in patients with this condition.

Notes

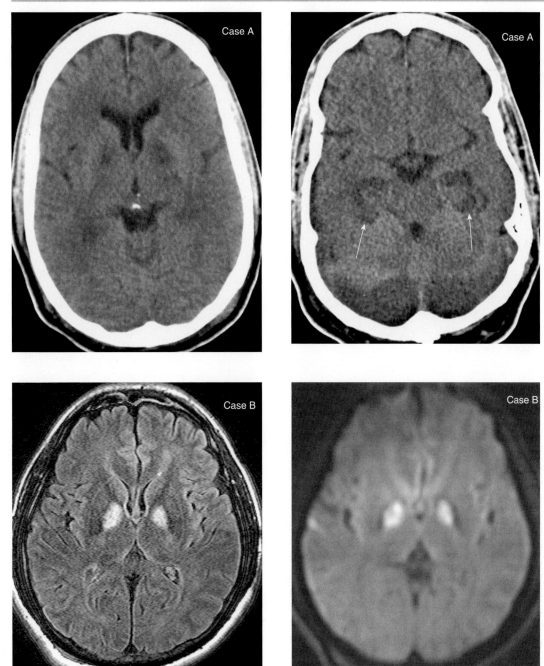

1. What basal ganglionic structures are involved in these cases?

2. What toxic exposures may result in injuries or infarction to the globus pallidus?

3. What structures are shown (*arrows,* Case A)?

4. What movement disorders may be associated with pallidal lesions?

Carbon Monoxide Poisoning

1. The globus pallidus.

2. The most common is carbon monoxide poisoning. Other exposures that affect the globus pallidus include cyanide and manganese (hyperalimentation).

3. The hippocampi.

4. Slow initiation and execution of voluntary movements (akinesia), dystonia, and increased rigidity.

Reference

Sener RN: Acute carbon monoxide poisoning: diffusion MR imaging findings, *AJNR Am J Neuroradiol* 24: 1475–1477, 2003.

Cross-Reference

Neuroradiology: THE REQUISITES, 2nd ed, pp 206, 354, 358.

Comment

Injury to the brain with a particular predilection for the basal ganglia may be seen in a variety of toxic exposures, neurodegenerative processes, and metabolic disorders. Of the toxic insults, carbon monoxide, cyanide, and trichloroethane (typewriter correction fluid) poisoning have a particular predilection to involve the globus pallidus bilaterally. The pathologic and microscopic correlate of the abnormal hypodensity on CT or T2W hyperintensity on MR imaging within the bilateral globus pallidus is that of necrosis caused by anoxic injury. Although carbon monoxide toxicity has a characteristic imaging appearance, the diagnosis is usually established by the clinical circumstances in which the patient is found. The diagnosis of carbon monoxide toxicity is confirmed by identification of carboxyhemoglobin in the blood.

In addition to CT density and MR intensity alterations in the globus pallidus bilaterally, other imaging manifestations of diffuse anoxic brain injury may be identified, including injury to the hippocampus (Ammon's horn) bilaterally (as in Case A, *arrows*) and global cerebral swelling manifested as sulcal effacement and accentuation of the gray–white matter differentiation. Abnormalities in the cerebellum may also be noted (as in Case A). Patients with carbon monoxide poisoning may experience sudden neurologic deterioration and coma approximately 2 to 3 weeks after the initial injury. Imaging often shows accompanying white matter disease, which may be extensive and which pathologically represents acute demyelination. On delayed imaging performed months to years after carbon monoxide injury, T2W hypointensity in the deep gray matter, especially the putamen, may be present and is likely due to iron deposition.

Notes

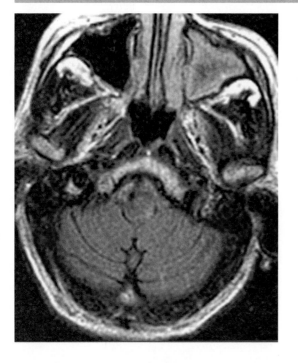

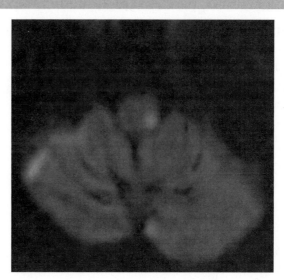

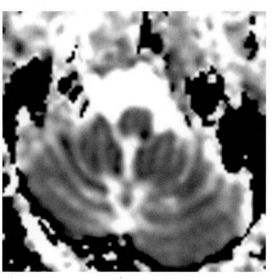

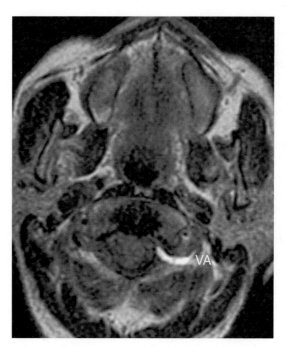

1. What is the radiologic diagnosis?

2. What are the symptoms associated with Wallenberg's syndrome?

3. The posterior inferior cerebellar artery supplies perforating vessels to what part of the brainstem?

4. What is the cause of the left posterior inferior cerebellar artery infarct?

Lateral Medullary Syndrome—Wallenberg's Syndrome

1. An acute infarct in the left lateral and posterior medulla.

2. Loss of pain and temperature sensation on the contralateral side of the body and the ipsilateral side of the face. Other symptoms may include ataxia, cranial nerve IX and X neuropathies, nystagmus, and vertigo.

3. The lateral and posterior medulla in the retro-olivary region.

4. Left vertebral artery dissection (VA). Note the high signal intensity in the vessel and the lack of vascular flow void.

Reference

Min WK, Kim YS, Kim JY, Park SP, Suh CK: Athero-thrombotic cerebellar infarction: vascular lesion-MRI correlation of 31 cases, *Stroke* 30:2376–2381, 1999.

Cross-Reference

Neuroradiology: THE REQUISITES, 2nd ed, pp 88–90, 174–196.

Comment

Infarction in the posterior inferior cerebellar artery territory can produce the lateral medullary syndrome (Wallenberg's) illustrated in this case, which causes loss of pain and temperature sensation on the contralateral side of the body and the ipsilateral side of the face. Other symptoms may include ataxia, cranial nerve IX and X neuropathies, nystagmus, and vertigo.

In older patients, the most common cause of posterior circulation ischemia is thromboembolic disease resulting from accelerated atheromatous disease or embolic disease from a cardiac source. However, because the vasculature (including the vertebral arteries) becomes more tortuous as a patient ages, in the elderly population, in the setting of embolic disease from a systemic source, it is less common to have embolic disease isolated to the posterior fossa (usually patients also have embolic disease to the anterior circulation). In my experience, isolated posterior fossa embolic disease is more common in young patients in whom the vertebral arteries course vertically with little tortuosity. In young patients with posterior fossa ischemia, in addition to embolic disease, the diagnosis of a dissection should also be considered. This can be evaluated with MR imaging and MR angiography, or with CT angiography. MR imaging should include unenhanced axial T1W images through the distal vertebral arteries with fat suppression, when possible, to look for clot in the vessel wall, which is hyperintense due to

methemoglobin. In addition, the dissected vessel may be enlarged due to mural hematoma, and occlusion (absence of signal void) or luminal narrowing (reduced size of the signal void) may be seen. In this case, the patient's ischemic disease was related to thrombosis of the distal left vertebral artery due to dissection.

Notes

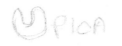

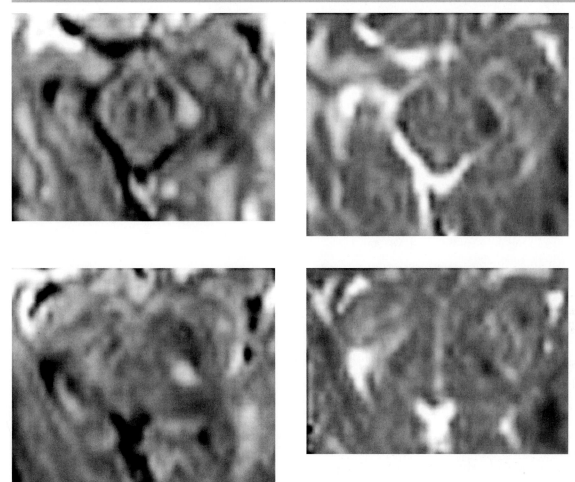

1. What is the pertinent finding in the brainstem?

2. What are causes of this finding?

3. What is the salient finding of this entity in its chronic stage?

4. What is the most common cause of this entity?

Wallerian Degeneration

1. There is restricted diffusion in the left corticospinal tract.

2. Infarction, trauma, demyelinating disease, and neurodegenerative processes.

3. Atrophy.

4. Cerebral infarction.

References

Mazumdar A, Mukherjee P, Miller JH, Malde H, McKinstry RC: Diffusion-weighted imaging of acute corticospinal tract injury preceding Wallerian degeneration in the maturing human brain, *AJNR Am J Neuroradiol* 24:1057–1066, 2003.

Uchino A, Sawada A, Takase Y, Egashira R, Kudo S: Transient detection of early Wallerian degeneration on diffusion weighted MRI after an acute cerebrovascular accident, *Neuroradiology* 46:183–188, 2004.

Cross-Reference

Neuroradiology: THE REQUISITES, 2nd ed, p 358.

Comment

Wallerian degeneration is a secondary manifestation of brain injury from a spectrum of causes. Secondary antegrade degenerative changes of axons and their myelin sheaths occur along the distal axonal segment as a result of injury to the proximal axon or neuronal cell body. Among the causes of degeneration of the corticospinal tract pathways, the most common is cortical infarction. Other injuries and neurodegenerative processes (eg, amyotrophic lateral sclerosis) may result in wallerian degeneration. It may occur as a result of trauma (as in this patient); hemorrhage; white matter disease, including demyelination; or neoplasia and its treatment (radiation injury). Histologically, wallerian degeneration represents several stages of progressive axonal degradation, ultimately resulting in gliosis and volume loss.

Magnetic resonance imaging is superior to CT in detecting wallerian degeneration, especially in the acute stages. CT may show the later changes of atrophy of the involved corticospinal pathways within the brainstem, but it does not show the earlier changes. On MR imaging, signal alteration on T2W or T1W images may be seen as early as 4 weeks after injury (some studies have shown these changes even earlier), and in the late stages (weeks to months), signal alteration and atrophy are invariably present. In the late stages, T2W hyperintensity is accompanied by hypointensity on corresponding T1W images. More recent work has shown that diffusion-weighted imaging and corresponding apparent diffusion coefficient (ADC) maps may reflect the changes of acute wallerian degeneration within a week, manifest as restricted diffusion (hyperintensity on diffusion-weighted images) and hypointensity on corresponding ADC images (low ADC values), as in this case.

Notes

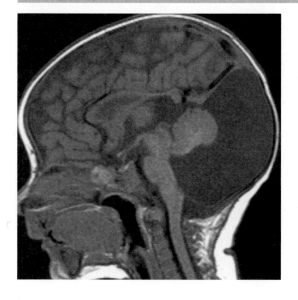

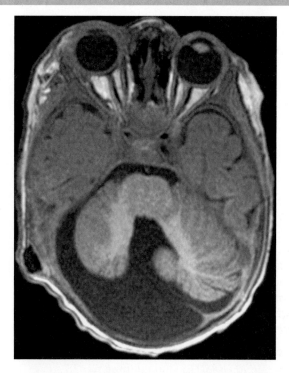

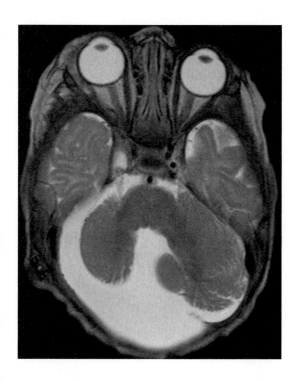

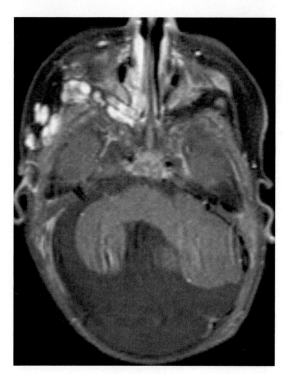

1. What is the differential diagnosis of a nonneoplastic cystic mass in the posterior fossa?

2. Which of these cystic masses is associated with supratentorial developmental anomalies?

3. What is the diagnosis in this case?

4. EYE TEST: What other finding and condition does this pediatric patient have?

Dandy-Walker Malformation

1. Arachnoid cyst, Dandy-Walker malformation, and giant cisterna magna.

2. Dandy-Walker malformation.

3. Dandy-Walker malformation.

4. A plexiform neurofibroma involving the right face including the periorbital region, zygomatic masticator space, and pterygopalatine fossa. This is best appreciated on the fat-suppressed enhanced T1-weighted MR image. The patient has neurofibromatosis type 1. Do you need glasses?

Reference

Glenn OA, Barkovich J: Magnetic resonance imaging of the fetal brain and spine: an increasingly important tool in prenatal diagnosis: part 2, *Am J Neuroradiol* 27:1807–1814, 2006.

Cross-Reference

Neuroradiology: THE REQUISITES, 2nd ed, pp 432–438.

Comment

The Dandy-Walker complex (which includes Dandy-Walker malformation and its variants) is a congenital anomaly believed to be related to an in utero insult to the fourth ventricle leading to complete or partial outflow obstruction of CSF. As a result, there is cyst-like dilation of the fourth ventricle, which protrudes up between the cerebellar hemispheres to prevent their fusion, and there is incomplete formation of all or part of the inferior vermis. The spectrum of Dandy-Walker variant depends on the time in utero at which the insult occurs, as well as the severity of the insult (the degree of fourth ventricular outflow obstruction). Dandy-Walker malformations are associated with hydrocephalus in approximately 75% of cases that usually develops in the postnatal period. Dandy-Walker malformations may be associated with atresia of the foramen of Magendie and, possibly, the foramen of Luschka; however, atresia of the cerebellar outlet foramina is not an essential feature of the condition. In addition, 70% of patients have associated supratentorial anomalies, including dysgenesis of the corpus callosum, migrational anomalies, and encephaloceles.

This case demonstrates characteristic MR findings of a Dandy-Walker malformation including a large retrocerebellar cyst, enlargement of the posterior fossa with osseous remodeling, abnormally high position of the straight sinus, torcular herophili, and tentorium, and torcular lambdoid inversion. The radiologic hallmark of Dandy-Walker malformation is communication of the retrocerebellar cyst with the fourth ventricle, which is readily appreciated on the sagittal MR image.

A mega cisterna magna consists of an enlarged posterior fossa secondary to an enlarged cisterna magna, but with a normal cerebellar vermis and fourth ventricle. Retrocerebellar arachnoid cysts of developmental origin are clinically important. They displace the fourth ventricle and cerebellum anteriorly and show significant mass effect. Differentiation of posterior fossa arachnoid cyst from Dandy-Walker malformation is essential as surgical therapy differs between the two entities.

Notes

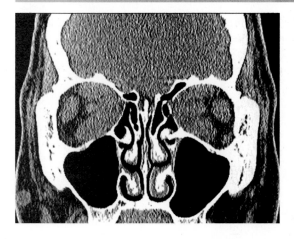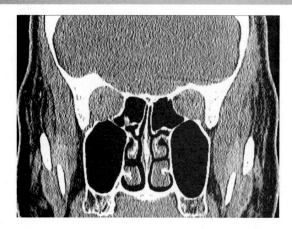

1. What are the most common patterns of extraocular muscle involvement in this disease?

2. What are vascular causes of enlargement of the extraocular muscles?

3. Isolated involvement of what extraocular muscle is extremely rare in thyroid ophthalmopathy?

4. In thyroid eye disease, what portion of the extraocular muscles is characteristically spared?

Thyroid Ophthalmopathy—with Optic Nerve Compression in the Orbital Apex

1. Enlargement of all of the extraocular muscles or of the inferior and medial rectus muscles only.

2. Carotid–cavernous fistula, thrombosis of the superior ophthalmic vein, cavernous sinus thrombosis, and arteriovenous malformation.

3. The lateral rectus muscle.

4. The tendinous insertions.

Reference

Aydin K, Guven K, Sencer S, Cikim A, Gul N, Minareci O: A new MRI method for the quantitative evaluation of extraocular muscle size in thyroid ophthalmopathy, *Neuroradiology* 45:184–187, 2003.

Cross-Reference

Neuroradiology: THE REQUISITES, 2nd ed, pp 503–504.

Comment

Thyroid ophthalmopathy is more common in women by a ratio of 4:1 and is frequently asymptomatic; however, when present, it may be seen in euthyroid or hyperthyroid states. Clinical signs and symptoms may include proptosis, lid retraction, decreased ocular range of motion, visual loss resulting from compression of the optic nerve in the orbital apex, and corneal exposure caused by eyelid retraction. Pain is uncommon. The most common cause of unilateral or bilateral exophthalmos in adults is thyroid ophthalmopathy. The incidence of bilateral disease may be as high as 90% of cases. Most patients evaluated with CT or MR imaging carry a known diagnosis of thyroid ophthalmopathy, and the role of imaging is to assess for the presence of optic nerve compression in the orbital apex by enlarged muscles, as in this case. When there is compromise of vision in patients who do not respond to medical therapy, orbital decompression by removal of the osseous walls around the orbital apex may be necessary.

Magnetic resonance imaging may also be useful in evaluating patients with ophthalmopathy without laboratory or clinical evidence of thyroid disease. The most common patterns of extraocular muscle involvement are enlargement of all of the extraocular muscles or of the inferior and medial rectus muscles only. Isolated involvement of the lateral rectus muscle is unusual, and when present, it should raise suspicion for a different disease process, such as myositis or pseudotumor. Characteristically, in thyroid ophthalmopathy, there is enlargement of the muscle bellies, with sparing of the tendinous insertions. In late stages of disease, fibrosis resulting in contraction of the muscle bellies may be evident, and there may be fatty replacement of the muscles.

Notes

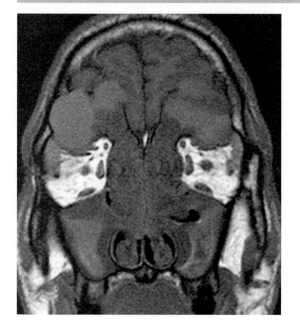

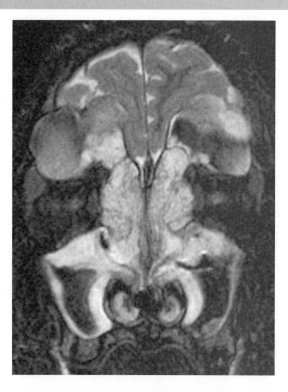

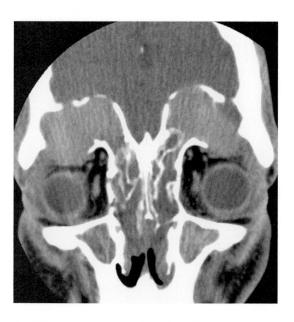

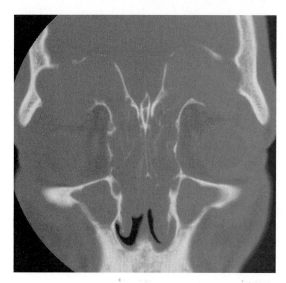

1. What determines the signal characteristics of these lesions on MR imaging?

2. What causes these lesions to develop?

3. What underlying risk factors contribute to this condition?

4. These lesions are most common in what paranasal sinus?

Bilateral Frontal Sinus Mucoceles

1. Their protein concentration, water content, viscosity, and cross-linking of glycoproteins. They are often hyperintense on both T1W and T2W images, as in this case.

2. Obstruction of a sinus ostium or a compartment of a septated sinus.

3. Risk factors for the development of mucoceles include a history of sinusitis, trauma, allergies, or instrumentation.

4. The frontal sinus.

References

Ishibashi T, Kikuchi S: Mucocele-like lesions of the sphenoid sinus with hypointense foci on T2-weighted magnetic resonance imaging, *Neuroradiology* 43: 1108–1111, 2001.

Tassel P, Lee YY, Jing BS, De Pena CA: Mucoceles of the paranasal sinuses: MR imaging with CT correlation, *AJR Am J Roentgenol* 153:407–412, 1989.

Cross-Reference

Neuroradiology: THE REQUISITES, 2nd ed, p 510.

Comment

This case shows multiple, expansile, slow-growing lesions in the bilateral frontal sinuses (the remainder of the paranasal sinuses are opacified in this patient with chronic, recurrent sinus infections). The material within the expansile lesions is hyperdense on unenhanced CT, consistent with mucoid material, and corresponding MR images show the material to be hyperintense on T1W (very common) and heterogeneous on T2W images.

Mucoceles develop from obstruction of the sinus ostia or septated compartments of a sinus and represent mucoid secretions encased by mucus-secreting epithelium (sinus mucosa). In more than 90% of cases, mucoceles occur in the frontal sinuses or the ethmoid air cells (the anterior is more common than the posterior). Although the reported literature suggests that they are least common in the sphenoid sinus, in my experience, mucoceles are least common in the maxillary sinus. Patients frequently have a history of chronic sinusitis, trauma, or sinus surgery. When symptomatic, mucoceles present with signs and symptoms related to mass effect, including frontal bossing, headache, and orbital pain. Orbital extension, as in this case, may result in proptosis and diplopia. Secondary infection (mucopyocele) and direct extension into the anterior cranial fossa are not infrequent complications. Extension into the anterior cranial fossa or orbit is more likely if there is an associated fracture of an involved sinus wall. Alternatively, as a mucocele expands, it may directly erode a sinus wall, allowing for extrasinus extension. Advances in endoscopic sinus surgery have led to an acceptance of simple drainage procedures, even for some seemingly very complicated mucoceles.

In the radiologic evaluation of mucoceles, CT best demonstrates the osseous changes of the sinus walls, which may be remodeled and expanded, thinned, and with large mucoceles, partially dehiscent. However, MR imaging best detects the interface of the mucocele with the intraorbital and intracranial structures. When necessary, enhanced MR imaging is useful in distinguishing a mucocele (which shows peripheral enhancement) from a neoplasm (which typically shows solid enhancement).

Notes

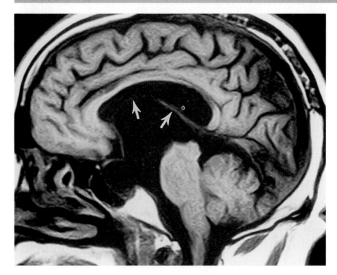

1. Localization of a lesion to the suprasellar cistern rather than the third ventricle may be determined by looking at the relation of the lesion to what structure?

2. When large, posterior fossa arachnoid cysts typically present with what symptoms?

3. What percentage of intracranial arachnoid cysts arise in the suprasellar region?

4. When symptomatic, what is the most common clinical presentation of arachnoid cysts in the quadrigeminal cistern?

Suprasellar Cistern Arachnoid Cyst

1. The third ventricle.

2. Symptoms related to hydrocephalus (headache, nausea, ataxia).

3. Approximately 10%.

4. Obstructive hydrocephalus related to compression of the aqueduct.

Reference

Miyajima M, Arai H, Okuda O, Hishii M, Nakanishi H, Sato K: Possible origin of suprasellar arachnoid cysts: neuroimaging and neurosurgical observation in nine cases, *J Neurosurg* 93:62–67, 2000.

Cross-Reference

Neuroradiology: THE REQUISITES, 2nd ed, pp 542–543.

Comment

Arachnoid cysts are common and frequently asymptomatic, especially when located in the middle cranial fossa or over the cerebral convexities. Arachnoid cysts positioned in strategic locations are the lesions most likely to be symptomatic. Large cysts in the posterior fossa may present with ataxia or other symptoms of mass effect related to hydrocephalus. Similarly, when large enough, cysts in the quadrigeminal cistern may cause hydrocephalus by compressing the aqueduct of Sylvius. As in this case, arachnoid cysts in the region of the suprasellar cistern or third ventricle may cause headache, visual symptoms (related to compression of the optic chiasm), or symptoms related to mass effect and hydrocephalus. Arachnoid cysts of the suprasellar cistern may be mistaken for third ventricular cystic masses, such as seen with parasitic infection (cysticercosis), ependymal cysts, or epidermoid cysts.

Usually, arachnoid cysts follow the signal characteristics of CSF on all MR pulse sequences and are isodense to CSF on CT. Occasionally, CSF stasis or protein within the cyst may result in different intensities on MR imaging. These are nonenhancing lesions. When looking at a lesion in this location, localization to the suprasellar cistern rather than the third ventricle may be determined by looking for elevation of the floor of the third ventricle (*arrows*). Arachnoid cysts should have smooth margins, and calcification is rarely present. Most asymptomatic arachnoid cysts are left alone. In cases of strategically positioned cysts that result in symptoms, shunting or surgical resection may be necessary.

Notes

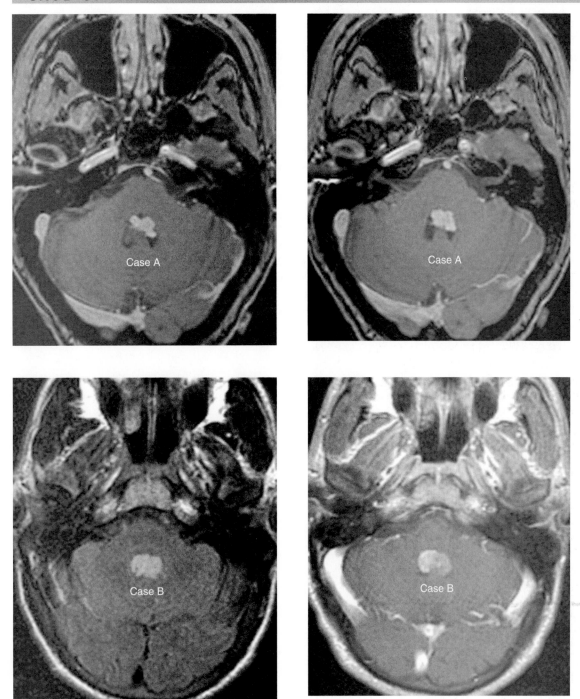

1. Where anatomically is the abnormality in these cases?

2. What is the differential diagnosis in these cases?

3. Where do ependymomas classically occur?

4. What is the most common location of choroid plexus papillomas in children?

Fourth Ventricular Neoplasms—Choroid Plexus Papilloma and Ependymoma

1. The fourth ventricle.

2. Meningioma, choroid plexus papilloma, ependymoma, metastasis, and occasionally, hemangioma. The age of the patient will usually help in limiting the playing field. In the pediatric population, ependymoma is the best choice. The other types of neoplasms are more common in adults.

3. The posterior fossa is most common. Ependymomas may also arise in the supratentorial compartment, the filum terminale, and the central canal of the spinal cord.

4. The trigone of the lateral ventricle.

Reference

Koeller KK, Sandberg GD: From the archives of the AFIP: cerebral intraventricular neoplasms. Radiologic-pathologic correlation, *RadioGraphics* 22:1473–1505, 2002.

Cross-Reference

Neuroradiology: THE REQUISITES, 2nd ed, pp 111–114, 127–128.

Comment

Choroid plexus papillomas (Case A) are epithelial tumors arising from the surface of the choroid plexus. They occur most commonly in the lateral ventricles (45%). They may also arise within the fourth ventricle (40%) and the third ventricle (10%). In adults, the majority of choroid plexus papillomas occur in the fourth ventricle, whereas in children, 80% arise in the atria or trigone of the lateral ventricles. Choroid plexus papillomas may cause hydrocephalus as a result of overproduction of CSF or obstructive hydrocephalus related to adhesions from proteinaceous or hemorrhagic material blocking the subarachnoid cisterns or ventricular outlets. In addition, large tumors will cause focal expansion of the ventricle they fill; they may also cause trapping. These tumors are composed of vascularized connective tissue and frond-like papillae lined by a single layer of epithelial cells.

Intracranial ependymomas occur above or below the tentorium. The tumor arises in rests of ependymal cells lining the ventricles that extend into adjacent white matter. Infratentorial ependymomas occur in approximately two thirds of cases, and 75% of these posterior fossa tumors are located in the fourth ventricle (Case B). Approximately 15% arise in the cerebellopontine angle, and the remaining small percentage within the cerebellar hemisphere. Approximately 50% of infratentorial ependymomas extend into the cerebellopontine angle cisterns and foramen magnum via the lateral recesses of the fourth ventricle (foramina of Magendie and Luschka). Of infratentorial ependymomas, 12% present with subarachnoid seeding, especially those demonstrating anaplastic histology.

Calcification, hemorrhage, and cysts are frequently present in both choroid plexus papillomas and ependymomas. Calcification is readily identified on CT, as are large regions of cyst formation. On MR imaging, hypointensity may correspond to calcium, vessels, or blood products. Tumors that are very cystic will be hyperintense on T2W images, whereas those with large areas of old blood products may be hypointense. Both neoplasms may enhance avidly or heterogeneously, depending on the degree of cyst formation, calcification, and hemorrhage. When contained in the fourth ventricle, choroid plexus papillomas and ependymomas may be identical in appearance, as in these cases. Age is the best clinical distinguishing factor.

Notes

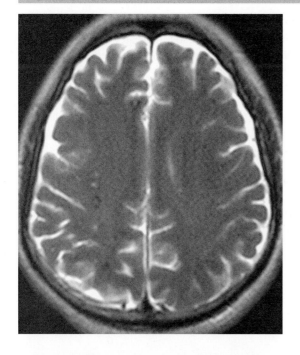
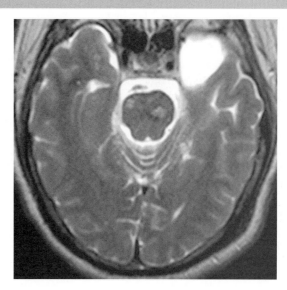
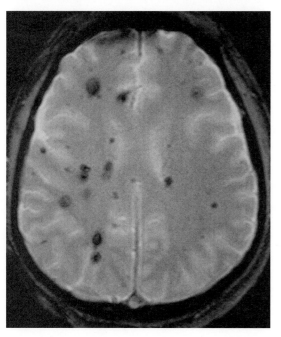
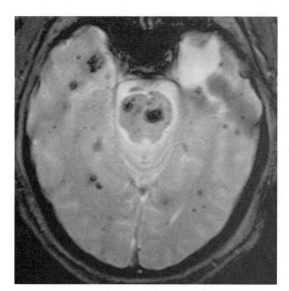

1. What is the differential diagnosis?

2. The higher sensitivity to susceptibility effects of gradient echo imaging is due to what feature of the pulse sequence?

3. In gradient echo imaging, what factors contribute to T1 and T2 weighting?

4. Gradient echo imaging for detection of blood products is achieved by using what type of flip angle and time to echo?

Multiple Cavernous Malformations—Familial Pattern

1. Multiple cavernous malformations, hypertension, and amyloid angiopathy. Hemorrhagic metastases and metastatic melanoma are included in the differential diagnosis, but are less likely, given the absence of associated edema.

2. Gradient echo imaging is more sensitive to magnetic field inhomogeneities and susceptibility due to the lack of a 180-degree rephasing pulse.

3. The flip angle and the time to echo.

4. The lower the flip angle and the longer the time to echo, the greater the sensitivity will be to susceptibility effects.

References

Mori T, Fujimoto M, Sakae K, et al: Familial presumed cerebral cavernous angiomas diagnosed by MRI: three generations, *Neuroradiology* 38:641–645, 1996.

Rigamonti D, Hadley MN, Drayer BP, et al: Cerebral cavernous malformations: incidence and familial occurrence, *N Engl J Med* 319:343–347, 1988.

Cross-Reference

Neuroradiology: THE REQUISITES, 2nd ed, pp 231–234.

Comment

Cavernous malformations have a characteristic appearance on MR imaging. Specifically, they have central high signal intensity on unenhanced T1W and T2W imaging and are surrounded by a rim of hemosiderin that is hypointense on T2W and blooms on gradient echo imaging. In approximately 25% of cases, these lesions are multiple, and in a small percentage, there is a familial pattern. Many patients with multiple cavernomas have lesions too numerous to count. As in this case, many of the lesions may be quite small and only identifiable on gradient echo susceptibility images. Although cavernomas are believed to be congenital lesions, de novo development is not uncommon in patients with a familial pattern, as well as after radiation therapy and in association with developmental venous anomalies (venous angiomas).

Gradient echo imaging has increased sensitivity to magnetic susceptibility due to the lack of a 180-degree rephasing pulse. Therefore, blood products (hemosiderin), calcium, iron, and other ions are more readily seen on this sequence as areas of marked hypointensity. The T1 or T2 weighting of a gradient echo scan may be determined by selection of the flip angle and the time to echo. A small flip angle and a long time to echo will result in more T2 weighting. Similarly, a smaller flip angle and a longer time to echo will result in greater sensitivity to susceptibility effects. In addition to increased sensitivity to magnetic field inhomogeneities, gradient echo scanning has several useful features. It is generally faster than conventional spin-echo imaging. In addition, flow-related enhancement (bright blood) may be attained and is the basis of MR angiography. Another advantage of gradient echo scanning is that three-dimensional imaging allows for very thin sections. Such thin sections may also be acquired with three-dimensional fast spin-echo imaging.

Notes

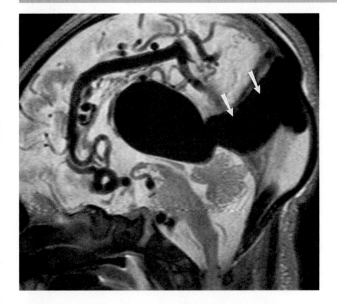 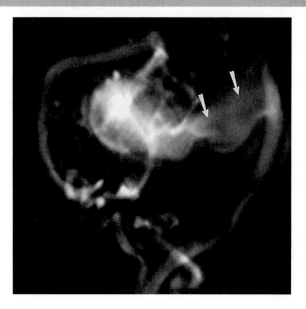

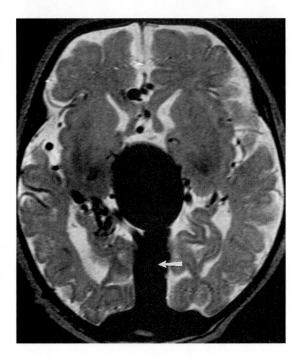

1. What is the diagnosis?

2. What are the classic clinical presentations for this entity?

3. What are the two major types of vascular abnormalities associated with this entity?

4. What anatomic structure or variant is denoted by the arrows?

Vein of Galen Aneurysm

1. Vein of Galen aneurysm.

2. High-output congestive heart failure, hydrocephalus, or macrocephaly.

3. The two major types of vascular abnormalities are true arteriovenous malformations (AVMs) and direct arteriovenous fistulas (between choroidal arteries and the vein of Galen).

4. The falcine sinus. In the setting of a persistent median prosencephalic vein, the straight sinus may not develop because the median prosencephalic vein provides diencephalic venous drainage. Instead, a falcine sinus is frequently noted, as in this case (*arrows*).

Reference

Hassan T, Timofeev EV, Ezura M, et al: Hemodynamic analysis of an adult vein of Galen aneurysm malformation by use of 3D image-based computational fluid dynamics, *AJNR Am J Neuroradiol* 24:1075–1082, 2003.

Cross-Reference

Neuroradiology: THE REQUISITES, 2nd ed, p 236.

Comment

The CT appearance of a vein of Galen aneurysm in an infant is characteristic. On unenhanced images, the vein of Galen appears as a hyperdense, demarcated mass at the level of the posterior third ventricle and diencephalon. After intravenous contrast administration, there is marked homogeneous enhancement of the malformation. MR imaging not only confirms the presence of flow within this abnormality, but also better delineates both the arterial and venous anatomy. In combination with MR angiography, MR imaging may show large choroidal arteriovenous fistulas or the presence of a parenchymal AVM. In this case, a vein of Galen aneurysm is associated with a large AVM confirmed by MR angiography. Because many women undergo obstetric ultrasound as part of their prenatal care, many of these malformations are detected in utero with color flow Doppler sonography.

Early in embryologic development, the deep brain structures and diencephalon are drained by the median prosencephalic vein. As the internal cerebral veins begin to develop, this vein slowly regresses. A caudal remnant of the median prosencephalic vein will become the normal vein of Galen. In patients with vein of Galen aneurysms related to either a parenchymal AVM or a direct arteriovenous fistula between the choroidal vessels, a persistent median prosencephalic vein may occur. Because this provides diencephalic venous drainage, the straight sinus may not form. Instead, a falcine sinus is frequently noted, as in this case (*arrows*). Vein of Galen malformations resulting from direct arteriovenous fistulas are frequently associated with venous obstruction and venous hypertension. High-output heart failure in newborns and hydrocephalus due to obstruction of the aqueduct of Sylvius by the enlarged vein of Galen with macrocephaly are common clinical scenarios in infants.

Treatment of these malformations is catheter angiography and glue embolization of the shunt. Several embolization procedures may be necessary to completely obliterate the vascular shunts and communications. This is often done over a several-month period before the child is a toddler.

Notes

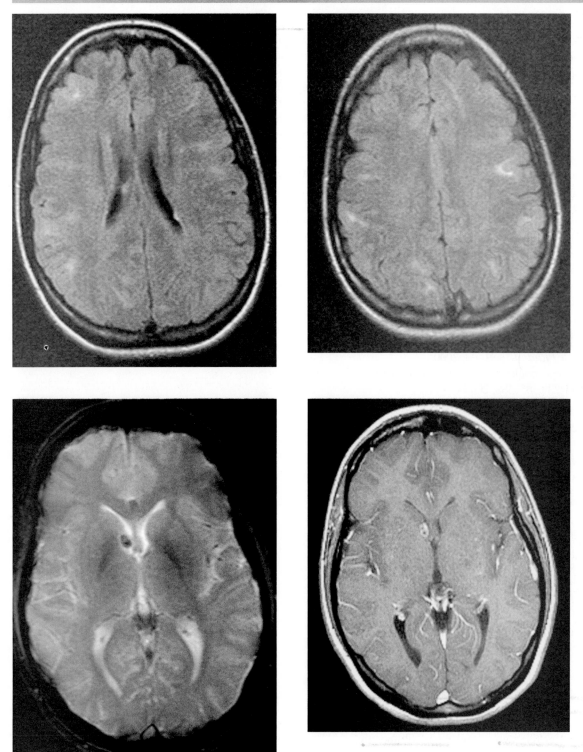

1. How might this pediatric patient have presented clinically?

2. What benign neoplasm is associated with this syndrome?

3. What is the CNS imaging hallmark seen in 98% of patients with this disorder?

4. What organ systems in addition to the CNS are affected in patients with tuberous sclerosis?

Tuberous Sclerosis (Bourneville's Disease)

1. With seizures, mental retardation, or adenoma sebaceum. Other clinical signs include skin lesions (ash-leaf spots, shagreen patches, and subungual fibromas).

2. Subependymal giant cell astrocytoma.

3. Subependymal nodules (tubers).

4. The kidneys may have hamartomas (angiomyolipomas), cysts, and rarely, renal cell carcinoma; the retina may have hamartomas; rhabdomyomas may occur along the ventricular septum in the heart; the lungs may be affected by angiomyomatosis; and the liver and pancreas may have adenomas. A variety of skeletal lesions (bone islands and cysts) and, occasionally, vascular lesions (aneurysms or stenoses) may be present.

References

Evans JC, Curtis J: The radiological appearances of tuberous sclerosis, *Br J Radiol* 73:91–98, 2000.

Lonergan GJ, Smirniotopoulos JG: Case 64: Tuberous sclerosis, *Radiology* 229:385–388, 2003.

Cross-Reference

Neuroradiology: THE REQUISITES, 2nd ed, pp 453–454.

Comment

Tuberous sclerosis most commonly occurs as a sporadic mutation (chromosome 11); it may also be an autosomal dominant disorder transmitted by a mutation on chromosome 9. There are a spectrum of clinical signs and symptoms in these patients; however, the imaging manifestations should be sufficient to make the diagnosis in the majority of cases. Seizures, mental retardation, and adenoma sebaceum are the classic clinical triad described in tuberous sclerosis; however, the three together are seen in fewer than 50% of patients with this diagnosis.

The CNS manifestations of tuberous sclerosis are numerous and include subependymal nodules, cortical tubers, white matter lesions (believed to represent dysplastic white matter or foci of hypomyelination), subependymal giant cell astrocytomas, and ventriculomegaly. Subependymal nodules are seen in essentially all patients with tuberous sclerosis, and more than 75% are calcified. Because of the high incidence of calcification, subependymal nodules are easily detected on CT, but they can be difficult to detect on MR imaging. Gradient echo and unenhanced T1W imaging are best for detection of these lesions, which are hypointense and often mildly hyperintense to brain, respectively.

Cortical tubers are present in approximately 50% of these patients, and approximately half are calcified. Cortical tubers are hyperintense on long TR images and are frequently bilateral and symmetric (as in this case). They affect the frontal, parietal, occipital, and temporal lobes, in descending order of frequency. Up to 33% of subependymal nodules and 5% of cortical tubers may enhance.

Notes

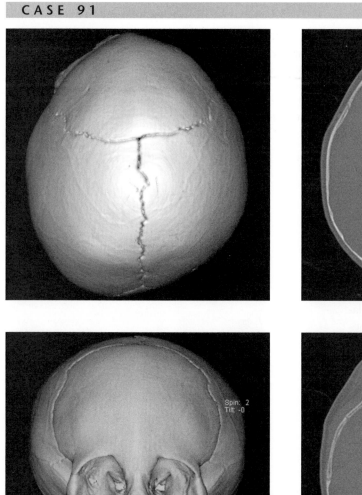

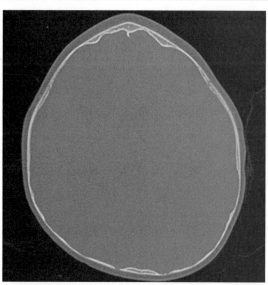

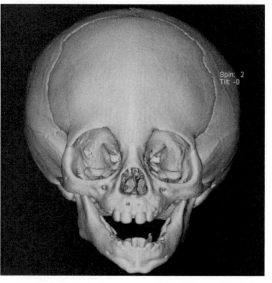

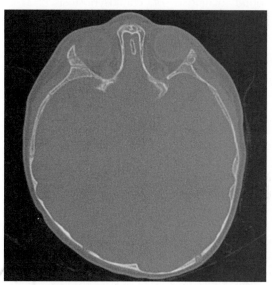

1. What is meant by cranial synostosis?

2. What is the most common suture to close prematurely?

3. Trigonocephaly and hypotelorism are characteristic of premature closure of which suture?

4. Plagiocephaly refers to what pattern of craniosynostosis?

Craniosynostosis—Metopic Suture

1. Premature closure of one or more cranial sutures.

2. The sagittal suture.

3. The metopic suture.

4. Premature closure of one of the paired sutures (coronal, lambdoid or, much less frequently, temporosquamosal).

References

Aviv RI, Rodger E, Hall CM: Craniosynostosis, *Clin Radiol* 57:93–102, 2002.

Medina LS: Three-dimensional CT maximum intensity projections of the calvaria: a new approach for diagnosis of craniosynostosis and fractures, *AJNR Am J Neuroradiol* 12:1951–1954, 2000.

Ngo AV, Sze RW, Parisi MT, et al: Cranial suture simulator for ultrasound diagnosis of craniosynostosis, *Pediatr Radiol* 34:535–540, 2004.

Cross-Reference

Neuroradiology: THE REQUISITES, 2nd ed, pp 438–440.

Comment

Craniostenosis, or craniosynostosis, refers to premature closure of one or more of the cranial sutures. Isolated premature closure of the sagittal suture is most common, occurring in more than 50% of cases of craniosynostosis. Unilateral or bilateral premature closure of coronal sutures is the next most common, followed by premature closure of the metopic suture. The lambdoid suture undergoes premature closure in fewer than 1% of cases of craniosynostosis. Depending on the sutures involved, there are characteristic deformities of the skull and orbit. Premature closure of the sagittal suture results in a head that has limited growth in the transverse dimension. This results in dolichocephaly (scaphocephaly), in which there is an increase in head size in the anteroposterior dimension.

Plagiocephaly refers to premature closure of a single coronal or lambdoid suture (or, occasionally, a temporosquamous suture). In the majority of cases, plagiocephaly is seen with closure of a single coronal suture, resulting in elevation of the lesser wing of the sphenoid bone and leading to a "harlequin" appearance of the orbit. Premature closure of both coronal sutures results in brachycephaly. Early fusion of the metopic suture in the frontal region results in trigonocephaly, or simply a "triangular" configuration of the head, as in this case. Craniosynostosis is usually an isolated abnormality, although it may be associated with a variety of congenital syndromes. Such conditions include Apert's syndrome, which is associated with a "cloverleaf" deformity of the skull resulting from closure of the coronal, lambdoid, and sagittal sutures. Other syndromes associated with craniostenosis are hypophosphatasia, Crouzon's disease (craniofacial dysostosis), and Treacher Collins syndrome (mandibulofacial dysostosis).

Notes

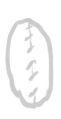

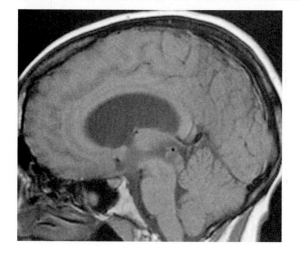

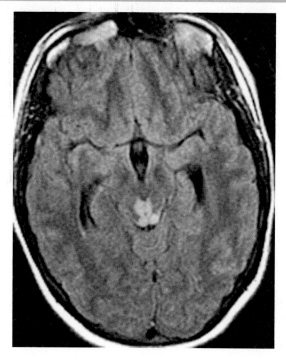

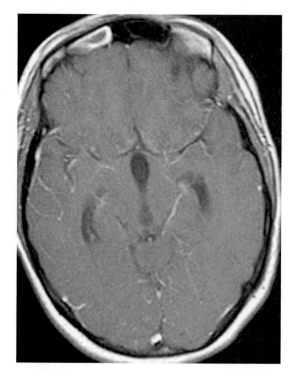

1. From what structure does the lesion arise?

2. What are the secondary imaging findings due to this lesion?

3. The tectum, or roof, of the midbrain contains what paired structures?

4. What congenital anomaly is usually associated with "beaking" of the tectum?

Glioma of the Tectum (Quadrigeminal Plate)

1. Tectum (quadrigeminal plate).

2. Obstructive hydrocephalus due to compression of the aqueduct of Sylvius.

3. The superior and inferior colliculi.

4. Chiari II malformation.

References

Sherman JL, Citrin CM, Barkovich AJ, Bower BJ: MR imaging of the mesencephalic tectum: normal and pathologic variations, *AJNR Am J Neuroradiol* 8:59–64, 1987.

Sun B, Wang CC, Wang J: MRI characteristics of midbrain tumours, *Neuroradiology* 41:158–162, 1999.

Cross-Reference

Neuroradiology: THE REQUISITES, 2nd ed, pp 40, 372–373.

Comment

These images show a mildly expansile mass lesion of the tectal plate that is predominantly cystic. There is no significant pathologic enhancement after contrast administration. There is resultant compression of the aqueduct of Sylvius, as is typically seen in patients with tectal gliomas. In many patients, the clinical presentation is that of obstructive hydrocephalus. Gliomas arising from the tectum are usually low-grade astrocytomas. They may be solid or cystic masses and have a wide spectrum of enhancement characteristics, ranging from none to prominent. Because most of these are low-grade neoplasms, the absence of enhancement is not surprising.

The midbrain is separated into the tegmentum and the tectum, which are portions of the midbrain anterior and posterior to the aqueduct of Sylvius, respectively. The tectum (roof) consists of the quadrigeminal plate that contains the paired superior and inferior colliculi. The tectum is affected more frequently by extrinsic rather than intrinsic lesions. It is often compressed (particularly the superior colliculi), along with the aqueduct of Sylvius, by pineal region masses, such as meningiomas in adults, germ cell tumors (germinoma, embryonal carcinoma, choriocarcinoma, and teratoma), tumors of pineal origin (pineoblastoma and pineocytoma), and aneurysms of the vein of Galen, which may result in Parinaud's syndrome. In this case, * denotes the normal pineal gland. Occasionally, the tectum may be affected by demyelinating disease, vascular abnormalities, or trauma. In addition, the tectum may be abnormal in congenital malformations, most notably, Chiari II malformation, in which there may be a spectrum of abnormalities, ranging from collicular fusion to tectal beaking.

Notes

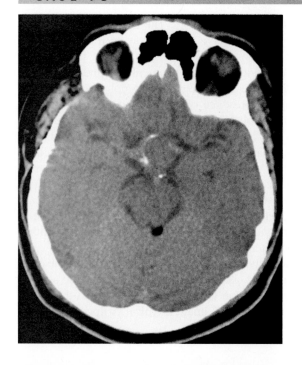

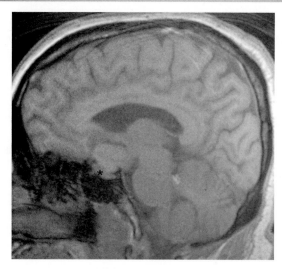

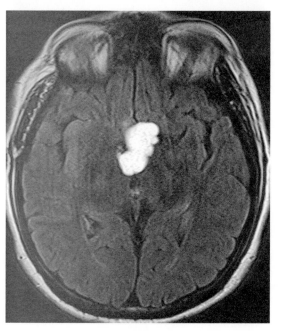

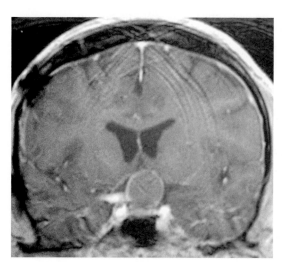

1. What is the best diagnosis in this case?

2. What is the typical age of presentation for this entity?

3. What are the characteristic imaging findings in craniopharyngioma?

4. How do squamous papillary craniopharyngiomas differ from adamantinomatous craniopharyngiomas radiologically?

Craniopharyngioma—Recurrent Adamantinomatous Type

1. Suprasellar craniopharyngioma. The * on the sagittal image denotes the pituitary gland. The mass is separate from the gland, making a pituitary macroadenoma unlikely. Did you notice the remote right craniotomy? This is recurrent tumor 8 years later.

2. The age distribution is bimodal. Those in children between the ages of 5 and 10 years are of the adamantinomatous type. The second peak occurs in the fifth and sixth decades of life.

3. Cystic or cystic and solid mass, calcification, and enhancement.

4. Squamous papillary craniopharyngiomas are typically solid, do not calcify, and are frequently present within the third ventricle rather than in the suprasellar cistern. The majority are seen in men.

References

Nagahata M, Hosoya T, Kayama T, Yamaguchi K: Edema along the optic tract: a useful MR finding for the diagnosis of craniopharyngiomas, *AJNR Am J Neuroradiol* 19:1753–1757, 1998.

Sartoretti-Schefer S, Wichmann W, Aguzzi A, Valavanis A: MR differentiation of adamantinous and squamous-papillary craniopharyngiomas, *AJNR Am J Neuroradiol* 18:77–87, 1997.

Cross-Reference

Neuroradiology: THE REQUISITES, 2nd ed, pp 545–548.

Comment

Craniopharyngiomas arise from metaplastic squamous epithelial rests (Rathke's pouch) along the hypophysis or from ectopic embryonic cell rests, and are seen in children and adults. Histologically, they are characterized by palisading adamantinous epithelium, keratin, and calcification. They account for 1% to 3% of all intracranial neoplasms and 10% to 15% of all supratentorial tumors. They are more common in boys and men. The majority of craniopharyngiomas arise within the suprasellar cistern (80%–90%), as in this case; however, they also may arise within the sella turcica and, occasionally, the third ventricle. Clinical presentation includes visual disturbances related to compression of the optic chiasm, pituitary hypofunction related to compression of the gland or hypothalamus, and symptoms of increased intracranial pressure.

Imaging findings typically include a cystic or a solid and cystic mass lesion. Approximately 80% to 90% of all craniopharyngiomas have a cystic component. Smaller lesions may be purely solid. The majority (90%) of craniopharyngiomas have calcification or regions of avid homogeneous enhancement (in solid portions of tumor) or peripheral enhancement (around cystic portions). Because MR imaging may not be sensitive in detecting the presence of calcification, CT may be quite useful in establishing the diagnosis of craniopharyngioma. On MR imaging, the signal characteristics may be quite variable, depending on the contents and viscosity within the cysts. Whereas the cystic portion is frequently hyperintense on T2W and FLAIR imaging, it may be hypointense, isointense, or hyperintense on T1W imaging. High signal intensity on T1W images may be due to high concentrations of protein or methemoglobin (rather than cholesterol or lipid products).

Incidentally noted, there is a small lipoma in the perimesencephalic cistern on the left adjacent to the tectum. It is hypodense on CT, and hyperintense on the unenhanced sagittal T1 W images, typical of lipomas.

Notes

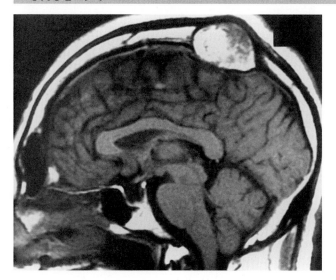
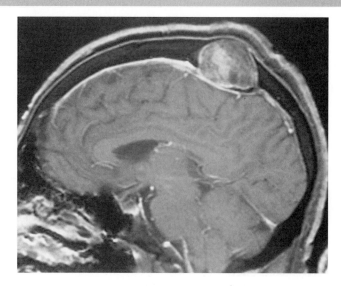

1. How would this lesion appear on plain film radiographs of the skull?

2. Osseous hemangiomas occur most frequently in what part of the skeleton?

3. What is the classic appearance of a calvarial hemangioma on plain film?

4. What are the proposed causes of epidermoid cysts of the skull?

Intradiploic Epidermoid Cyst

1. As a well-circumscribed, lytic lesion.

2. The vertebral column.

3. A radiating sunburst or honeycomb pattern.

4. Inclusion of ectodermal cell rests during embryonic development; less commonly, it has been suggested that they may be acquired by traumatic implantation of ectodermal tissue into the bone.

Reference

Arana E, Latorre FF, Revert A, et al: Intradiploic epidermoid cysts, *Neuroradiology* 38:306–311, 1996.

Cross-Reference

Neuroradiology: THE REQUISITES, 2nd ed, pp 115–119.

Comment

Epidermoid and dermoid cysts of the skull are rare. Both are proposed to occur as a result of inclusion of epithelial cells during closure of the neural tube between the third and the fifth week of gestation. However, development of epidermoid cysts secondary to implantation of epithelial cells after trauma has been suggested as the cause in approximately 25% of cases. Epidermoid cysts account for fewer than 2% of intracranial and cranial tumors. Approximately 25% occur in the skull, whereas the remaining 75% are intradural. Dermoid cysts are even less common. Epidermoid cysts tend to present in young adults, whereas dermoid cysts present in children and young adolescents.

Approximately 10% of calvarial epidermoid cysts are incidental lesions; the remaining 90% are symptomatic. The most common presentation is an enlarging scalp mass; however, pain or headache is present in approximately 20% of cases. The most common location of these cysts is the parietal bone, followed by the frontal and temporal bones. Approximately 70% of these lesions involve both the inner and outer tables of the skull. Involvement of only the outer cortical table or, less commonly, the inner table may occur. On plain films, epidermoid cysts typically appear as lytic lesions with sclerotic borders. The differential diagnosis includes hemangioma, eosinophilic granuloma, and leptomeningeal cysts, especially in childhood. Other lytic lesions, particularly in adults, cannot be definitively differentiated on plain films alone. These lesions are typically hyperintense on T2W imaging; however, on unenhanced T1W imaging, their signal characteristics are variable. High T1W signal intensity may be due to the presence of blood products, protein, debris, crystals, or fat.

Notes

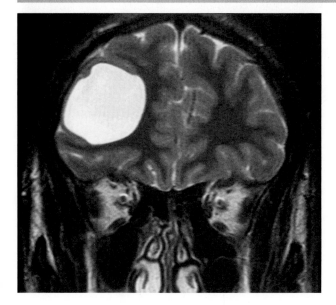 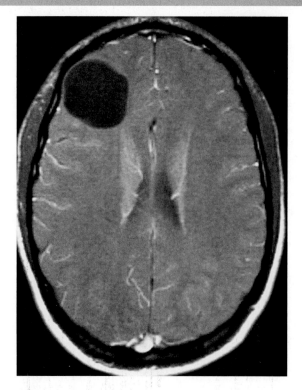

1. What tissue lines the CSF-filled open-lip schizencephaly?

2. What lines the cystic cavity in this entity?

3. What are the causes of this entity?

4. What is neonatal alloimmune thrombocytopenia, and what are the associated findings on neuroimaging?

Porencephalic Cyst

1. Gray matter.

2. White matter that is frequently gliotic.

3. An old insult usually related to infarction, infection, or trauma.

4. Neonatal alloimmune thrombocytopenia is a serious fetal disorder resulting from platelet–antigen incompatibility between mother and fetus. The diagnosis is usually made after the discovery of unexpected neonatal thrombocytopenia. Antenatal or early postnatal neuroimaging has shown that intracranial hemorrhage and porencephalic cysts should raise concern for this entity. Between 10% and 20% of affected fetuses have intracranial hemorrhages, and 25% to 50% occur in utero. Porencephalic cysts are also very common.

Reference

Dale ST, Coleman LT: Neonatal alloimmune thrombocytopenia: Antenatal and postnatal imaging findings in the pediatric brain, *Am J Neuroradiol* 23:1457–1465, 2002.

Cross-Reference

Neuroradiology: THE REQUISITES, 2nd ed, p 390.

Comment

Porencephalic cysts occur in regions of encephalomalacic brain. Insults that occur in utero after development of the brain, postnatally, or in childhood, such as infarction, trauma, or infection (especially viral agents, such as herpes and cytomegalovirus) involving the cerebral cortex and underlying subcortical white matter, typically predispose to this entity. The porencephalic cyst often communicates with the ventricles and extends to the surface of the brain. However, in some instances, intervening tissue between the ventricle and the cyst may be present. Transmission of CSF pulsations from the ventricles into the cyst or development of adhesions within the cyst, resulting in a ball-valve mechanism, leads to ventricular and cystic enlargement, which may result in remodeling or expansion of the inner table of the calvarium, as is seen with large superficial arachnoid cysts.

Another entity that extends from the superficial surface of the cerebrum to the ventricular margin is open-lip schizencephaly, which may resemble a porencephalic cyst on quick initial observation. Schizencephaly is a developmental migrational abnormality (unlike a porencephalic cyst, which is destruction of normally developed brain). Schizencephaly can be distinguished from porencephaly in that the schizencephalic CSF cleft is lined by gray matter, whereas the porencephalic cyst is lined by white matter.

Notes

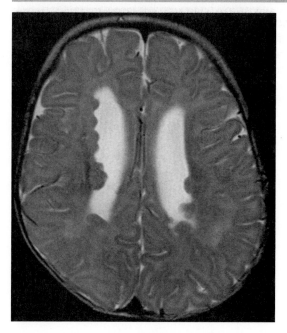 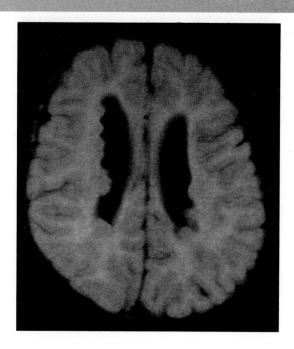

1. How did this 5-month-old infant present clinically?
2. What percentage of subependymal tubers in tuberous sclerosis are calcified?
3. What is the diagnosis in this case?
4. What heritable pattern has been described in some cases of this entity?

Subependymal Heterotopia

1. This infant presented with seizures.

2. Approximately 98%.

3. Subependymal heterotopia.

4. Some cases have X-linked inheritance.

References

Barkovich AJ: Morphologic characteristics of subcortical heterotopia: MR imaging study, *AJNR Am J Neuroradiol* 21:290–295, 2000.

Mitchell LA, Simon EM, Filly RA, Barkovich AJ: Antenatal diagnosis of subependymal heterotopia, *AJNR Am J Neuroradiol* 21:296–300, 2000.

Cross-Reference

Neuroradiology: THE REQUISITES, 2nd ed, p 427.

Comment

This case illustrates multiple subependymal heterotopias that consist of clusters of disorganized neurons and glial cells that are located in close proximity to the ventricular walls. In subependymal heterotopia, nodules are often bilaterally symmetric along the length of the lateral ventricles, as in this case, or there may be just a few lesions. Heterotopias appear as masses that are isointense to gray matter on all pulse sequences and do not enhance. High signal intensity in the parenchyma surrounding the heterotopia should not occur. The differential diagnosis for subependymal heterotopia is limited, and the diagnosis is usually easily established by the stereotypical imaging appearance. Subependymal nodules in tuberous sclerosis are readily differentiated because they do not follow the signal characteristics of gray matter, and the vast majority are calcified (hypointense on T2W and gradient echo susceptibility images and mildly hyperintense on unenhanced T1W images). In addition, other sequelae of tuberous sclerosis are commonly present. Metastatic masses are uncommon and typically enhance after contrast administration. Other signs of metastatic disease are frequently present in the intracranial compartment.

Periventricular heterotopia represents failed migration from the germinal region; however, some cases may result from abnormal proliferation of neuroblasts in the periventricular region, failure of regression, or apoptosis of neuroblasts within the germinal matrix. Heterotopia may be associated with a spectrum of other congenital anomalies, including Chiari malformations, ventral induction defects (holoprosencephaly, dysgenesis of the corpus callosum), other migrational abnormalities, and encephaloceles. Some cases have X-linked inheritance, and early antenatal diagnosis is important for appropriate management. In this patient, there is ex vacuo enlargement of the occipital horns of the lateral ventricles (colpocephaly) as a result of underdevelopment of the surrounding deep white matter and dysgenesis of the splenium of the corpus callosum.

Notes

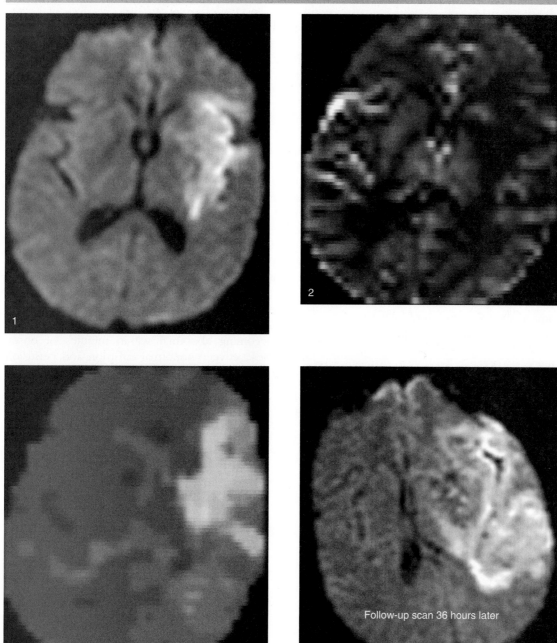

Follow-up scan 36 hours later

1. What is meant by the term penumbra?

2. What functional MR imaging techniques may be used to detect ischemic tissue in the setting of acute stroke?

3. Which type of MR imaging assesses the transit of intravenous gadolinium during the first pass of this contrast agent through the brain?

4. What is the diagnosis?

Acute Middle Cerebral Artery Stroke

1. Normal brain tissue surrounding a region of infarcted brain that is at increased risk for ischemic injury.

2. Diffusion-weighted and perfusion imaging.

3. Perfusion imaging. Perfusion may also be assessed using CT.

4. Acute left middle cerebral artery infarction with extension of the infarct on follow-up MR imaging. The first diffusion-weighted (DW) image shows high signal intensity in the left MCA territory, consistent with an acute stroke. Note the "mismatch" between this DW image and perfusion imaging (image 3 = rCBF; image 3 = TTP). The perfusion imaging shows a much larger region of decreased blood flow (hypointensity on image 3 rCBF) around the acute stroke, consistent with brain at risk. Follow-up DW image shows extension of infarct in the region of "brain at risk" identified on perfusion imaging.

References

Liu YJ, Chen CY, Chung HW, et al: Neuronal damage after ischemic injury in the middle cerebral arterial territory: deep watershed versus territorial infarction at MR perfusion and spectroscopic imaging, *Radiology* 229:366–374, 2003.

Neumann-Haefelin T, du Mesnil de Rochemont R, Fiebach JB, et al: Effect of incomplete (spontaneous and post-thrombolytic) recanalization after middle cerebral artery occlusion: a magnetic resonance imaging study, *Stroke* 35:109–114, 2004.

Cross-Reference

Neuroradiology: THE REQUISITES, 2nd ed, pp 86–88, 183–187.

Comment

An unenhanced CT scan of the head remains the first imaging study for the emergent evaluation of acute stroke because it is readily available, rapidly performed, and sensitive in identifying acute intracranial hemorrhage and mass effect that may require immediate and urgent surgical intervention.

Magnetic resonance imaging is more sensitive than CT in detecting acute infarcts and showing extension of infarctions on follow-up examinations, as in this case. It is identification of this "penumbra" (brain tissue at risk for irreversible ischemia) that is at the heart of further development of MR imaging techniques. It is important to protect this tissue from ischemia by applying appropriate interventions. Furthermore, to deliver protective agents, perfusion to this tissue is necessary. Tissue perfusion may be assessed with perfusion imaging. Rapid imaging is performed both before and during the bolus intravenous injection of gadolinium. On first pass through the cerebral vasculature, there is a drop in measured signal intensity due to the T2* effects of this agent. Mathematic models can be used to convert this decrease in signal intensity to concentration of contrast over time. Tissue perfusion may also be assessed with diffusion imaging, which measures movement of water molecules. In this sequence, a 180° pulse is flanked by strong diffusion gradients. The greater the distance a water molecule travels, the more signal loss will occur due to dephasing. In the CNS, water molecules have a predilection to move more readily in the direction of axons. This directional preference is termed anisotropic diffusion. The direction in which a diffusion gradient is applied will determine the end result. Diffusion imaging is the most sensitive indicator of ischemia, with the image becoming abnormal within minutes of onset. Mismatches between abnormal diffusion and perfusion imaging may indicate brain at risk, as in this case.

Notes

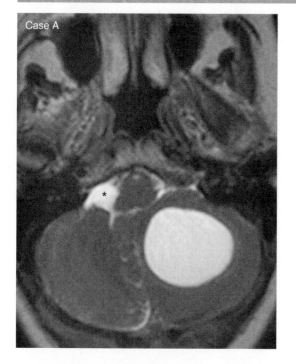

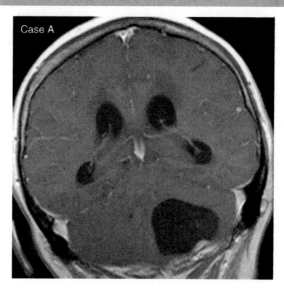

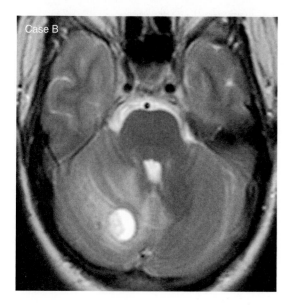

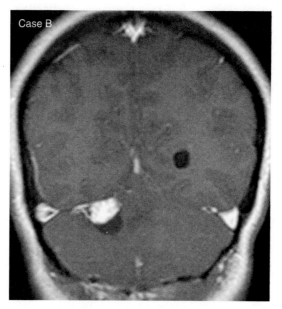

1. What is the differential diagnosis in these adults?

2. What is the most common cerebellar "mass" in adults?

3. What clinical factor helps to distinguish a hemangioblastoma from a pilocytic astrocytoma?

4. What neurocutaneous syndrome is associated with multiple hemangioblastomas?

C A S E   9 8

Hemangioblastoma

1. Hemangioblastoma, pilocytic astrocytoma, and vascular metastasis. ·

2. A stroke is the most common "mass"! The most common cerebellar neoplasm in an adult is a metastasis, whereas the most common primary cerebellar neoplasm is a hemangioblastoma.

3. The age of the patient. Pilocytic astrocytomas tend to occur in children, whereas isolated cerebellar hemangioblastomas usually present in young adults.

4. von Hippel-Lindau disease.

References

Quadery FA, Okamoto K: Diffusion-weighted MRI of hemangioblastomas and other cerebellar tumours, *Neuroradiology* 45:212–219, 2003.

Slater A, Moore NR, Huson SM: The natural history of cerebellar hemangioblastomas in von Hippel-Lindau disease, *AJNR Am J Neuroradiol* 24:1570–1574, 2003.

Cross-Reference

Neuroradiology: THE REQUISITES, 2nd ed, pp 131–132.

Comment

Cerebellar hemangioblastomas are benign neoplasms that represent the most common primary infratentorial neoplasm in adults. They are more common in men, and presentation is typically during adulthood (except when associated with von Hippel-Lindau disease, where presentation may occur in late adolescence). Patients may present with headache, nausea and vomiting, ataxia, and vertigo. Although these neoplasms typically have a vascular nidus, subarachnoid hemorrhage is an uncommon presentation. More than 80% of posterior fossa hemangioblastomas occur in the cerebellum. They may also occur in the spinal cord or medulla (in the region of the area postrema). Cerebral hemangioblastomas are unusual, representing fewer than 2% of all hemangioblastomas, and are usually indicative of von Hippel-Lindau disease (posterior fossa tumors are also usually present in this neurocutaneous syndrome).

There are two characteristic imaging appearances of cerebellar hemangioblastomas. The first is that of a solid and cystic mass (>50% of cases). In most cases, there is no enhancement around the cyst wall. The solid vascular mural nodule associated with the cyst avidly enhances, and the nodule usually abuts the pial surface, as in these cases. Alternatively, hemangioblastomas may present as poorly demarcated, avidly enhancing masses typically associated with numerous vascular flow voids (up to 40% of cases). In Case A, the * represents an incidental arachnoid cyst in the right cerebellomedullary angle.

Management is typically surgical resection, which is considered curative. Recurrence may occur if there has been incomplete resection of the solid vascular nidus.

Notes

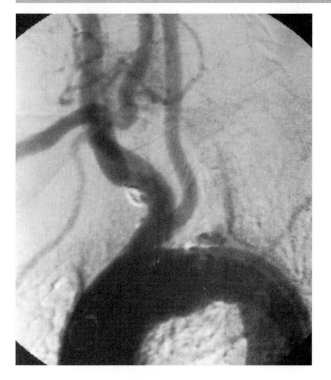 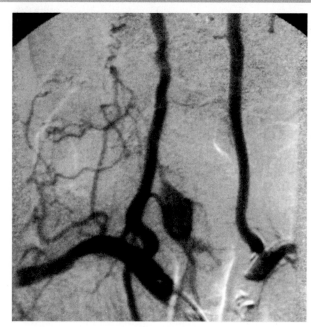

1. What vessel is selected on the second image?

2. What is the pertinent finding on the brachiocephalic injection?

3. What is the name of this entity, and is it more frequently found on the left or the right?

4. To confirm the diagnosis of "subclavian steal" on two-dimensional time-of-flight MR angiography, what is the best place to position the stationary saturation pulse?

Posterior Circulation Ischemia due to Subclavian Steal

1. The bracheocephalic artery.

2. Retrograde flow down the left vertebral artery. The first image, an arch aortogram, shows that the origin of the left subclavian artery is occluded.

3. "Subclavian steal" and on the left, respectively.

4. On standard two-dimensional time-of-flight MR angiography, there is usually a stationary superior saturation pulse that is used to suppress the signal from the neck veins. Because in subclavian steal there is retrograde flow in the involved vertebral artery, this saturation pulse has to be removed or an inferior saturation pulse should be applied.

References

Al-Mubarak N, Liu MW, Dean LS, et al: Immediate and late outcomes of subclavian artery stenting, *Cathet Cardiovasc Intervent* 46:169–172, 1999.

Malek AM, Higashida RT, Phatouros CC, et al: Treatment of posterior circulation ischemia with extracranial percutaneous balloon angioplasty and stent placement, *Stroke* 30:2073–2085, 1999.

Cross-Reference

Neuroradiology: THE REQUISITES, 2nd ed, pp 178–180, 183.

Comment

Subclavian steal results from occlusion or a hemodynamically significant stenosis of the subclavian artery proximal to the origin of the vertebral artery, or stenosis of the brachiocephalic artery. Subclavian steal occurs much more commonly on the left than on the right. There is retrograde flow of blood down the ipsilateral vertebral artery (stealing blood from the circle of Willis) to provide collateral blood supply to the arm (bypassing the occlusion or stenosis of the proximal subclavian artery).

In patients with subclavian steal, symptoms and signs may be related to decreased blood flow to the arm (decreased pulse, reduced blood pressure, decreased temperature, or claudication) or to neurologic symptoms due to periodic ischemia in the posterior circulation (as was the case in this patient) from decreased antegrade flow (not "stealing" of blood from the circle of Willis). Neurologic symptoms include transient attacks, dizziness, and visual symptoms. Similar neurologic symptoms may occur with high-grade stenoses or occlusions of the proximal vertebral artery; however, the arm is not symptomatic. Subclavian stenosis can often be diagnosed on physical examination. Imaging studies that may help to confirm the diagnosis include Doppler ultrasound and MR angiography studies, which may correctly demonstrate retrograde flow down the involved vertebral artery. On arch aortography, early arterial films show occlusion or stenosis of the proximal left subclavian artery, whereas delayed films demonstrate retrograde flow. Neurointerventional techniques may be used to treat symptomatic patients and include percutaneous transluminal angioplasty or positioning of stents.

Notes

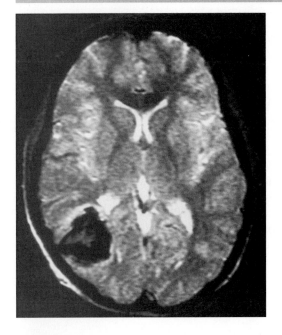

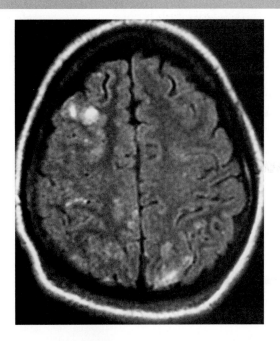

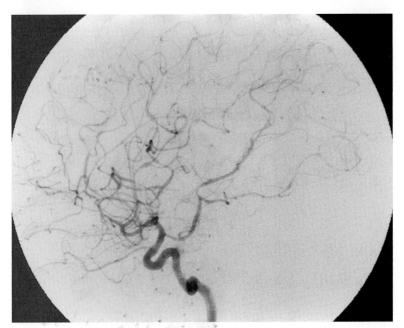

1. What are the findings on MR imaging and conventional catheter angiogram?

2. What is the differential diagnosis for segmental regions of narrowing of the cerebral arteries?

3. What diagnosis best ties all of the imaging findings together?

4. What rare intravascular neoplasm may mimic CNS vasculitis?

CNS Vasculitis—Cerebral Hemorrhage and Infarcts

1. Magnetic resonance imaging shows a right parietal lobe hemorrhage and multifocal regions of increased signal intensity involving the cerebral cortex and gray–white matter interface consistent with infarcts. Note diffuse segmental narrowing with alternating regions of dilation involving the cerebral vessels.

2. Vasculitis, intracranial atherosclerosis, hypercoagulable state (antiphospholipid antibodies), and vasospasm. Neoplasms may cause segmental narrowing due to encasement of the vessel by tumor; however, this tends to be more focal in distribution.

3. CNS vasculitis.

4. Rarely, intra-arterial lymphoma may simulate vasculitis.

References

Campi A, Benndorf G, Filippi M, Reganati P, Martinelli V, Terreni MR: Primary angiitis of the central nervous system: serial MRI of brain and spinal cord, *Neuroradiology* 43:599–607, 2001.

Wasserman BA, Stone JH, Hellmann DB, Pomper MG: Reliability of normal findings on MR imaging for excluding the diagnosis of vasculitis of the central nervous system, *AJR Am J Roentgenol* 177:455–459, 2001.

Cross-Reference

Neuroradiology: THE REQUISITES, 2nd ed, pp 196–206.

Comment

The clinical presentation of CNS vasculitis is variable, ranging from headache, changes in mental status, and meningitis to stroke and intracranial hemorrhage, as in this case. The vasculitides that can affect the CNS include infectious and noninfectious causes. Infectious etiologies include tuberculosis, which frequently involves the vessels around the basal cisterns. Neurosyphilis may cause a basilar meningitis and vasculitis; however, it may also affect more distal cerebral vessels, and it is especially likely to affect the middle cerebral arteries. There are several classifications of noninfectious vasculitis that result from inflammatory infiltrates, both within and surrounding the vessel walls, that lead to regions of segmental narrowing and dilation on conventional catheter angiography. Among the noninfectious causes of vasculitis are the necrotizing vasculopathies, such as primary angiitis, periarteritis nodosa, sarcoidosis, and Wegener's granulomatosis. Vasculitis is occasionally associated with collagen vascular diseases, such as systemic lupus erythematosus and rheumatoid arthritis; however, this is less frequent than is reported. More often, the cause of ischemic events in these patients is related to a hypercoagulable state, such as antiphospholipid antibodies (lupus anticoagulant and anticardiolipin antibodies). Certain recreational drugs have also been associated with vasculitis and infarcts, including amphetamines, ecstasy, and cocaine.

Even with the technical advances in MR angiography and CT angiography, conventional catheter angiography is still best for showing the changes of vasculitis in the cerebral arteries. A normal (negative) finding on angiogram does not exclude CNS vasculitis. If vasculitis is highly suspect clinically, biopsy is indicated to make the diagnosis. Even in cases in which angiography findings are positive, biopsy may still be necessary to confirm the diagnosis.

Notes

✱ vasculitis :

= infection (TB , syphilis ...)
- non infection
SLE
RA
Cocaine / amphetamine
Anti ph Ab
sarcoid
wegner
periartiris nodosa

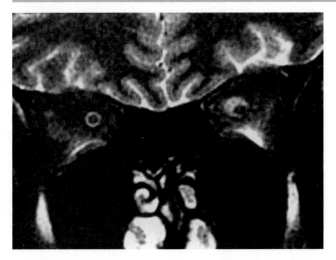 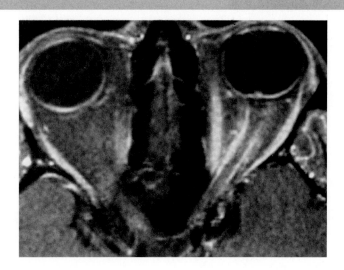

1. What is the differential diagnosis?

2. What is pneumosinus dilatans?

3. When this lesion involves the optic nerve sheath complex bilaterally, from what area does it usually arise?

4. What is the typical clinical presentation of this lesion?

Optic Nerve Meningioma

1. Meningioma, sarcoid, lymphoma, metastatic disease, and pseudotumor may result in this "tram-track" enhancement pattern of the optic nerve sheath (enhancing sheath around a filling defect that represents the optic nerve).

2. Pneumosinus dilatans is characterized by expansion of a paranasal sinus that contains only air. Pneumosinus dilatans involving the sphenoid sinus has been associated with optic nerve meningiomas.

3. The tuberculum sellae or planum sphenoidale.

4. Vision loss.

Reference

Jackson A, Patankar T, Laitt RD: Intracanalicular optic nerve meningioma: a serious diagnostic pitfall, *Am J Neuroradiol* 24:1167–1170, 2003.

Cross-Reference

Neuroradiology: THE REQUISITES, 2nd ed, pp 496–497.

Comment

Optic nerve sheath meningiomas typically present first with vision loss. If the lesion goes undetected or misdiagnosed and enlarges, it may present later with proptosis and optic atrophy. These tumors most commonly present in middle-aged women; however, they may also be present in children with neurofibromatosis in whom they are also frequently bilateral. Bilateral orbital meningiomas also may rarely occur when they arise from the tuberculum sellae or planum sphenoidale. In this situation, meningiomas normally grow anteriorly along the optic nerves, from the optic canal into the orbit. In every patient with suspected optic meningioma, it is important to assess both eyes and the region of the tuberculum sellae on imaging.

On imaging, "tram-tracking" is the term that has been used to describe both the pattern of enhancement and the pattern of calcification. On CT, 20% to 50% of optic nerve meningiomas have calcification along the nerve sheath. Linear enhancement may be seen on both sides of the optic nerve. Other findings to assess on CT include secondary bony changes (erosion or hyperostosis) of the optic canal, sphenoid sinus, and planum sphenoidale. There may be enlargement of the optic canal. A major advantage of MR imaging is its ability to evaluate the optic nerve separately from the surrounding nerve sheath. This is extremely helpful in differentiating lesions arising from the optic nerve itself (optic neuritis, gliomas) from those arising from the nerve sheath (meningiomas, metastases, and granulomatosis disorders). In addition, because of artifact arising from the bones, MR imaging is better than CT in evaluating the nerve within the optic canal as well as spread into the intracranial compartment. When performing orbital MR imaging, it is important to use fat suppression so that the full extent of the tumor around the optic nerve can be assessed. Limitations of MR imaging include its inability to detect small calcifications and artifacts (chemical shift or susceptibility from the aerated paranasal sinuses) in the orbit that may obscure small lesions.

Notes

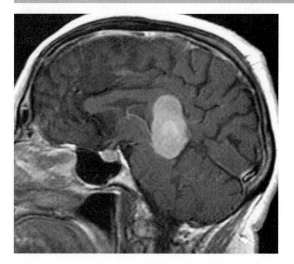

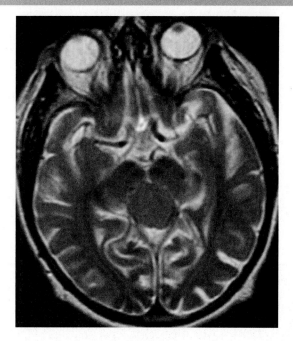

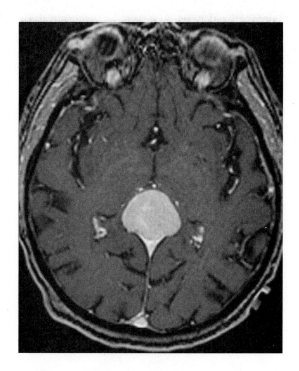

1. What vascular structures course above the pineal gland?

2. Pineal neoplasms arise from what two cells of origin?

3. Which pineal neoplasm is most frequently associated with tumor seeding of the subarachnoid spaces?

4. What are the two most common neoplasms in the peripineal region in adults?

Peripineal Meningioma

1. The internal cerebral veins and vein of Galen.

2. Tumors of germ cell origin and tumors arising from pineal cells.

3. Pineoblastoma. When large enough, pineoblastomas may directly invade the brain parenchyma.

4. Meningioma and primary glioma.

References

Nakamura M, Saeki N, Iwadate Y, Sunami K, Osato K, Ymaura A: Neuroradiological characteristics of pineocytoma and pineoblastoma, *Neuroradiology* 42:509–514, 2000.

Smirniotopoulos JG, Rushing EJ, Mena H: Pineal region masses: differential diagnosis, *RadioGraphics* 12:577–596, 1992.

Cross-Reference

Neuroradiology: THE REQUISITES, 2nd ed, p 160.

Comment

This case shows a well-demarcated, avidly enhancing cellular mass in the peripineal region. There is elevation of the internal cerebral veins and splenium of the corpus callosum, and compression of the tectal plate. There is no acute hydrocephalus. On T2W imaging, the mass is isointense to gray matter because of its dense cellularity.

Tumors of pineal cell origin (pineoblastoma and pineocytoma) account for only 15% of pineal region masses. Unlike germ cell tumors, which show a marked predilection for boys and men, tumors of pineal cell origin occur equally among men and women. Tumors of pineal origin frequently calcify. Calcification of the pineal gland in a child younger than 7 years of age should raise suspicion of tumor until proven otherwise. After 7 years of age, the pineal gland begins to show calcification, which increases with age. Up to 10% of people have calcification in the pineal gland by adolescence, and up to 50% have pineal gland calcification by the age of 30 years. In cases in which the calcification is small and more central, it may be difficult to determine whether it is the natural calcification of the pineal gland or calcification within the tumor matrix.

Magnetic resonance imaging is most useful in characterizing masses in the pineal region. Tumors arising in the peripineal region in a child are usually gliomas arising from the tectal plate, whereas tumors arising in the peripineal region in adults may represent gliomas or meningiomas arising from the tentorium, as in this case. Imaging findings and the patient's age and sex together may be useful in suggesting the correct histologic features of the tumor. Pineal tumors of germ cell origin occur in children, as do pineoblastomas, whereas pineocytomas generally are seen in adults.

Notes

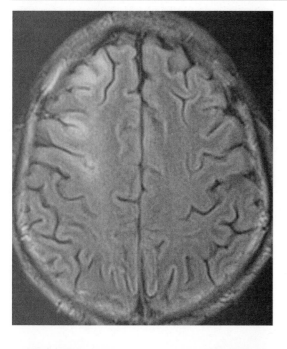
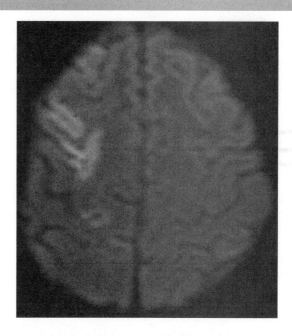
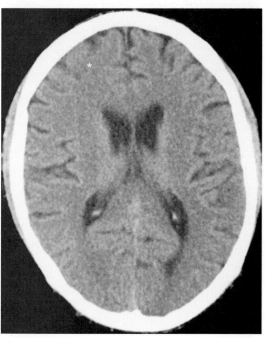
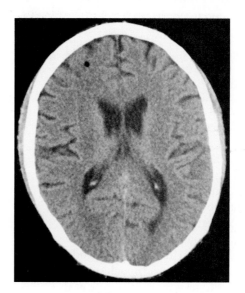

1. What does the * represent?

2. What is the diagnosis?

3. What are the signs and symptoms of this entity?

4. What are the direct complications related to central venous catheters?

Air Embolism with Acute Right Cerebral Infarct

1. Intracranial air.

2. Cerebral infarction due to air embolus.

3. Signs and symptoms of air embolism include cyanosis, respiratory distress, hypotension, gasp reflex, cardiac arrhythmias, elevated central venous pressure, elevated pulmonary artery pressure, loss of consciousness, and neurologic deficits.

4. Air embolism, catheter dislodgement, infection, and thrombus formation.

References

Hiraki T, Fujiwara H, Sakurai, et al: Nonfatal systemic air embolism complicating percutaneous CT-guided transthoracic needle biopsy, *Chest* 132:684–690, 2007.

Peter DA, Saxman C: Preventing air embolism when removing CVCs: an evidence-based approach to changing practice, *Medsurg Nurs* 12:223–228, 2003.

Cross-Reference

Neuroradiology: THE REQUISITES, 2nd ed, pp 174–175, 263–264, 286–287.

Comment

Cerebral air embolism is a known complication of trauma, surgical procedures, and central line catheterization. Cerebral and cardiac air emboli are also a known complication of thoracic instrumentation, initially reported many years ago during pneumothorax therapy and pleurodesis for the treatment of tuberculosis. More recently, it has been associated with CT-guided percutaneous needle biopsy for pulmonary tumors. The mechanism by which air emboli occur in this scenario includes both the presence of a fistula between a bronchus and a pulmonary vein and a transthoracic pressure gradient in which intrathoracic pressure is lower than atmospheric pressure, as when coughing or taking a deep breath, that allows air to flow into a pulmonary vein from the bronchus. From there, air may enter the systemic circulation.

Venous air embolism is an underrecognized, potentially fatal, but preventable complication of central lines. It can result in cardiovascular, pulmonary, and CNS infarcts and dysfunction. Cerebral air embolism may result from a paradoxical intracardiac shunt (patent foramen ovale) or intrapulmonary right-to-left shunt. Insertion, accidental disconnection, or removal of a central venous catheter may result in cerebral air embolism, as it did in this patient. Cerebral air emboli usually occur on the right side because air preferentially flows into the first branch of the aortic arch, the brachiocephalic artery.

When a cerebral air embolism is suspected, the patient's head should be quickly lowered (Trendelenburg position), and the patient should be turned to the left lateral decubitus position to trap air in the apex of the ventricle and prevent further ejection into the pulmonary arterial system. Oxygen should be administered. Of course, the best treatment is prevention. Central lines should be removed with the patient in the Trendelenburg position. An occlusive dressing should be applied.

Notes

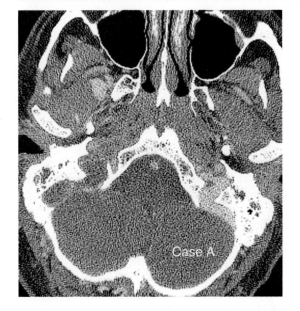

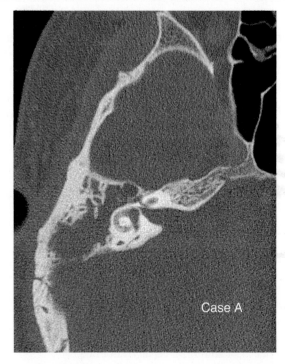

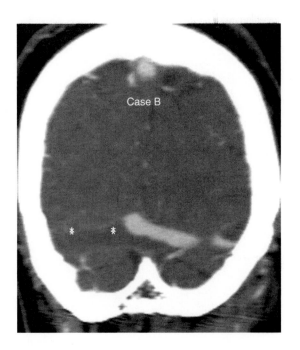

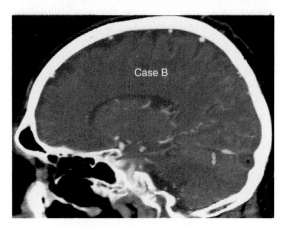

1. What is the diagnosis in these two patients?

2. What systemic disorders are associated with this condition?

3. What is the cause of this condition in Case A

4. What is the most serious complication associated with venous thrombosis?

Venous Sinus Thrombosis Complicating Otomastoiditis

1. Sinus thrombosis of the right sigmoid and distal transverse sinuses in Case A, and thrombosis of the right transverse sinus in Case B. In Case B, the filling defect in the sinus is shown (*).

2. Dehydration, hypercoagulable states (deficiency of antithrombin-III, protein C or S, nephrotic syndrome, use of oral contraceptives, antiphospholipid antibodies, homocystinuria, L-asparaginase), underlying malignancy, pregnancy, and infection (meningitis).

3. Coalescent mastoiditis.

4. Hemorrhagic venous infarction.

References

Rodallec MH, Krainik A, Feydy A, et al: Cerebral venous thrombosis and multidetector CT angiography: tips and tricks, *RadioGraphics* 26:S5–S18, 2006.

Stolz E, Trittmacher S, Rahimi A, et al: Influence of recanalization on outcome in dural sinus thrombosis: a prospective study, *Stroke* 35:544–547, 2004.

Cross-Reference

Neuroradiology: THE REQUISITES, 2nd ed, pp 217, 219–220.

Comment

Dural sinus thrombosis and venous infarction are commonly underdiagnosed because of lack of consideration of these entities. Sinus thrombosis has a spectrum of clinical presentations, including headache and papilledema related to increased intracranial pressure, as well as focal neurologic deficits and seizures in cases complicated by intraparenchymal hemorrhage or venous infarction. Venous thrombosis is associated with a variety of underlying systemic disorders, as discussed earlier. In the differential diagnosis of intracerebral hemorrhage in the absence of known risk factors (eg, trauma, hypertension), the presence of bilateral or subcortical hemorrhages that are not in arterial vascular distributions should raise suspicion for sinus thrombosis complicated by venous infarction.

Diagnosing venous thrombosis has become easier with noninvasive techniques, especially with advanced MR imaging sequences and CT venography (CTV) performed using multidetector CT. On CTV, thrombosis is readily identified as filling defects in the affected venous sinuses. I prefer CTV to MR imaging, which is an excellent technique, but requires more experience and an understanding of some physics. In the setting of acute thrombosis, deoxyhemoglobin is hypointense on T2W imaging and may be mistaken for normal blood flow. In the acute setting, flow-sensitive gradient echo imaging may distinguish normal blood flow, which is of high signal intensity, from acute thrombosis, which is hypointense because of lack of flow. In subacute thrombosis, methemoglobin within the clot appears hyperintense on both T1W and T2W images. Flow-sensitive time-of-flight gradient echo images often are not helpful because both the methemoglobin in the thrombus and blood flow are hyperintense. In this situation, phase-contrast MR angiography is helpful because it provides suppression of high signal from the hemorrhage such that only flow is shown on these images.

Notes

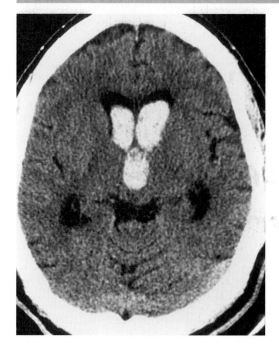 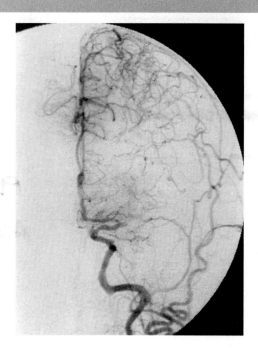

1. What are the major imaging findings?

2. What is the major risk factor for intraventricular hemorrhage related to germinal matrix bleeds in newborns?

3. What aneurysm may present with fourth ventricular hemorrhage?

4. In adults, what are the most common clinical presentations of moyamoya?

Intraventricular Hemorrhage

1. Diffuse intraventricular hemorrhage with acute hydrocephalus.

2. Prematurity or low birth weight.

3. Rupture of a posterior inferior cerebellar artery aneurysm.

4. Acute intracranial hemorrhage and stroke.

References

Blankenberg FG, Loh NN, Bracci P, et al: Sonography, CT, and MR imaging: a prospective comparison of neonates with suspected intracranial ischemia and hemorrhage, *AJNR Am J Neuroradiol* 21:213–218, 2000.

Gentry LR, Thompson B, Godersky JC: Trauma to the corpus callosum: MR features, *AJNR Am J Neuroradiol* 9:1129–1138, 1988.

Cross-Reference

Neuroradiology: THE REQUISITES, 2nd ed, pp 254–258.

Comment

This case shows an intraventricular blood clot with thrombus casting the lateral, third, and fourth ventricles. There is secondary acute hydrocephalus. Intraventricular hemorrhage is common in the setting of closed head injury, occurring in 2% to 40% of patients, depending on the severity of injury. Traumatic intraventricular hemorrhage is most commonly associated with diffuse axonal injury, particularly of the corpus callosum, and may also be seen with injury to the septum pellucidum due to tearing of small subependymal veins.

Nontraumatic causes of intraventricular hemorrhage include rupture of large parenchymal hematomas, as is seen with hypertension or amyloid angiopathy in the elderly. In patients with intraventricular hemorrhage, in the absence of other findings to suggest a cause, vascular abnormalities, such as choroidal arteriovenous malformations must be excluded, and CT angiography, MR imaging or MR angiography or conventional angiography is usually indicated for further evaluation. Ruptured aneurysms of the posterior inferior cerebellar artery may also present with intraventricular hemorrhage, although the hemorrhage is usually located preferentially in the fourth ventricle. Isolated intraventricular hemorrhage in the absence of a parenchymal bleed is unusual. In this case, angiography shows chronic occlusion of the proximal left middle cerebral artery, narrowing of the supraclinoid internal carotid artery with enlarged lenticulostriate collaterals, and filling of some distal middle cerebral artery branches through meningeal collaterals. This patient presented with hypertension (220/110 mm Hg), and it is presumed that the intraventricular hemorrhage is related to hypertension complicating moyamoya disease.

Notes

PICA   4th vent

Acomm lat

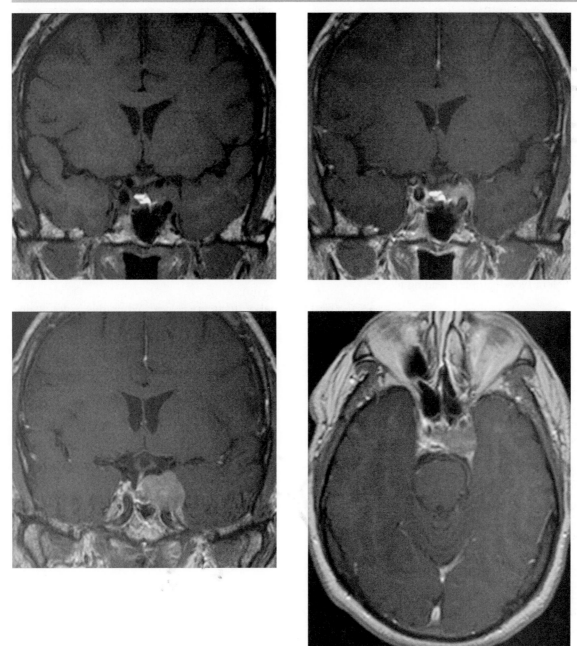

1. What anatomic area is this mass primarily involving?

2. What was the clinical presentation of this patient?

3. What is the differential diagnosis?

4. What is pituitary apoplexy?

Pituitary Macroadenoma Invading the Left Cavernous Sinus

1. The left cavernous sinus.

2. Third and sixth cranial neuropathies caused by invasion of the left cavernous sinus.

3. Pituitary macroadenoma, meningioma, schwannoma, lymphoma, and metastasis.

4. Pituitary apoplexy results from infarction or sudden hemorrhage within the pituitary, more often in macroadenomas. This presents as a medical emergency, with headache, sudden collapse, and shock. Administration of stimulatory agents such as thyroid-stimulating hormone or gonadotropin-releasing hormone have been postulated to lead to increased metabolic needs by the macroadenoma (which has deficient blood supply), leading to necrosis.

References

Riedl M, Clodi M, Kotzmann H, et al: Apoplexy of a pituitary macroadenoma with reversible third, fourth, and sixth cranial nerve palsies following administration of hypothalamic releasing hormones: MR features, *Eur J Radiol* 36:1–4, 2000.

Scotti G, Yu CY, Dillon WP, et al: MR imaging of cavernous sinus involvement by pituitary adenomas, *AJR Am J Roentgenol* 151:799–806, 1988.

Cross-Reference

Neuroradiology: THE REQUISITES, 2nd ed, p 534.

Comment

Approximately 75% of pituitary adenomas present as a result of endocrine dysfunction. Macroadenomas often present with compressive signs and symptoms related to mass effect. These include headache, visual symptoms (characteristically bitemporal hemianopsia), increased intracranial pressure, and cranial nerve palsies, as in this case. The challenging part of this case is determining where the mass arises because this case illustrates predominantly lateral growth into the cavernous sinus of a macroadenoma, with a small portion in the left lateral sella and mild deviation of the pituitary stalk from left to right. Pituitary macroadenomas may encase the cavernous internal carotid artery, but unlike meningiomas, they usually do not result in significant narrowing. In a study examining cavernous sinus involvement by pituitary adenomas, Scotti and colleagues found that invasion was unilateral in all cases and most commonly occurred with prolactin or adrenocorticotropic hormone–secreting adenomas located laterally in the gland. The most specific

sign of cavernous sinus invasion was encasement of the carotid artery.

Pituitary adenomas arise from epithelial pituitary cells and account for 10% to 15% of all intracranial tumors. Tumors larger than 10 mm are defined as macroadenomas, and those smaller than 10 mm are considered microadenomas. Most pituitary adenomas are microadenomas. The exact pathophysiology leading to the development of pituitary adenomas is unknown. Some pituitary tumors may occur as part of a clinical syndrome. In multiple endocrine neoplasia type I, an autosomal dominant genetic disorder, pituitary adenomas (most often prolactinomas) occur in association with tumors of the parathyroid and pancreatic islet cells. In McCune-Albright syndrome, skin lesions and polyostotic fibrous dysplasia occur with hyperfunctioning endocrinopathies (most commonly somatotropinomas resulting in acromegaly).

The goal of treatment is cure. When this is not attainable, reducing tumor size, restoring hormone function, and restoring normal vision are attempted using drug therapy, surgery, and radiation therapy. Macroadenomas often require surgical intervention; however, macroprolactinomas frequently have an excellent response to medical therapy.

Notes

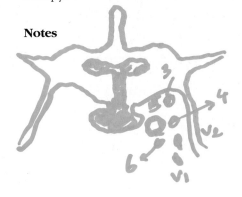

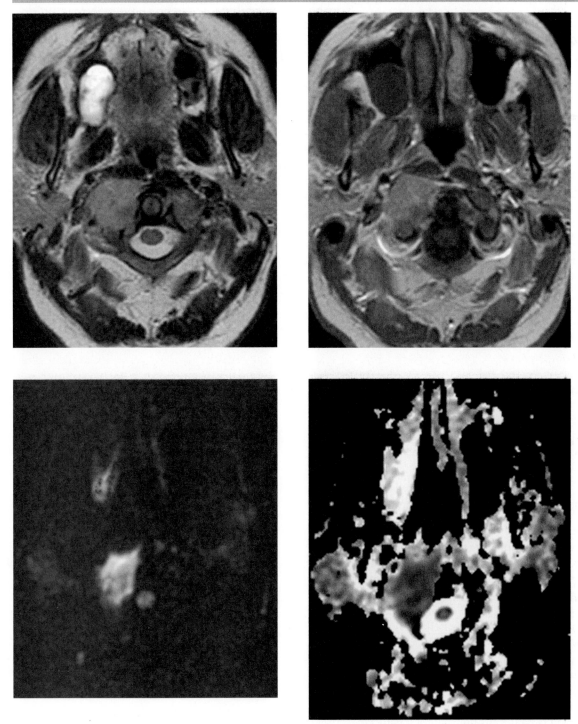

1. What structures attach the dens of vertebra C2 to the occipital condyles?

2. Extension of skull base disease into the hypoglossal canal may result in what cranial nerve palsy?

3. What is the mechanism of injury in occipital condyle fractures?

4. What type of lymphoma is most commonly associated with blastic metastases?

Lymphoma of the Occipital Condyle and C1

1. Right and left alar ligaments arise from the odontoid process of C2 and attach to their respective occipital condyles.

2. Cranial nerve XII palsy, including tongue fasciculations, deviation, and weakness.

3. Axial loading injury with associated ipsilateral flexion.

4. Hodgkin disease is more commonly associated with blastic metastases compared with non-Hodgkin's subtypes.

References

Loevner LA, Yousem DM: Overlooked metastatic lesions of the occipital condyle: a missed case treasure trove, *RadioGraphics* 17:1111–1121, 1997.

Pavithran K, Doval DC, Hukku S, Jena A: Isolated hypoglossal nerve palsy due to skull base metastasis, *Australas Radiol* 45:534–535, 2001.

Cross-Reference

Neuroradiology: THE REQUISITES, 2nd ed, p 560.

Comment

In children, abnormalities of the craniovertebral junction may be congenital (Chiari malformations) or acquired (traumatic, inflammatory, neoplastic). In adults, acquired craniovertebral and occipital condyle lesions may result from trauma (fractures due to axial loading with ipsilateral flexion), inflammatory disorders (such as rheumatoid arthritis), and metabolic disorders (such as Paget's disease and hyperparathyroidism), and may result in basilar invagination. In my experience, primary hematologic malignancies and metastatic disease to the craniovertebral junction, and more specifically, the occipital condyles, are not uncommon and probably are often overlooked. In addition to prostate, breast, and lung carcinoma, primary malignancies affecting the gastrointestinal tract may metastasize to the condyles. Spread is most likely hematogenous.

The occipital condyles and pathology affecting them are often overlooked because it is unusual for a clinician to specifically request evaluation of these structures and because they are frequently seen only at the edge of films (the inferior sections of an axial brain MR imaging or CT scan and the lateral sections of a sagittal MR imaging scan).

Most patients present with occipital headaches or neck pain, as was the case with this patient, which may be associated with cranial neuropathies related to extension of tumor into the hypoglossal canal (resulting in tongue weakness or fasciculations) or jugular foramen (resulting in neuropathies of cranial nerves IX through XI). Secondary thrombosis of the sigmoid and transverse sinuses may also be present. Sagittal and axial unenhanced T1W images are most useful in identifying abnormalities of the craniovertebral junction and condyles because the hyperintense fat within the marrow is an excellent intrinsic "contrast agent" and replacement of this fat with abnormal hypointense tissue is easily seen. In this case, the right inferior occipital condyle and the lateral mass of C1 are replaced by a very cellular tumor. Lesions are less conspicuous on T2W and enhanced T1W images without fat saturation. The axial diffusion-weighted image shows restricted diffusion, with marked hypointensity on the corresponding apparent diffusion coefficient map, consistent with cellularity and highly suggestive of lymphoma.

Notes

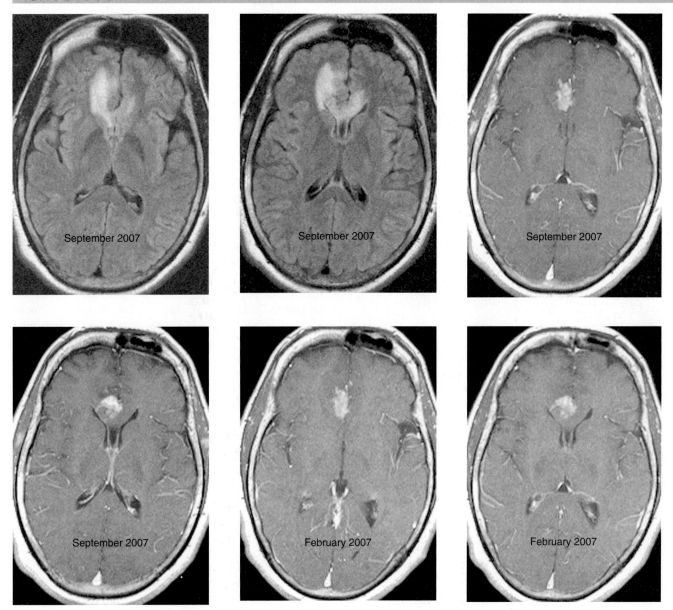

September 2007

September 2007

September 2007

September 2007

February 2007

February 2007

1. What neoplasms typically affect the corpus callosum?

2. What findings may be present in the CSF in CNS sarcoidosis?

3. What is the characteristic enhancement pattern of primary CNS lymphoma?

4. What is the characteristic pathologic finding in sarcoidosis?

Central Nervous System Sarcoidosis

1. Primary glial neoplasms and lymphoma. Other tumors, such as metastatic disease, occur in the corpus callosum, but are relatively rare.

2. CSF findings are nonspecific for sarcoidosis, but include elevated protein levels, increased cell counts (predominantly lymphocytes), and decreased glucose levels.

3. Solid enhancement. However, in immunocompromised patients, a spectrum of enhancement patterns may occur, including only peripheral enhancement. This is because such patients may not be able to mount the inflammatory reaction that impairs the integrity of the blood–brain barrier to allow contrast in.

4. Sarcoidosis is a systemic disorder characterized pathologically by noncaseating granulomas.

References

Dumas JL, Valeyre D, Chapelon-Abric C, et al: Central nervous system sarcoidosis: follow-up at MR imaging during steroid therapy, *Radiology* 214:411–420, 2000.

Smith JK, Matheus MG, Castillo M: Imaging manifestations of neurosarcoidosis, *AJR Am J Roentgenol* 182: 289–295, 2004.

Cross-Reference

Neuroradiology: THE REQUISITES, 2nd ed, pp 198, 320–322, 541–542.

Comment

This case is an example of CNS sarcoid with leptomeningeal disease and secondary parenchymal extension. There is FLAIR hyperintensity in the anterior genu of the corpus callosum, with contiguous FLAIR signal abnormality in the right greater than left frontal lobes. There is solid, ill-defined enhancing tissue along the medial right frontal lobe. On initial inspection, the clinician might suspect a high-grade primary glial neoplasm or lymphoma as the etiology of these findings. However, on close inspection of the images, the pattern of enhancement is seen to be that of primary leptomeningeal disease, with secondary extension into the brain parenchyma. There is encasement of cerebral veins along the surface of the medial right frontal lobe by the enhancing tissue. In addition, two enhanced images are shown from a previous examination. There is essentially no significant change between the findings on the two examinations separated in time by 9 months. A high-grade glial neoplasm or lymphoma would almost certainly have shown a change between studies. Patients with CNS sarcoid are managed with steroid therapy. Response patterns over 1- to 2-year follow-up intervals show a spectrum of MR imaging findings ranging from regression to progression, including stable disease without significant imaging changes, as in this case.

Multiple patterns of CNS involvement in sarcoidosis have been described. The most common of these is chronic meningitis with a predilection for the leptomeninges of the basal cisterns. These patients may present with chronic meningeal symptoms, cranial neuropathies (especially involving the facial and optic nerves), or symptoms related to involvement of the hypothalamus and pituitary stalk. Imaging findings are best demonstrated with MR and include thick, nodular enhancement of the involved leptomeninges. There may be enhancing tissue around the hypothalamus and pituitary stalk. Parenchymal brain involvement with regions of abnormality may occur as a result of direct extension from leptomeningeal disease (as in this case) or disease along the Virchow-Robin spaces, or less commonly, there may be granulomas in the brain. White matter lesions mimicking multiple sclerosis may be present because of disease extension along the perivascular spaces or related to sarcoid-induced small vessel vasculitis. Less commonly, dural-based disease may be the predominant imaging finding and may be mistaken for a meningioma.

Notes

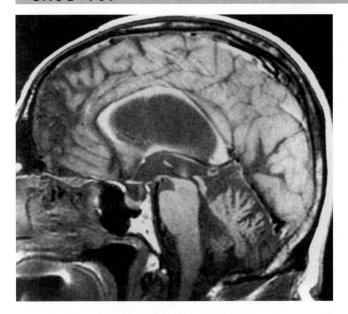

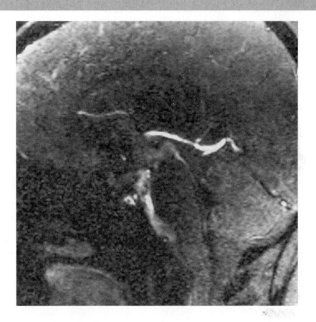

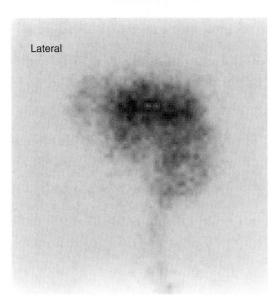

Lateral

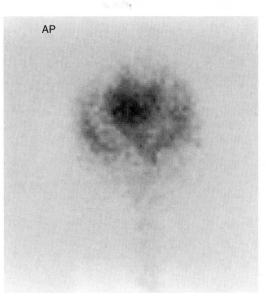

AP

1. What is the diagnosis?

2. What clinical triad may be present in this elderly patient?

3. In normal pressure hydrocephalus (NPH), what are the imaging findings on a positive isotope (indium-DTPA) cisternogram?

4. Who gets external hydrocephalus, and what are the radiologic findings?

Normal Pressure Hydrocephalus

1. Communicating hydrocephalus.

2. Gait disturbance, urinary incontinence, and dementia.

3. Reflux of isotope into the ventricular system and, to a lesser extent, the sylvian cisterns, and no ascent of the radiotracer over the cerebral convexities at 24 hours.

4. Typically, it is seen in children younger than 2 years of age and results from decreased resorption of CSF at the arachnoid villi. Imaging typically shows enlargement of the cerebral sulci (especially in the frontal region and along the interhemispheric fissure). In contrast to NPH and other types of communicating hydrocephalus, the ventricles are relatively normal in size; this may be because the cranial sutures are still open (instead there may be mild enlargement of the head circumference in external hydrocephalus).

References

Fishman RA, Dillon WP: Normal pressure hydrocephalus: new findings and old questions, *Am J Neuroradiol* 22:1640–1641, 2001.

Tullerg M, Jensen C, Ekholm S, Wikkelso C: Normal pressure hydrocephalus: vascular white matter changes on MR images must not exclude patients from surgery, *Am J Neuroradiol* 22:1665–1673, 2001.

Cross-Reference

Neuroradiology: THE REQUISITES, 2nd ed, pp 375–377.

Comment

Normal pressure hydrocephalus, a form of communicating hydrocephalus, is characterized by normal mean CSF pressure. In NPH, the lateral and third ventricles are enlarged in comparison with the fourth ventricle. Distention of the lateral ventricles may result in thinning and elevation of the corpus callosum, whereas enlargement of the third ventricle may result in dilation of the infundibular and optic recesses, which may be displaced inferiorly. Patients typically have accentuation of the flow void in the aqueduct of Sylvius on spin-echo images, and CSF flow in the aqueduct may be seen on flow-sensitive gradient echo imaging, as in this case. Transependymal CSF spread may be present, or NPH may have an MR imaging presentation of a more chronic, compensated communicating hydrocephalus.

Although the cause of NPH is still debated, it is believed to result most often from remote intracranial hemorrhage or meningeal infection. Some investigators have suggested that ischemic injury or edema in the periventricular white matter reduces the tensile strength of the ventricles, resulting in their enlargement. Some patients with NPH have marked improvement of their symptoms after shunting. Response to shunting is most favorable when ataxia is the predominant symptom, the patient has had symptoms for only a short time, findings on isotope cisternography are positive, the patient has a known history of intracranial hemorrhage or infection, MR imaging shows a prominent CSF flow void in the aqueduct, and there is relative absence of deep periventricular white matter atrophy. Lumbar puncture with removal of 15 mL or more of CSF and subsequent improvement of clinical symptoms may also indicate a patient who may have a favorable response to shunting.

There are no MR imaging findings that have been reliably shown to predict the outcome of shunt surgery in patients with NPH. It is unclear if the presence of foci of high signal intensity in the deep and subcortical white matter (small vessel ischemic disease) in patients with NPH can predict a lesser outcome from shunt surgery; however, when there is associated significant white matter volume loss, long-term outcomes may be diminished. Care must be used to separate foci of high signal intensity related to small vessel ischemic disease from irregular hyperintensity around the frontal and occipital horns that may be attributable to transependymal flow of CSF. The major diagnostic challenge is to differentiate NPH from cerebral atrophy and deep white matter ischemia, both far more common causes of the clinical triad than NPH. The decision to perform shunt surgery should be based largely on clinical findings and MR imaging studies that indicate that brain atrophy is not responsible for the ventriculomegaly.

Notes

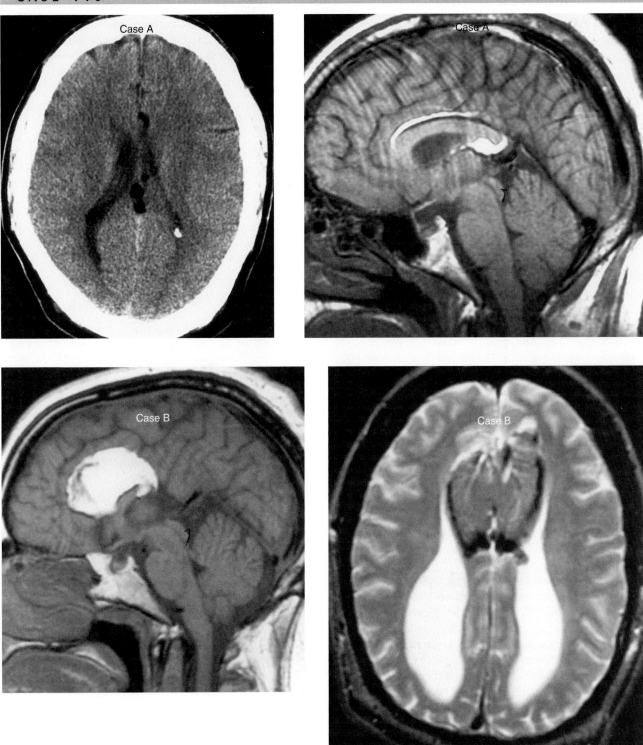

Case A

Case A

Case B

Case B

1. These lesions are believed to develop from what embryologic structure?

2. What structures may be responsible for the presence of signal voids in these masses?

3. It is possible to confirm that an intracranial mass is composed of fat by identifying what other MR imaging finding?

4. Underdevelopment of what structure may occur with lipomas in the quadrigeminal cistern?

Lipomas Associated with the Corpus Callosum

1. They are believed to arise from abnormal differentiation of the embryologic meninx primitiva (a mesodermal derivative of the neural crest).

2. Vessels or calcifications.

3. Chemical shift artifact on T2W images (which results in hypointensity at the periphery of the lesion along the frequency encoded axis, although the contralateral edge is hyperintense). Another approach is to perform a quick fat-suppressed T1W sequence, such as fast multiplanar spoiled gradient echo, to assess for loss of signal with application of fat suppression.

4. The inferior colliculus.

References

Demaerel P, Van de Gaer P, Wilms G, et al: Interhemispheric lipoma with variable callosal dysgenesis: relationship between embryology, morphology, and symptomatology, *Eur Radiol* 6:904–909, 1996.

Utsunomiya H, Ogasawara T, Hayashi T, Hashimoto T, Okazaki M: Dysgenesis of the corpus callosum and associated telencephalic anomalies: MRI, *Neuroradiology* 39:302–310, 1997.

Cross-Reference

Neuroradiology: THE REQUISITES, 2nd ed, pp 424–425.

Comment

A widely accepted theory for the development of intracranial lipomas is that they arise from abnormal differentiation of embryologic meninx primitiva (a mesodermal derivative of the neural crest). The meninx primitiva encases the CNS, and its inner lining is resorbed to allow formation of the subarachnoid spaces. Intracranial lipomas are not neoplasms, but rather disorders of the development of subarachnoid spaces. Because lipomas are believed to develop from the inner layer of the meninx primitiva that forms the subarachnoid space, pericallosal arteries in interhemispheric lipomas and cranial nerves in cerebellopontine angle lipomas, respectively, often course through the lesions.

Intracranial lipomas most often occur in the interhemispheric fissure (up to 50%), followed by the quadrigeminal cistern (25%), the suprasellar cistern (15%), and the cerebellopontine cistern (10%). They are frequently associated with underdevelopment or dysgenesis of adjacent brain tissue. Lipomas along the posterior corpus callosum, especially the splenium (Case A), are "ribbon-like" in appearance. In these cases, the corpus callosum is relatively normally developed. Lipomas along the anterior corpus callosum within the interhemispheric fissure (Case B) are often "tumefactive" (mass-like in configuration) and are associated with partial agenesis of the corpus callosum. Lipomas in the quadrigeminal cistern may be associated with underdevelopment of the inferior colliculus.

Notes

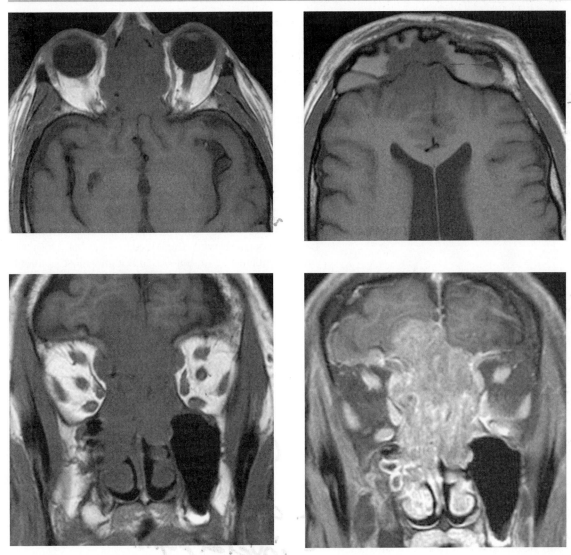

1. What determines the signal characteristics of secretions in the paranasal sinuses?

2. What is a nasal glioma?

3. What is the risk of malignant transformation of an inverting papilloma into squamous cell carcinoma?

4. What is the most common histology of maxillary sinus malignancies?

Sinonasal Undifferentiated Carcinoma with Intracranial Extension

1. Free water content, protein concentration, viscosity, and cross-linking of glycoproteins.

2. The term nasal glioma is a misnomer in that it is benign mass composed of heterotopic glial tissue. Unlike meningoceles (encephaloceles), nasal gliomas do not have CSF spaces that communicate with the intracranial subarachnoid spaces. In 15% of cases, nasal gliomas are connected to the intracranial compartment via fibrous or glial bands.

3. Approximately 5% to 10%.

4. Squamous cell carcinoma.

References

Eisen MD, Yousem DM, Loevner LA, et al: Preoperative imaging to predict orbital invasion by tumor, *Head Neck* 22:456–462, 2000.

Loevner LA, Sonners A: Imaging of neoplasms of the paranasal sinuses, *Neuroimaging Clin N Am* 14:625–646, 2004.

Cross-Reference

Neuroradiology: THE REQUISITES, 2nd ed, pp 634–635.

Comment

This case shows a large, aggressive mass in the bilateral sinonasal cavity involving the nasal vault and ethmoid air cells, with extension into the frontal sinus. There is extension into the anterior cranial fossa through the cribriform plate, with elevation of the frontal lobes (T2W images [not shown] showed no edema in the frontal lobes). There is lateral bowing of the bilateral lamina papyracea, with findings highly suggestive of invasion of the periorbita. On the second unenhanced axial T1W image, the hyperintense material filling the frontal sinus is proteinaceous, inspissated secretions, whereas the central material isointense to muscle in the frontal sinus is neoplasm.

Malignant tumors of the sinonasal tract are rare, accounting for 3% of head and neck cancers. The majority arise in the maxillary sinus, approximately 20% arise in the ethmoid sinuses, and the remainder (<1%) originate in the frontal and sphenoid sinuses. Squamous cell carcinoma is the most common histologic type. Nickel and chrome refining processes have been implicated in the development of all types of malignancy of the paranasal sinuses, and exposure to wood dust has been associated specifically with adenocarcinoma of the ethmoid. Up to a fivefold increased risk of sinonasal carcinoma has been observed with heavy smoking. Clinical presentation of sinus malignancies is nonspecific and often mimics benign disease. Approximately 10% of patients are asymptomatic. Delay in diagnosis is common. Up to 75% of all paranasal sinus tumors are stage T3 or T4 at the time of diagnosis. Resectability and treatment are determined by the presence of orbital invasion, intracranial spread, dural invasion, and perineural spread.

Sinonasal undifferentiated carcinoma is a rare cancer of the nasal cavity or paranasal sinuses. Initial symptoms range from bloody nose, runny nose, double vision, and bulging eye to chronic infections and nasal obstruction. It has been associated with papillomas in the nasal cavity, which are benign, but can undergo malignant degeneration. A history of radiation therapy for other cancers has been associated with the development of sinonasal undifferentiated carcinoma, although most patients have not had previous radiation therapy.

Notes

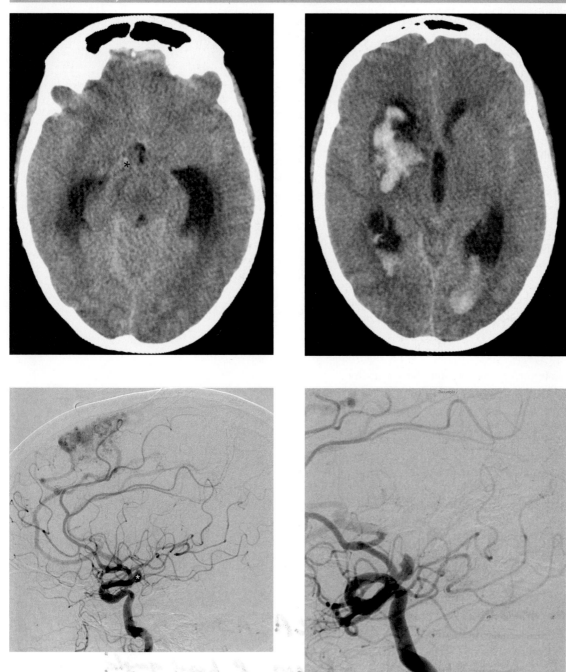

1. What are the major imaging findings on CT?

2. What does the hypodensity in the periventricular white matter represent?

3. What is the best diagnosis (etiology) for the CT imaging findings?

4. What other incidental finding is seen on the angiogram?

Intracerebral Rupture of a Posterior Communicating Artery Aneurysm

1. Acute hemorrhage in the right basal ganglia, acute subarachnoid hemorrhage, acute intraventricular hemorrhage, and acute hydrocephalus.

2. Transependymal flow of CSF in the setting of acute hydrocephalus.

3. Rupture of a right posterior communicating artery aneurysm (*).

4. An arteriovenous malformation in the frontal lobe.

Reference

Abbed KM, Ogilvy CS: Intracerebral hematoma from aneurysm rupture, *Neurosurgery* 15:1–5, 2003.

Cross-Reference

Neuroradiology: THE REQUISITES, 2nd ed, pp 225–230.

Comment

Saccular aneurysms frequently rupture into the subarachnoid space, accounting for 70% to 80% of spontaneous subarachnoid hemorrhages. Aneurysmal rupture also may result in intraparenchymal, intraventricular, or subdural hemorrhage. Patients who present with cerebral hemorrhage associated with aneurysm rupture may require acute hematoma evacuation in addition to obliteration of the aneurysm. Although most ruptured aneurysms present with acute subarachnoid hemorrhage, associated parenchymal hemorrhage is not uncommon. The presence of an intraparenchymal hemorrhage has a negative effect on clinical presentation, patient course, and outcome. The incidence of intracerebral hematoma associated with acute subarachnoid hemorrhage on initial head CT ranges from 4% to 20%. The most commonly ruptured aneurysms associated with acute intracerebral hematoma are the middle cerebral artery, followed by aneurysms of the anterior communicating artery. In this case, an acutely ruptured posterior communicating aneurysm (*) was responsible for the right basal ganglionic hematoma.

Management of patients with acute parenchymal hematomas in association with subarachnoid hemorrhage from aneurysm rupture has been controversial. Based on available evidence in the literature, patients with aneurysmal subarachnoid hemorrhage, a large cerebral hematoma, and a poor clinical grade at presentation have a poor outcome, regardless of therapy. The controversy is mainly as to whether, when, and how (craniotomy or burr hole) to evacuate the hematoma. Studies have shown that in patients in whom the hematomas have been evacuated mortality rates are lower if the aneurysm is clipped at the same time (during the same operation) as the evacuation.

Notes

MCA – Acom
Pcom R basal ganglia

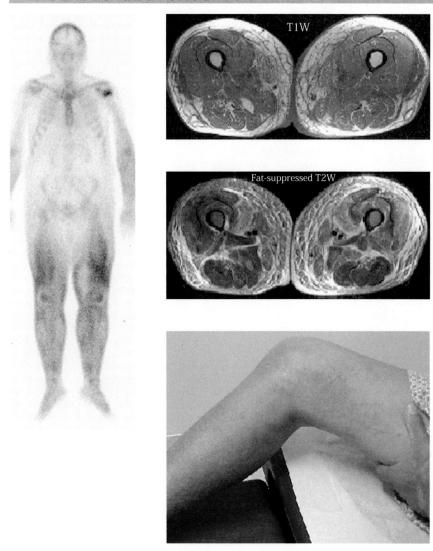

1. What organ system does nephrogenic systemic sclerosis primarily affect?

2. What systemic condition does nephrogenic systemic fibrosis mimic?

3. What are the early symptoms and signs of this condition?

4. What are the late symptoms and signs of this condition?

Figures in Cases 113 and 114 courtesy of Dale Broome.

C A S E   1 1 3

Gadolinium-Associated Nephrogenic Systemic Fibrosis—Part I

1. It primarily affects the skin, but may affect other organs.

2. Scleroderma.

3. Extremity edema and swelling, arthralgias, myalgias, and weakness.

4. Extremity contractures, myopathy, and weakness.

Reference

Broome DR, Girguis MS, Baron PW, Cottrell AC, Kjellin I, Kirk GA: Gadodiamide-associated nephrogenic systemic fibrosis: why radiologists should be concerned, *Am J Roentgenol* 188:586–592, 2007.

Cross-Reference

Neuroradiology: THE REQUISITES, 2nd ed, pp 17–18, 20–22.

Comment

Nephrogenic systemic fibrosis is a rare fibrosing disorder that primarily affects the skin, but may affect other organs in patients with renal insufficiency. To date, approximately 200 cases have been reported to the International Center for Nephrogenic Fibrosing Dermopathy Research. Originally, this fibrosing skin condition was termed nephrogenic fibrosing dermopathy because it occurred exclusively in patients with renal failure. The skin changes can mimic progressive systemic sclerosis, or scleroderma, with a predilection for peripheral extremity involvement. Specific histologic findings include thickened collagen bundles with surrounding clefts, mucin deposition, and increased numbers of fibrocytes and elastic fibers. Systemic manifestations may include fibrosis of the skeletal muscle, bone, lungs, pleura, pericardium, myocardium, kidneys, and dura. Thus, the terminology has changed from nephrogenic fibrosing dermopathy to nephrogenic systemic fibrosis to reflect this systemic involvement. This condition can be very disabling because the skin and musculotendinous involvement results in contractures that reduce range of motion. Some patients are bedridden or wheelchair-bound.

Most signs and symptoms are bilateral and symmetric, usually starting in the extremities and spreading proximally. Lower extremity involvement is most common, followed by involvement of the upper extremities, as in this case. Less commonly, the torso may be affected. The face and neck appear to be spared. Early signs and symptoms seen within the first 2 weeks after gadolinium injection include extremity edema and swelling, arthralgias, myalgias, and extremity weakness. In this case, bone scan shows symmetric increased radionuclide skin and muscle uptake in the lower extremities and distal upper extremities. MR imaging of the thighs shows skin thickening and edema with soft tissue stranding in the subcutaneous fat and muscles. Late signs and symptoms (usually 2 weeks to 8 weeks after gadolinium injection) include skin fibrosis, thickening, and tightening. Skin findings include slightly raised and erythematous or brawny nodular plaques, linear striations, or confluent regions of fibrosis. Extremity contractures, myopathy, and weakness are common.

Notes

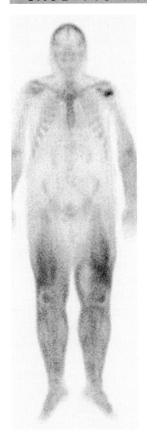

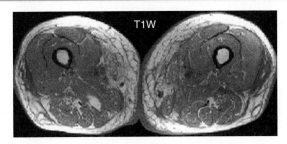

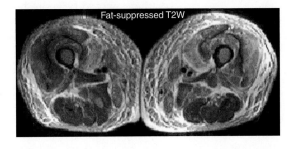

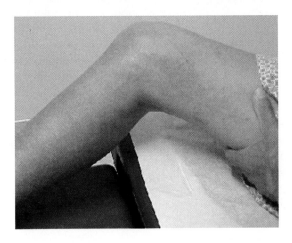

1. What clinical settings have been associated with nephrogenic systemic fibrosis (NSF)?

2. What is the typical interval between gadolinium injection for MR imaging and the onset of symptoms in NSF?

3. What is transmetallation?

4. What is the treatment for NSF?

CASE 114

Gadolinium-Associated Nephrogenic Systemic Fibrosis—Part II

1. Intravenous gadodiamide injection for MR imaging in the setting of renal failure managed with dialysis, and hepatorenal syndrome.

2. Symptoms develop within 2 to 8 weeks after gadolinium injection.

3. Transmetallation is the release of free gadolinium from the chelate, with subsequent binding to endogenous ions.

4. There is no proven consistent effective treatment.

References

Kalb RE, Helm TN, Sperry H, Thakral C, Abraham JL, Kanal E: Gadolinium-induced nephrogenic systemic fibrosis in a patient with an acute and transient kidney injury, *Br J Dermatol* 158:607–610, 2008.

Cross-Reference

Neuroradiology: THE REQUISITES, 2nd ed, pp 17–18, 20–22.

Comment

The exact cause of NSF is unclear. There is no convincing evidence that it is caused by specific drugs, infections, or dialysis itself. It has been specifically associated with intravenous gadodiamide injection in the setting of renal failure managed with dialysis, and hepatorenal syndrome. The only gadolinium-based contrast agent to date reported to be associated with NSF is gadodiamide. Symptoms in most reported cases have developed within 2 to 8 weeks after gadolinium injection for MR imaging, although cases have been reported with longer time intervals. It has been suggested that a combination of factors leads to the development of NSF, beginning with renal disease, followed by allergen deposition, leading to circulating fibrocyte deposition. Fibrinocytes are very important in wound healing and fibrosis. The idea that endothelial damage and elevated levels of cytokines may lead to the development of NSF is supported by the fact that vascular surgery, deep venous thrombosis, and coagulopathies have been noted to occur in the interval between gadodiamide injection and the development of skin fibrosis.

Five different gadolinium chelates have received U.S. FDA approval as paramagnetic contrast agents for diagnostic MR imaging. Intravenous gadolinium at standard doses of 0.1 mmol/kg has relatively few adverse reactions in healthy and renally impaired patients. Double and even triple dosing of gadodiamide, increasingly used in abdominal MR imaging and MR angiography examinations, has been reported to be safe, with a similar incidence of adverse reactions as with the standard dose. It has been postulated that NSF may result from a toxic reaction to free gadolinium (Gd^{3+}) liberated from the chelate but not adequately excreted due to impaired renal function. Transmetallation, the release of free gadolinium from the chelate, with subsequent binding to endogenous ions, is dependent on the molecular conditional thermodynamic stability. Gadolinium agents with lower conditional stability constant values, such as gadodiamide, would be more likely to undergo transmetallation and result in NSF.

Most institutions now have policies regarding the use of these agents. Gadolinium is usually not given to patients with end-stage renal disease or to those receiving dialysis. To screen patients scheduled for contrast-enhanced MR scans, a recent serum creatinine level and calculated creatinine clearance should be obtained in patients who have a history of kidney disease or diabetes and in those older than 60 years of age. At our institution, patients with GFRs over 60 receive a calculated dose based on weight in kilograms; patients with GFRs between 30 and 60 receive a half dose of multihance; in patients with GFRs under 30, a radiologist must approve the administration of contrast, and a half dose of multihance is administered when approved.

There is no consistently effective treatment or prevention regimen. Dialysis immediately after gadodiamide injection has not prevented NSF.

Notes

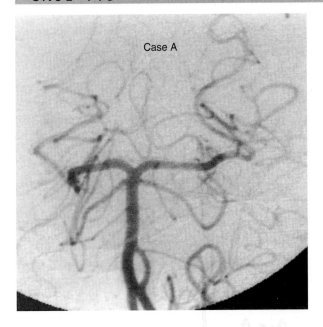

Case A

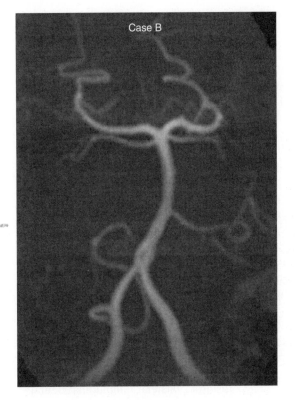

Case B

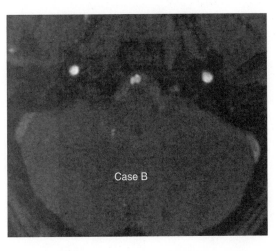

Case B

1. What branch of the basilar artery may extend into the internal auditory canal?

2. What arteries of the posterior circulation give rise to midbrain perforating arteries?

3. What primitive vessels fuse to form the basilar artery?

4. What aneurysm may rupture into the fourth ventricle?

Fenestration of the Basilar Artery

1. The anterior inferior cerebellar artery.

2. The basilar artery and the proximal posterior cerebral arteries (P1 segments).

3. The longitudinal neural arteries.

4. Aneurysms of the posterior inferior cerebellar artery.

Reference

Sanders WP, Sorek PA, Mehta BA: Fenestration of intracranial arteries with special attention to associated aneurysms and other anomalies, *AJNR Am J Neuroradiol* 14:675–680, 1993.

Cross-Reference

Neuroradiology: THE REQUISITES, 2nd ed, pp 88–89.

Comment

Fenestration of a cerebral artery is defined as a division of the vessel lumen that results in two separate vascular channels that are frequently not equal in size. Each of the channels is lined by endothelium. Pathologic evaluation of basilar artery fenestrations shows that the vascular channels may or may not share a common adventitial layer. Histologically, there are short segmental regions at both the proximal and distal ends of the fenestration in which there are defects in the media, similar to bifurcations of cerebral arteries.

Fenestrations are more common in the posterior circulation, reported in up to 0.6% of cerebral angiograms. In comparison, the angiographic incidence of fenestrations in the anterior circulation has been reported in up to 0.2% of cases. On postmortem examination, fenestrations in the posterior and anterior circulation have been reported in 6% to 7% of cases. The discrepancy between pathologic and angiographic incidence is likely due to the increased sensitivity at pathology. The basilar artery is formed by early fusion of bilateral longitudinal neural arteries. Fenestrations occur along regions where there is failure of complete fusion of the medial aspects of these longitudinal arteries. Aneurysms may arise from a fenestration; however, when considering all fenestrations (anterior and posterior circulation), the incidence is approximately 3%, not significantly different from the incidence of aneurysms arising at the circle of Willis. Aneurysms arising from fenestrations of the posterior circulation may occur more frequently (in up to 7% of cases). Aneurysms arise most commonly at the proximal end of the fenestration.

The vertebral arteries are formed by fusion of primitive cervical segmental arteries and basivertebral anastomotic vessels. Extracranial duplications of a vertebral artery are most likely related to failure of regression of the cervical segmental arteries, whereas intracranial duplications likely arise as a result of persistence of basivertebral anastomoses.

Notes

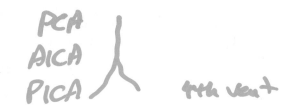

PCA
AICA
PICA

4th vent

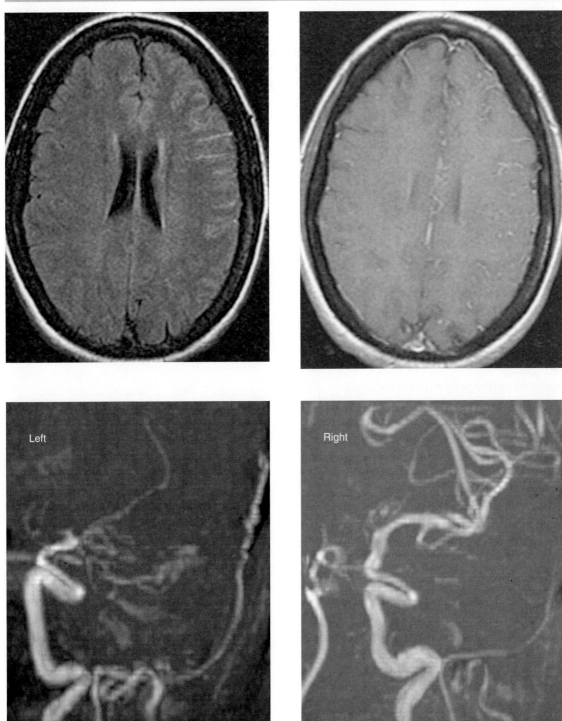

1. What disorders have been associated with these angiographic findings?

2. What is the characteristic clinical presentation in children with this disorder?

3. What is the most common clinical presentation in adults with this disorder?

4. From what vessels do transdural collaterals arise?

Moyamoya Disease

1. Sickle cell disease, neurofibromatosis type 1, atherosclerosis, chronic infection, and radiation therapy. However, in many cases, these findings are idiopathic.

2. Transient ischemic attacks or strokes.

3. Intracranial hemorrhage is probably the most common, and stroke is seen as well.

4. Transdural collaterals most commonly arise from the external carotid artery (ophthalmic and middle meningeal arteries).

Reference

Yamada I, Matsushima Y, Suzuki S: Moyamoya disease: diagnosis with three-dimensional time-of-flight MR angiography, *Radiology* 184:773–778, 1992.

Cross-Reference

Neuroradiology: THE REQUISITES, 2nd ed, pp 202–203.

Comment

This case shows marked narrowing of the left supraclinoid internal carotid artery and occlusion of the proximal left anterior and middle cerebral arteries. There are collateral vessels from the external carotid circulation, leptomeningeal collaterals from the cerebral arteries (best appreciated as the FLAIR hyperintensity in the left cerebral subarachnoid spaces, with corresponding enhancement), as well as collaterals from the perforators in the basal ganglia. On the right, there is no flow in the proximal anterior cerebral artery. There is good flow in the middele cerebral artery without significant narrowing of the middle cerebral circulation. Mildly prominent perforators at the basal ganglia are noted.

Moyamoya refers to slow, progressive occlusive disease of the distal intracranial internal carotid arteries and its proximal branches, including the anterior and middle cerebral arteries. There may also be involvement of the posterior cerebral arteries. Moyamoya disease is predominantly an idiopathic arteriopathy. However, a moyamoya pattern has been associated with a variety of conditions, including neurofibromatosis type 1, sickle cell disease, radiation therapy, chronic infection, and atherosclerosis. Because of the slowly progressive development of high-grade stenoses or occlusions of the distal internal carotid arteries or its proximal branches, collateral circulation develops through a number of pathways, including leptomeningeal collaterals from the cerebral arteries; parenchymal collaterals through the perforating arteries (particularly the basal ganglia); and transdural collaterals, which most commonly arise from the external carotid artery (ophthalmic and middle meningeal arteries).

Moyamoya disease is more symptomatic when it presents in childhood, typically with transient ischemic attacks and stroke. In adults, the disease is less frequently symptomatic, but when it is, it more commonly presents with intracranial hemorrhage.

Notes

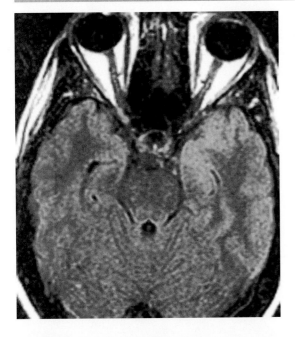

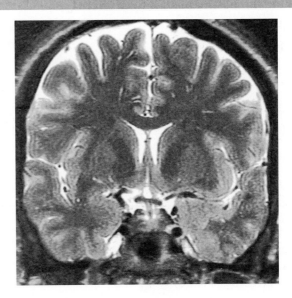

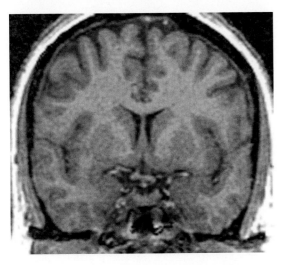

1. What was this patient's clinical presentation?

2. What is the differential diagnosis?

3. From what embryologic structure is the cerebral cortex derived?

4. Along what fibers do neurons migrate from the germinal matrix along the lateral ventricles to the cerebral cortex?

Focal Cortical Dysplasia

1. Medically refractory epilepsy.

2. Focal cortical dyplasia versus low-grade infiltrating neoplasm in the medial left temoporal lobe.

3. The germinal matrix.

4. The radial glial fibers.

References

Barkovich AJ: Morphologic characteristics of subcortical heterotopia: MR imaging study, *Am J Neuroradiol* 21:290–295, 2000.

Taylor DC, Falconer MA, Bruton CJ, et al: Focal dysplasia of the cerebral cortex in epilepsy, *J Neurol Neurosurg Psychiatry* 34:369–387, 1971.

Cross-Reference

Neuroradiology: THE REQUISITES, 2nd ed, p 430.

Comment

Focal cortical dysplasia (aberrant cortical lamination) is found in approximately 50% of patients with medically refractory epilepsy. These lesions have also been reported as an incidental finding in 1% to 2% of brain autopsies. These lesions may involve only mild disorganization of the cortex, but they may also contain abnormal neuronal elements. Advances in neuroimaging have allowed better identification of these lesions. Surgery often results in significant reduction or cessation of seizures, especially if the entire lesion is resected.

Focal cortical dysplasias are part of a spectrum of disorders that have been referred to as disorders of cortical development, cortical dysplasias, cortical dysgenesis, and neuronal migration abnormalities. Classification of these disorders has been based on their pathologic features or on the origin of their pathologic elements (ie, neuronal migration). Histologic findings in cortical dysplasia include architectural abnormalities, such as cortical laminar disorganization. More severe forms are characterized by the presence of abnormal neuronal elements, such as immature neurons (round homogeneous cells with large nuclei), dysmorphic neurons (morphologically distorted cell bodies, axons, and dendrites), giant cells, and balloon cells. Balloon cells are considered a hallmark of focal cortical dyplasia, although they are not present in all cases. These cells have an eosinophilic cytoplasm and an eccentric nucleus.

Magnetic resonance imaging findings associated with cortical dyplasia may include focal areas of increased cortical thickening, as in this case, reduced demarcation of the gray–white matter junction, T2W hyperintensity of cortical gray matter and subcortical white matter, T1W hypointensity of subcortical white matter, lobar underdevelopment, or extension of cortical tissue, with increased signal intensity from the brain surface to the ventricle.

Notes

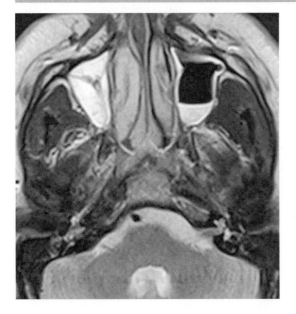 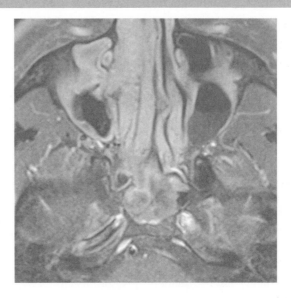

1. What is the diagnosis in this patient with facial pain?

2. What is the most common cause of new-onset acute sinusitis?

3. What sinus is most commonly affected by sinusitis?

4. What are the common bacterial pathogens responsible for acute sinusitis?

Acute Sinusitis

1. Acute sinusitis. There is mucosal disease in the maxillary sinuses, and a fluid level in the left maxillary sinus.

2. Most cases are related to antecedent upper respiratory tract infection. Mucosal edema results in mucosal apposition. These lead to obstruction of the normal sinus drainage, retained sinus secretions, and bacterial overgrowth with infection.

3. The ethmoid air cells.

4. *Streptococcus pneumoniae, Haemophilus influenzae,* β-hemolytic *streptococcus,* and *Moraxella catarrhalis.*

Reference

Yousem DM, Kennedy DW, Rosenberg S: Ostiomeatal complex risk factors for sinusitis: CT evaluation, *J Otorhinolaryngol* 20:419–424, 1991.

Cross-Reference

Neuroradiology: THE REQUISITES, 2nd ed, pp 616–624.

Comments

It is estimated that more than 30 million people in the United States have sinus inflammatory disease annually; more than half of these result in doctor visits. Approximately 0.5% of viral upper respiratory tract infections are complicated by sinusitis. Although many patients are treated for sinusitis based on clinical presentation, increasingly, CT imaging has become a part of the standard workup of these patients.

The radiologist should comment on the location of disease within the sinonasal cavity (mucosal thickening, air–fluid levels in specific parts of the sinuses), affected mucous circulatory passageways (such as the infundibulum of the ostiomeatal complex), and the presence (or absence) of the osseous structures confining the paranasal sinuses, such as the cribriform plate and medial orbital walls. The location of sinusitis is more significant in the production of symptoms than the extent of disease. Opacification of the infundibulum of the ostiomeatal complex is one of the best predictors for the development of maxillary sinusitis, with a positive predictive value of approximately 80%, whereas opacification of the middle meatus has greater than 90% specificity in predicting maxillary and ethmoid sinusitis. Obstruction of the sphenoethmoidal recess occurs in fewer than 10% of cases and may result in inflammation involving the sphenoid sinus and posterior ethmoid air cells.

In cases of acute sinusitis, an air–fluid level or sinus opacification is present in more than 50% of cases. These acute changes may be superimposed on chronic changes, including mucosal thickening, neo-osteogenesis, polyposis, and retention cysts. Sinusitis is a clinical diagnosis with supporting radiologic findings. The presence of sinus changes, including air–fluid levels, does not always equal sinusitis.

Notes

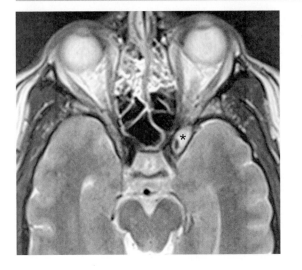
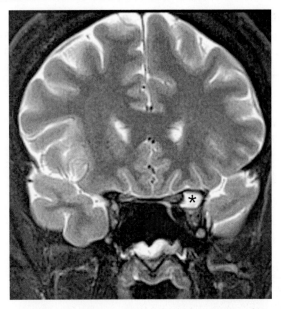
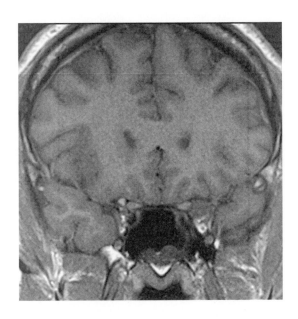
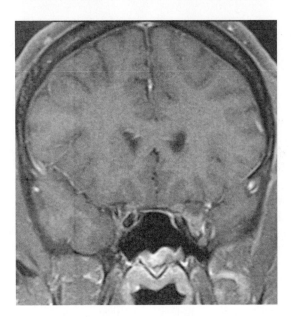

1. What structure is indicated by the *?

2. What cranial nerve sits medial to the structure denoted by the *?

3. What is the diagnosis?

4. Mucoceles occur least often in what major paranasal sinus?

Anterior Clinoiditis and Mucocele Formation Complicating Sinusitis

1. The * indicates the left anterior clinoid process.

2. The optic nerve.

3. Anterior clinoiditis with mucocele formation.

4. Mucoceles occur most commonly in the frontal or ethmoidal sinuses, followed by the sphenoid sinus. They are least common in the maxillary sinus.

Reference

Tchoyoson Lim CC, Dillon WP, McDermott MW: Mucocele involving the anterior clinoid process: MR and CT findings, *Am J Neuroradiol* 20:287–290, 1999.

Cross-Reference

Neuroradiology: THE REQUISITES, 2nd ed, pp 616–624.

Comments

These are additional images from the patient in the preceding case (118). These images show expansion and opacification of the left anterior clinoid process with material that is hyperintense on T2W and FLAIR (not shown) imaging, consistent with proteinaceous material. This demonstrates rim enhancement. The optic canal is mildly attenuated from the clinoid expansion. There is swelling in the orbital apex seen on the coronal images. The bony integrity along the medial margin of the left anterior clinoid or lateral margin of the optic canal cannot be assessed, and correlation with CT is necessary.

The greater and lesser wings of the sphenoid bone form the floor and the roof of the orbital apex, respectively. When these structures become pneumatized in the course of normal development, like the paranasal sinuses, they may be affected by obstructive inflammatory disease and mucocele formation. A mucocele represents chronic expansion with mucoid secretions of a sinus or previously aerated bone lined by respiratory epithelium. Mucoceles are uncommon in the posterior ethmoid and sphenoid sinuses, and may present with signs and symptoms referable to cranial nerves II to VI. Visual loss, visual field defects, and extraocular palsies and sensory deficits of the trigeminal nerve may occur. This patient presented with diplopia and chronic facial pain.

An Onodi cell is a posterior ethmoidal air cell that penetrates the sphenoid bone. The prevalence of Onodi cells on CT studies varies from 8% to 13%. The bones forming the orbital apex and anterior clinoid process may be aerated either by an Onodi cell or by the lateral recess of the sphenoidal sinus. Posterior ethmoidal air cells can grow into the upper sphenoid bone and may surround the optic canal. These may in turn become obstructed, resulting in mucocele formation. In a patient with signs and symptoms referable to the orbital apex, a mucocele of the paranasal sinus should be considered in the differential diagnosis.

Notes

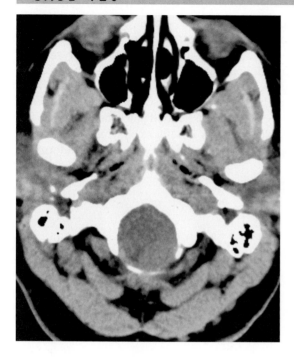
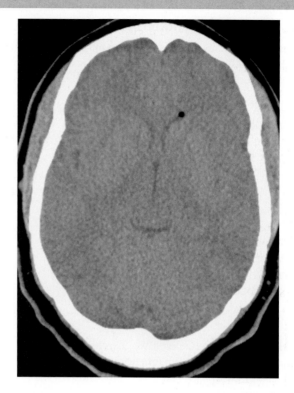

1. What are the pertinent imaging findings in this case?

2. What are this patient's symptoms?

3. What are causes of intracranial hypotension?

4. What is the differential diagnosis of diffuse dural enhancement?

Spontaneous Intracranial Hypotension

1. Low-lying cerebellar tonsils and a small amount of intraventricular air in the frontal horn of the left lateral ventricle.

2. Positional or postural headaches.

3. Thoracic diverticula due to focal thinning in the dura (MR imaging may detect these; if not, then postmyelography CT is useful in their identification), after trauma, and iatrogenic (after lumbar puncture or spinal surgery or instrumentation) causes.

4. Metastatic disease (breast and prostate carcinoma), lymphoma or leukemia, granulomatous disease (tuberculosis, sarcoidosis, Wegener's granulomatosis, Erdheim-Chester disease, lipid granulomatosis), spontaneous intracranial hypotension, and idiopathic hypertrophic pachymeningitis.

References

Moayeri NN, Henson JW, Schaefer PW, Zervas NT: Spinal dural enhancement on magnetic resonance imaging associated with spontaneous intracranial hypotension, *J Neurosurg* 88:912–918, 1998.

Sishman RA, Dillon WP: Dural enhancement and cerebral displacement secondary to intracranial hypotension, *Neuroradiology* 43:609–611, 1993.

Cross-Reference

Neuroradiology: THE REQUISITES, 2nd ed, pp 628–629.

Comment

This case illustrates low-lying cerebellar tonsils and intraventricular air in a patient who presented with postural headaches 2 weeks after a difficult epidural anesthesia for childbirth.

Spontaneous intracranial hypotension is caused by chronic, and often intermittent, leakage of CSF from the subarachnoid space. This leakage of CSF results in low intracranial pressure. Symptomatic patients typically present with headaches that are frequently postural in nature (exacerbated in the upright position, relieved when lying down). Trauma or spontaneous (rupture of Tarlov's cyst) or iatrogenic (after lumbar puncture or spine surgery or instrumentation) causes result in CSF leakage, which typically occurs somewhere along the spinal column. Imaging findings may be subtle and nonspecific such that in the absence of providing a history of postural headaches, the diagnosis of intracranial hypotension is frequently overlooked. Imaging findings include sagging of the posterior fossa contents, with low-lying cerebellar tonsils, elongation of the fourth ventricle, bilateral subdural effusions, and diffuse dural enhancement. In addition, prominent dural veins have been reported. Symptoms of intracranial hypotension may resolve spontaneously; however, further workup, including MR imaging, and if indicated, CT myelography or nuclear scintigraphy, is often necessary to identify the source of the CSF leak. If a source can be identified, positioning of an epidural blood patch can be performed and typically results in resolution of symptoms. Increasingly, prophylactic blood patches are being performed.

Notes

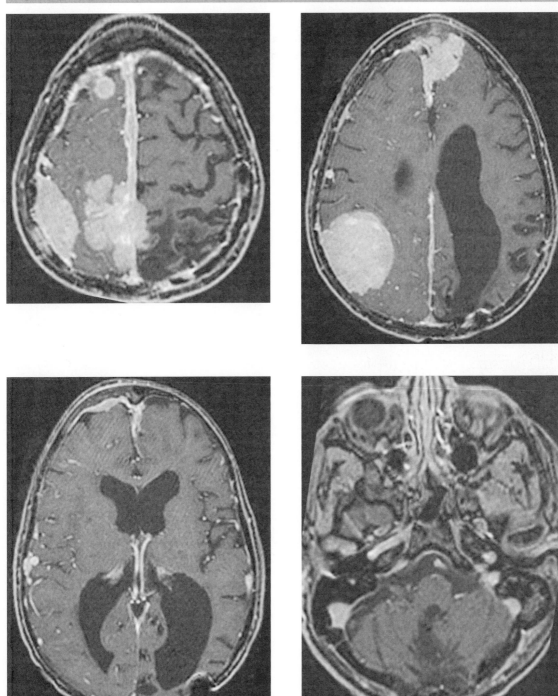

1. What are the imaging findings?

2. What is the best diagnosis?

3. What predisposed this patient to the development of this entity?

4. What are some radiation-induced intracranial neoplasms?

Multiple Meningiomas after Remote Whole-Brain Irradiation

1. There are multiple dural-based avidly enhancing masses; some are contiguous, whereas others are clearly separate.

2. Multiple meningiomas.

3. This patient has had an occipital craniotomy and brain radiation therapy for a posterior fossa neoplasm as a child (in this case, a primitive neuroectodermal tumor).

4. Meningiomas, sarcomas, schwannomas, and gliomas.

Reference
Sadetzki S, Flint-Richter P, Ben-Thal T, Nass D: Radiation-induced meningiomas: a descriptive study of 253 cases, *J Neurosurg* 97:1078–1082, 2002.

Cross-Reference
Neuroradiology: THE REQUISITES, 2nd ed, pp 104–105.

Comment

Balancing aggressive therapies that improve survival with efforts to decrease long-term side effects makes the treatment of brain tumors a major challenge in pediatric oncology. Pediatric brain tumors are a heterogeneous collection of lesions with 5-year survival rates ranging from 10% to 95%. Although standard care for most types of pediatric brain tumors continues to be surgery, often followed by radiation therapy with or without chemotherapy, there is increasing emphasis on trying to minimize the long-term effects of these treatments, such as cognitive deficits, as well as the risk of radiation-induced neoplasms.

The criteria for diagnosis of radiation-induced meningiomas (tumors) are the following: (1) there is a history of irradiation; (2) the tumors arise in a radiation field after a latency period of years; (3) there is proof of histologic difference between the secondary tumor and the originally irradiated tumor; and (4) there is no predisposition that may facilitate neoplastic growth. In the case of radiation-induced meningiomas, the patient cannot have other risk factors, such as neurofibromatosis type 2, that predisposes them to meningiomas. Meningiomas have been associated with low-dose irradiation treatment for tinea capitis and have a latency period of decades. Multiple meningiomas occur in up to 30% of patients with a remote history of radiation therapy and in 2% of nonirradiated patients with meningiomas. Recurrence rates are higher in radiation-induced tumors than in those occurring sporadically or in association with other entities, such as neurofibromatosis type 2. Radiation therapy induces up to five times as many meningiomas as it does sarcomas, schwannomas, or gliomas. The true risk of radiation-induced tumors is unknown.

Notes

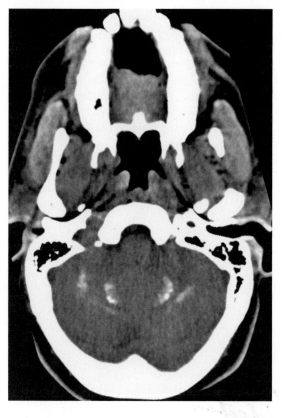
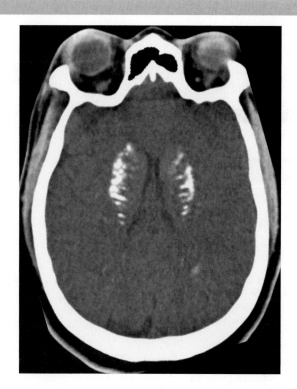

1. What are the nuclei of the basal ganglia?

2. What is the TORCH infection typically associated with periventricular calcification?

3. Carbon monoxide poisoning classically affects what deep gray matter?

4. What is the characteristic pattern of calcium deposition in Fahr disease?

Fahr Disease (Familial Cerebrovascular Ferrocalcinosis)

1. Globus pallidus, putamen, and caudate nuclei.

2. Cytomegalovirus.

3. The bilateral globus pallidus, which typically are affected by pallidal necrosis.

4. Bilaterally symmetric calcification within the basal ganglia, thalami, and dentate nuclei of the cerebellum.

References

Holland BA, Kucharcyzk W, Brant-Zawadzki M, et al: MR imaging of calcified intracranial lesions, *Radiology* 157: 353–356, 1985.

Scotti G, Scialfa G, Tampieri D, Landoni L: MR imaging in Fahr disease, *J Comput Assist Tomogr* 9:790–792, 1985.

Cross-Reference

Neuroradiology: THE REQUISITES, 2nd ed, p 396.

Comment

This case shows bilateral symmetric calcification within the basal ganglia (including the caudate and lentiform nuclei) and dentate nuclei of the cerebellum in a patient with progressive dementia. Mineral deposition is frequently noted to be hyperintense on unenhanced sagittal and axial T1W imaging. Fahr disease represents a relatively uncommon spectrum of neurologic disorders characterized by extensive abnormal calcium deposition in characteristic locations, such as the bilateral basal ganglia, with associated cell loss. This condition has been referred to as idiopathic basal ganglia calcification. Variable neurologic manifestations, including movement disorders such as athetosis (slow, involuntary movements) and chorea, dementia, and psychological impairment, occur. Calcification may also be seen in the dentate nuclei (as in this case), as well as within the white matter, including the centrum semiovale, corona radiata, and subcortical white matter.

Familial patterns of Fahr disease have been commonly noted in the literature. Transmission may be as an autosomal recessive trait, or may occur in large affected families as an autosomal dominant inheritance pattern.

The differential diagnosis of calcification within the deep gray matter of the cerebral hemispheres, particularly the basal ganglia, is extensive. Probably the most common cause is idiopathic. Calcification in the globus pallidus bilaterally may be noted as a normal finding, representing senescent calcification that occurs with advancing age. A variety of endocrine disorders, including abnormalities in phosphate and calcium metabolism, may result in calcification in these locations. Hypoparathyroidism has not infrequently been identified. Symptomatic patients may respond to correction of serum calcium phosphate abnormalities.

Another common cause of calcium deposition is in the postinflammatory setting. Specifically, calcification may be seen in infections, such as in utero cytomegalovirus exposure, tuberculosis, and cysticercosis, although in these instances, the pattern of calcification is not similar to that seen in Fahr disease. In recent years, calcification within the basal ganglia has been described in patients with in utero HIV infection. Some experts believe that Fahr disease in general may be the result of in utero infections.

Notes

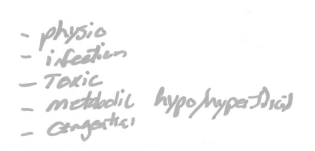

- physio
- infection
- Toxic
- metabolic   hypo/hyper thyroid
- Congenital

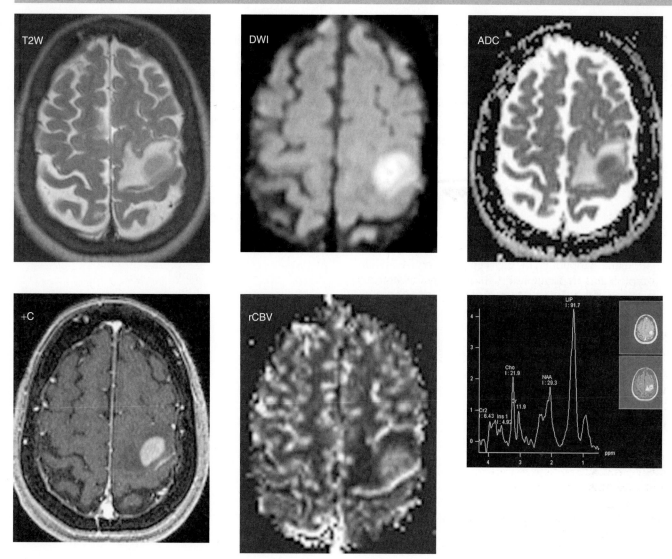

1. What is the differential diagnosis?

2. What is the best diagnosis?

3. What conditions predispose a patient to the development of primary CNS lymphoma?

4. Why does this mass have restricted diffusion?

Central Nervous System Lymphoma—Immunocompetent Patient

1. Lymphoma, metastasis, and primary glial tumor (glioblastoma multiforme).

2. CNS lymphoma. Because of the compact nature and the orientation of the white matter fibers.

3. Immunosuppression (particularly in patients with HIV infection) and immunosuppressive therapy for the treatment of cancer or after organ transplantation.

4. Because it has very dense cellularity.

References

Erdag N, Bhorade RM, Alberico RA, Yousuf N, Patel MR: Primary lymphoma of the central nervous system: typical and atypical CT and MR imaging appearances, *AJR Am J Roentgenol* 176:1319–1326, 2001.

Lai R, Rosenblum MK, DeAngelis LM: Primary CNS lymphoma: a whole-brain disease?, *Neurology* 59: 1557–1562, 2002.

Vazquez E, Lucaya J, Castellote A, et al: Neuroimaging in pediatric leukemia and lymphoma: differential diagnosis, *RadioGraphics* 22:1411–1428, 2002.

Cross-Reference

Neuroradiology: THE REQUISITES, 2nd ed, pp 153–155.

Comment

Primary CNS lymphoma is uncommon, but its incidence has increased significantly over the last decade as a result of its relatively common occurrence in patients with AIDS (affecting approximately 6%). The origin of lymphoma is unknown because the CNS does not have lymphoid tissue. It has been postulated that CNS lymphoma arises from microglial cells. Histologic evaluation of primary CNS lymphoma almost always shows intermediate- to high-grade extranodal non-Hodgkin's lymphoma of B-cell origin. It is most commonly seen in immunocompromised patients, but it has been increasingly recognized in immunocompetent patients. It usually presents in the sixth and seventh decades of life.

The supratentorial compartment is most commonly involved, although involvement of the brainstem and cerebellum is not rare. The most common imaging presentation of primary CNS lymphoma is multiple masses. Focal masses in the basal ganglia, thalami, and periventricular white matter are common. Alternatively, patients may present with a single mass with vasogenic edema, as in this case, in which a mass in the left precentral gyrus is seen. Conventional MR imaging, on a 3.0-Tesla unit in this case, shows features that favor lymphoma, including restricted diffusion and solid homogeneous enhancement.

Advanced MR imaging shows moderate elevation in relative cerebral blood volume on the perfusion study. Spectroscopy shows an elevated choline:creatine ratio, consistent with neoplasm, and decreased N-acetylaspartate. There is also marked elevation in the lipid and lactate peaks that have been described with lymphoma.

Although CNS lymphoma typically enhances solidly and avidly, in the setting of AIDS and other forms of immunosuppression, there is a spectrum of patterns of pathologic enhancement, ranging from solid to ring-like. The patient in this case is not immunocompromised. The T2W signal intensity characteristics may be quite variable, ranging from hyperintensity to marked hypointensity (isointense to brain) in cases of very cellular neoplasms. Hemorrhage is uncommon in lymphomatous masses.

Notes

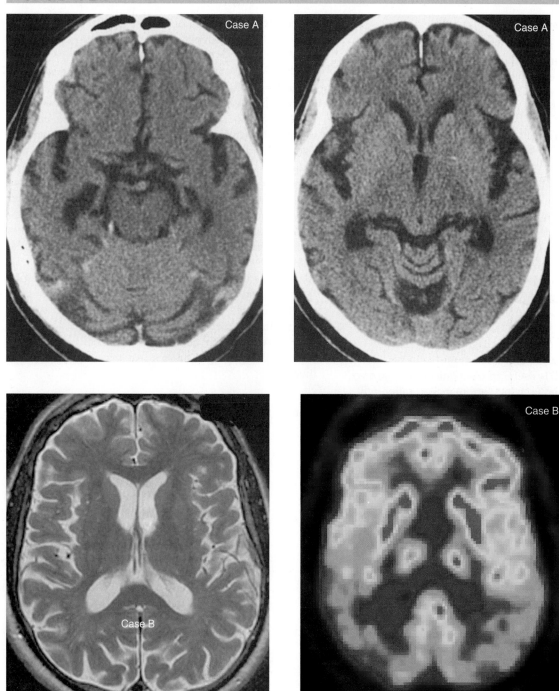

1. What are the pertinent CT findings in Case A?

2. What are the MR and fluorodeoxyglucose positron emission tomography (FDG PET) scan findings in Case B, a 55-year-old man with progressive dementia?

3. What are the FDG PET scan findings in Alzheimer's disease versus frontotemporal dementia?

4. In Parkinson's disease, the dopaminergic cells are abnormal in what structure?

Alzheimer's Disease

1. Global cortical atrophy, with enlargement of the basal cisterns and sylvian cisterns and dilation of the choroidal–hippocampal fissures, characteristic of Alzheimer's disease.

2. The FDG PET scan shows decreased metabolism in the bilateral temporal and parietal lobes, with relative preservation of metabolism in the frontal lobes and subcortical structures. The MR image shows cortical atrophy greater than expected for age.

3. In Alzheimer's disease, low activity is predominantly in the back part of the brain; in frontotemporal dementia (FTD), low activity is mostly in the front of the brain. FTD is a common cause of early-onset dementia among people 45 to 65 years old and is marked by behavioral changes and language difficulties. It can take years to develop and is incurable. Although FTD is a separate disorder, it often meets the clinical diagnostic criteria for Alzheimer's disease and often is misdiagnosed as such. FDG PET is useful in distinguishing these two causes of dementia, which are managed differently.

4. The pars compacta of the substantia nigra.

References

Kitagaki H, Mori E, Yamaji S, et al: Frontotemporal dementia and Alzheimer disease: evaluation of cortical atrophy with automated hemispheric surface display generated with MR images, *Radiology* 208: 431–439, 1998.

Matsuda H, Mizumura S, Nagao T, et al: Automated discrimination between very early Alzheimer disease and controls using an easy Z-score imaging system for multicenter brain perfusion single-photon emission tomography, *Am J Neuroradiol* 28:731–736, 2007.

Cross-Reference

Neuroradiology: THE REQUISITES, 2nd ed, pp 379, 381–382.

Comment

Each year, 1 in 500 people is diagnosed with dementia. Approximately 66% of these cases result from Alzheimer's disease that is characterized clinically by progressive memory loss and cognitive decline. As the disease progresses, it is often difficult for patients to carry out the daily tasks of living. Not uncommonly, depression accompanies Alzheimer's disease.

The most common imaging finding in Alzheimer's disease is diffuse cortical atrophy, which is often most pronounced in the temporal lobes. Approximately 70% of patients with Alzheimer's disease have dilation of the temporal horns. This is frequently accompanied by asymmetric dilation of the choroidal-hippocampal fissures (a response to medial temporal lobe and hippocampal atrophy). Other imaging findings, when compared with age-matched control subjects, include an increase in total CSF volume, enlargement of the sylvian cisterns, and an increase in ventricular size. In addition, longitudinal studies in patients with Alzheimer's disease compared with normal control subjects have demonstrated that atrophy progresses much more rapidly in patients with Alzheimer's disease. Deep white matter and periventricular regions of T2W hyperintensity are common in Alzheimer's disease. The literature suggests that there is no statistically significant difference in the extent of white matter disease between individuals with Alzheimer's disease and normal control subjects. Despite the radiologic findings in Alzheimer's disease, the findings are nonspecific and may be seen in a spectrum of other neurodegenerative processes. The major role of imaging in patients with dementia is to exclude underlying abnormalities, such as tumors that may be amenable to therapy.

Notes

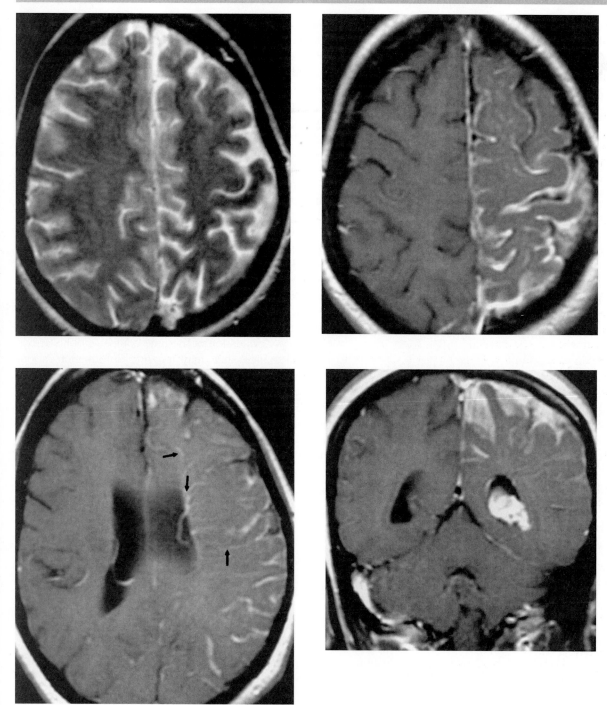

1. What is the cause of the intracranial lesion associated with this syndrome?

2. Where is the collateral venous drainage for this abnormality?

3. What is the inheritance pattern of this neurocutaneous disorder?

4. What is the classic cutaneous manifestation of this phakomatosis, and in what distribution does it typically occur?

Sturge-Weber Syndrome (Encephalotrigeminal Angiomatosis)

1. Leptomeningeal venous angiomatosis develops as a result of failure of development of normal cortical venous drainage in involved areas of the brain.

2. Collateral venous drainage occurs through an increase in the size and number of medullary and subependymal veins. There is also compensatory hypertrophy of the ipsilateral choroid plexus, and often there is enlargement of the internal cerebral veins.

3. Unlike most phakomatoses, Sturge-Weber syndrome occurs sporadically and has a relatively equal predilection in both men and women.

4. Port wine stain (nevus flammeus), which typically occurs in the trigeminal nerve distribution; the ophthalmic division (cranial nerve V1) is most common.

References

Griffiths PD, Blaser S, Boodram MB, Armstrong D, Harwood-Nash D: Choroid plexus size in young children with Sturge-Weber syndrome, *Am J Neuroradiol* 17:175–180, 1996.

Linn DD, Barker PB, Kraut MA, Comi A: Early characteristics of Sturge-Weber syndrome shown by perfusion MR imaging and proton MR spectroscopic imaging, *Am J Neuroradiol* 24:1912–1915, 2003.

Cross-Reference

Neuroradiology: THE REQUISITES, 2nd ed, pp 454, 456.

Comment

The pathogenesis of Sturge-Weber syndrome is uncertain; however, it is believed to result from persistence of the primitive vascular plexus as a result of failure of development of the normal cortical venous drainage in affected areas of the brain. A pial vascular malformation develops that is characterized pathologically by thin-walled, dilated capillaries and venules. The pial angiomatous malformation is usually ipsilateral to the facial port wine nevus and most commonly affects the posterior cerebral hemisphere (most frequently the occipital lobe, followed by the parietal and temporal lobes).

In patients older than 2 years of age, plain film radiographs or CT may show "tram-track" calcifications, representing cortical calcification. Enhanced MR imaging shows the extent of the angiomatous malformation because there is enhancement of the pia in regions involved with the vascular abnormality. Collateral venous drainage is manifested by an increase in both the size and number of medullary and subependymal veins. There is also compensatory hypertrophy of the ipsilateral choroid plexus from increased flow, and frequently, the internal cerebral veins are enlarged. Involved brain may have abnormal T2W hyperintensity within the white matter related to gliosis and demyelination, cortical enhancement related to anoxic injury, and atrophy. Secondary calvarial changes include compensatory hypertrophy of the diploic space and enlargement of the ipsilateral paranasal sinuses and mastoid air cells. This case shows many of these abnormalities, including the extent of the pial vascular malformation, cortical enhancement, dilated medullary and subependymal veins (*arrows*), and ipsilateral enlargement of the choroid plexus.

The finding of decreased N-acetylaspartate on proton MR spectroscopy has been observed in affected regions, suggesting neuronal dysfunction or loss. A decreased N-acetylaspartate level may be expected to develop in regions of significant hypoperfusion. MR perfusion imaging allows evaluation of the time course of bolus arrival and clearance that may provide information about abnormalities due to either the arterial or venous phase. A marked delay of venous clearance of contrast has been observed in areas of leptomeningeal angiomatous involvement. Venous stasis may be distinguished from hypoperfusion, which shows both delayed arrival and clearance of contrast.

Notes

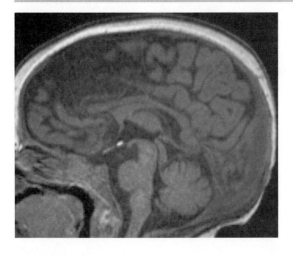
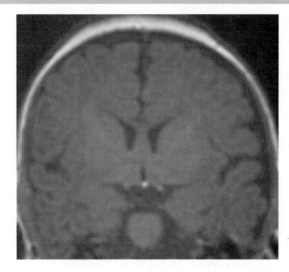

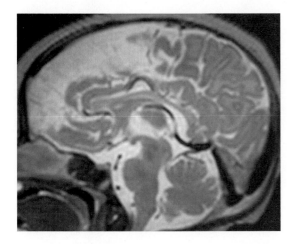

1. What was this child's clinical presentation?

2. What is the primary MR imaging finding?

3. What structure is not visualized?

4. What structure regulates pituitary endocrine function?

CASE 126

Ectopic Posterior Pituitary and Nonvisualization of the Infundibulum—Hypopituitarism

1. Hypopituitarism.

2. An ectopic posterior pituitary gland.

3. The infundibulum (pituitary stalk).

4. The hypothalamus.

References

Hamilton J, Blaser S, Daneman D: MR imaging in idiopathic growth hormone deficiency, *Am J Neuroradiol* 19:1609–1615, 1998.

Takahashi T, Miki Y, Takahashi JA, et al: Ectopic posterior pituitary high signal in preoperative and postoperative macroadenomas: dynamic MR imaging, *Eur J Radiol* 55:84–91, 2005.

Cross-Reference

Neuroradiology: THE REQUISITES, 2nd ed, pp 529–532.

Comment

The posterior pituitary develops from the neuroectoderm of the diencephalon. Pituitary gland function is controlled by the hypothalamus via the infundibular stalk. Nerve fibers from nuclei in the hypothalamus course into the infundibulum to reach the posterior pituitary gland. Normally, the anterior pituitary gland and the pituitary stalk are well defined. The posterior pituitary is usually identified as a hyperintense "bright" spot on T1W MR images. This hyperintensity has been attributed to lipids within pituicytes, the arginine vasopressin neurophysin complex, or phospholipids within the walls of the secretory vesicles containing the arginine vasopressin neurophysin complex.

An ectopic posterior pituitary gland may result from aberrant neuronal migration during embryogenesis, transection of the pituitary, or an insult to the pituitary stalk due to ischemia, anoxia, or compression leading to reorganization of the proximal neurons of the neurohypophysis. Breech delivery and perinatal anoxia have been associated with transection of the pituitary stalk and hypopituitarism. However, many patients with hypopituitarism and ectopic posterior pituitary have uncomplicated perinatal courses.

Growth hormone deficiency is a common cause of short stature. It may be idiopathic or acquired (tumors, instrumentation of the sellar region). Idiopathic growth hormone deficiency may occur in isolation or in association with other anterior pituitary hormone deficiencies. An ectopic posterior pituitary and nonvisualization of the stalk on MR imaging is associated with decreased function of the anterior pituitary (hypopituitarism). Posterior pituitary hormone deficiency in the presence of an ectopic posterior pituitary is uncommon, suggesting that this ectopic tissue functions normally to produce antidiuretic hormone. Nonvisualization of the pituitary stalk alone on MR imaging is associated with anterior pituitary hormone deficiencies limited to growth hormone and thyrotropin.

Notes

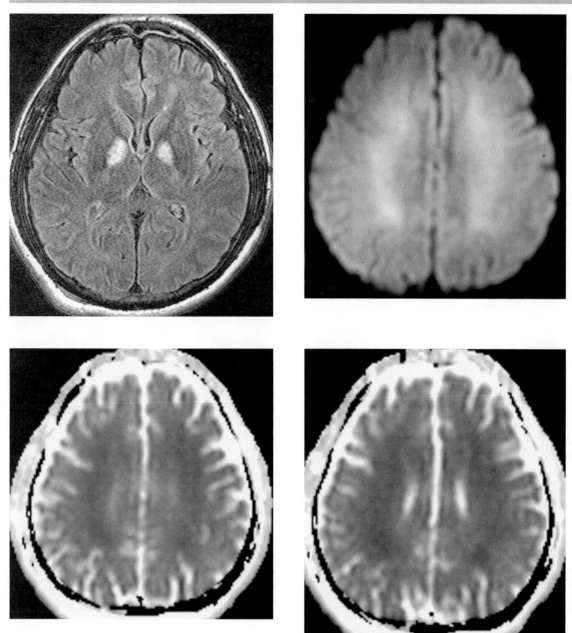

1. What are the imaging findings on the diffusion-weighted image?

2. What do the corresponding apparent diffusion coefficient (ADC) maps show?

3. What toxin was this patient exposed to?

4. What is your diagnosis?

Acute Toxic Demyelination—Carbon Monoxide Intoxication

1. Diffusion-weighted image shows bilaterally symmetric, confluent areas of high signal intensity in the periventricular white matter and centrum semiovale.

2. Corresponding ADC maps show signal in the involved white matter that is hypointense relative to normal white matter.

3. Carbon monoxide (CO).

4. Acute toxic demyelination.

Reference

Kim JH, Chang KH, Song IC, Kim KH, Kwon BJ, Kim HC: Delayed encephalopathy of acute carbon monoxide intoxication: diffusivity of cerebral white matter lesions, *AJNR Am J Neuroradiol* 24:1592–1597, 2003.

Cross-Reference

Neuroradiology: THE REQUISITES, 2nd ed, pp 206, 354, 358.

Comment

Patients with carbon monoxide poisoning may experience sudden neurologic deterioration. Delayed encephalopathy of CO poisoning is characterized by a recurrence of neurologic symptoms after an asymptomatic period of variable duration (usually 2–3 weeks) from the acute stage of CO intoxication. Similar delayed encephalopathies may also be seen with other insults that result in anoxia, such as respiratory arrest, strangling, drug overuse, and anesthesia. The course of the delayed encephalopathy varies with the severity of CO intoxication, ranging from recovery to progressive deterioration ending in coma or death. Clinical symptoms include altered mental status, urinary incontinence, and gait disturbance, as well as neuropsychiatric manifestations.

Initial imaging shows characteristic signal abnormality in the bilateral globus pallidus on the FLAIR image. Delayed imaging in patients with neurologic decline often shows white matter disease, which may be extensive and pathologically represents acute demyelination. The pathogenesis of acute demyelination is unclear. Conventional T2W MR imaging findings of delayed encephalopathy from CO intoxication show bilaterally symmetric, confluent areas of high-signal intensity in the periventricular white matter and centrum semiovale. Diffusion-weighted imaging shows bilateral areas of confluent high-signal intensity in the periventricular white matter and centrum semiovale, similar to those seen in this case. The hyperintensity can range from mild to marked. Corresponding ADC maps show signal in the involved white matter that may be normal, isointense, or hypointense. In this case, however, mean ADC values of the white matter lesions are significantly lower than those of normal-looking white matter, regardless of their intensity on ADC maps.

Notes

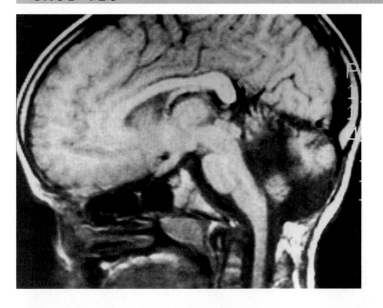

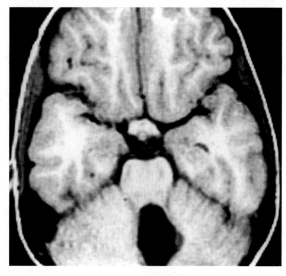

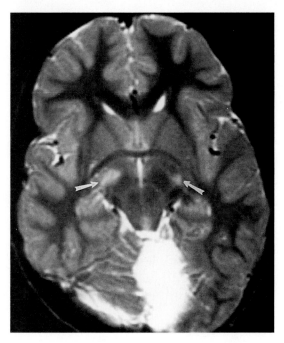

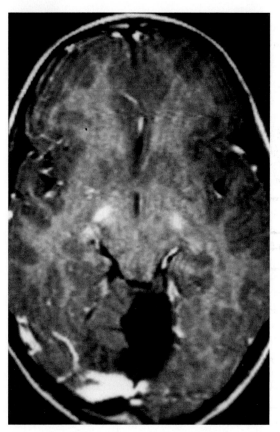

1. What anatomic structures (*arrows*) have abnormal T2W hyperintensity?

2. What are the common locations in which nonneoplastic T2W lesions may be identified in neurofibromatosis type 1?

3. What are the histologic features of optic pathway gliomas associated with neurofibromatosis type 1?

4. What chromosome has a mutation in neurofibromatosis type 1?

C A S E   1 2 8

Neurofibromatosis Type 1—Pilocytic Astrocytoma of the Optic Pathway

1. The posterior optic pathways (optic tracts and radiations).

2. The bilateral basal ganglia, brainstem, cerebellar peduncles, and dentate nuclei.

3. Pilocytic astrocytoma.

4. Chromosome 17.

References

DiMario FJ, Ramsby G: Magnetic imaging lesion analysis in neurofibromatosis type 1, *Arch Neurol* 55:500–505, 1998.

Thiagalingam S, Flaherty M, Billson F, North K: Neurofibromatosis type 1 and optic pathway gliomas: follow-up of 54 patients, *Ophthalmology* 111:568–577, 2004.

Cross-Reference

Neuroradiology: THE REQUISITES, 2nd ed, pp 493–496.

Comment

Neurofibromatosis type 1 (von Recklinghausen's disease) is caused by a mutation of chromosome 17. In one half of cases, this mutation is transmitted in an autosomal dominant pattern; in the other half, it is sporadic. Neurofibromatosis type 1 can be diagnosed when two or more of the following criteria are present: a first-degree relative with neurofibromatosis type 1, one plexiform neurofibroma or two or more neurofibromas of any type, six or more café-au-lait spots, two or more Lisch nodules (iris hamartomas), axillary or inguinal freckling, optic pathway glioma, and a characteristic bone abnormality (dysplasia of the greater wing of the sphenoid, overgrowth of a digit or limb, pseudarthrosis, lateral thoracic meningocele, or dural ectasia with vertebral dysplasia).

The most common CNS tumor in neurofibromatosis type 1 is a low-grade optic nerve pilocytic glioma, reported in 15% to 28% of patients. Growth along the optic tract, the lateral geniculate, and the optic radiations may occur. MR imaging is the best choice for assessing the extent of these tumors. Typically, when there is posterior extension along the optic tracts and radiations, there is enhancement. In this case, the optic chiasm is enlarged, with extension along the posterior optic pathways (*arrows*). Low-grade astrocytic tumors in other locations, such as the brainstem, are also seen with increased incidence in neurofibromatosis type 1. This patient had previous resection of a cerebellar astrocytoma. Neoplasms seen with increased incidence in neurofibromatosis type 1 include neurofibrosarcoma (malignant degeneration of a neurofibroma), seen in up to 5% of patients; leukemia; lymphoma; medullary thyroid carcinoma; pheochromocytoma; melanoma; and Wilms' tumor.

Neurofibromatosis type 1 may be associated with non-neoplastic hyperintense lesions on T2W sequences within the basal ganglia, cerebellar peduncles, dentate nuclei, brainstem, and white matter, and may be present in up to 60% of patients, especially in the pediatric age group. Mass effect is predominantly associated with lesions in the brainstem, thalamus, and cerebellar peduncles. Limited tissue specimens have confirmed many of these to represent spongiotic change or vacuolization. Serial T2W imaging shows regression in both the number and size of lesions over a 2- to 3-year period.

Notes

II: first degree relative
2 (at least) schwannoma, menangioma
ependymoma

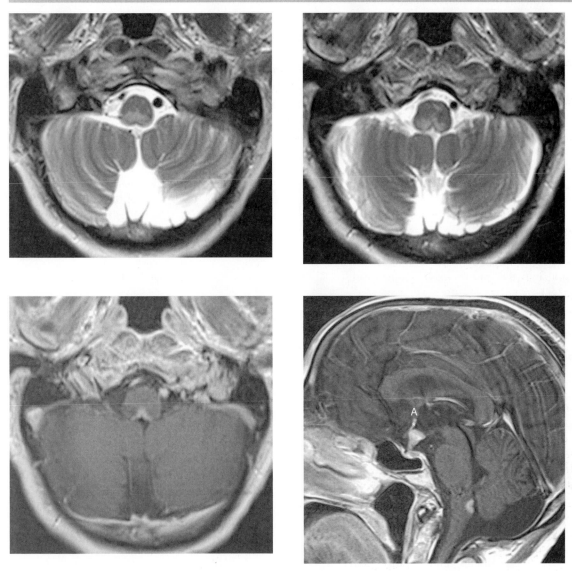

1. What area of the brainstem is involved with this entity?

2. What is the main differential diagnosis in an older adult?

3. The * represents what anatomic structure? The *A* represents what anatomic structure?

4. How did the patient present clinically?

Lymphoma Involving the Circumventricular Organs

1. The area postrema of the medulla (the "vomit center").

2. Lymphoma, sarcoid, tuberculosis, and carcinomatosis from systemic cancer.

3. The * represents the lamina terminalis, which is located behind the optic chiasm. The *A* represents the anterior commissure.

4. With diabetes insipidus.

References

Danchaivijitr N, Hesselink JR, Aryan HE, Herndier B: Cerebello-pontine angle (CPA) lymphoma with perineural extension into the middle fossa: case report, *Surg Neurol* 62:80–85, 2004.

Nozaki M, Tada M, Mizugaki Y, et al: Expression of oncogenic molecules in primary central nervous system lymphomas in immunocompetent patients, *Acta Neuropathol* 95:505–510, 1998.

Cross-Reference

Neuroradiology: THE REQUISITES, 2nd ed, pp 38–39, 40–43, 153–155.

Comment

This case shows abnormal T2W signal intensity involving the posterior medulla in the region of the area postrema, with avid enhancement along the surface of the medulla. There is also an avidly enhancing mass along the hypothalamus and infundibulum. The imaging findings are not specific for a particular disease entity. Correlation with the patient's clinical history is essential. Differential considerations include inflammatory disorders, such as sarcoidosis, and infectious etiologies, such as tuberculosis. Neoplastic conditions such as lymphoma, and carcinomatosis from a systemic cancer, such as breast or lung carcinoma, must also be strongly considered.

Circumventricular organs, such as the area postrema and the lamina terminalis, play critical roles as transducers of information among the blood, the neurons, and the CSF. They permit both release and sensing of hormones without disrupting the blood–brain barrier and hence participate in the regulatory control of multiple bodily physiologic functions. They have a documented role in the control of cardiovascular function, the regulation of body fluids, and the mediation of the central immune response, as well as in reproduction. The area postrema is the part of the brainstem that controls vomiting. It is located in the lateral reticular formation of the medulla oblongata. It is a circumventricular organ that detects toxins in the blood and, when necessary, induces vomiting. It connects to the nucleus of the solitary tract as well as other autonomic control centers in the brainstem. It is stimulated by visceral afferent sympathetic and vagal impulses arising from peripheral trigger areas, such as the gastrointestinal tract.

Notes

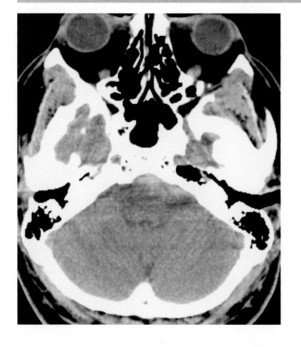

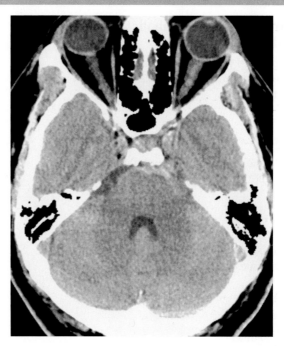

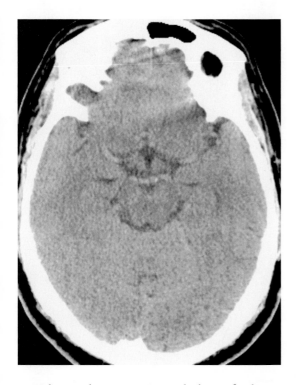

1. What is the pertinent radiologic finding?

2. What is the probability that an aneurysm will be found on catheter angiography?

3. What is believed to be the cause of this entity?

4. Fourth ventricular hemorrhage is frequently seen with what ruptured aneurysm?

Nonaneurysmal Perimesencephalic Subarachnoid Hemorrhage

1. Acute subarachnoid hemorrhage localized in the prepontine and perimesencephalic cisterns anterior to the brainstem.

2. Very low.

3. Rupture of small veins or capillaries.

4. Rupture of an aneurysm arising from the origin of the posterior inferior cerebellar artery.

PICA → 4th vent

Reference

Flaherty ML, Haverbusch M, Kissela B, et al: Perimesencephalic subarachnoid hemorrhage: incidence, risk factors and outcome, *J Stroke Cerebrovasc Dis* 14: 267–271, 2005.

Cross-Reference

Neuroradiology: THE REQUISITES, 2nd ed, pp 230–231.

Comment

Benign, nonaneurysmal subarachnoid hemorrhage with a distinct radiographic appearance was identified by van Gijn and associates in 1985. Nonaneurysmal perimesencephalic subarachnoid hemorrhage is an increasingly recognized cause of nontraumatic subarachnoid hemorrhage. These patients typically present in adulthood with an acute headache. On CT, acute subarachnoid hemorrhage is present and has a somewhat characteristic location. Specifically, hemorrhage is noted predominantly in the cisterns around the brainstem, including the prepontine, interpeduncular, and ambient cisterns. A small amount of hemorrhage may be present in the dependent portion of the sylvian cisterns. Significant intraventricular hemorrhage should not be present, and blood is not usually localized in the anterior interhemispheric fissure. Catheter angiography (which currently should still be performed, even in the presence of a characteristic localization of subarachnoid hemorrhage), shows no aneurysm. Subarachnoid hemorrhage in nonaneurysmal bleeds is believed to be related to venous or capillary rupture. In the presence of a characteristic pattern of subarachnoid hemorrhage and negative findings on high-quality conventional angiogram, follow-up angiography may not be necessary. Patients with this type of subarachnoid hemorrhage generally have an excellent prognosis.

Notes

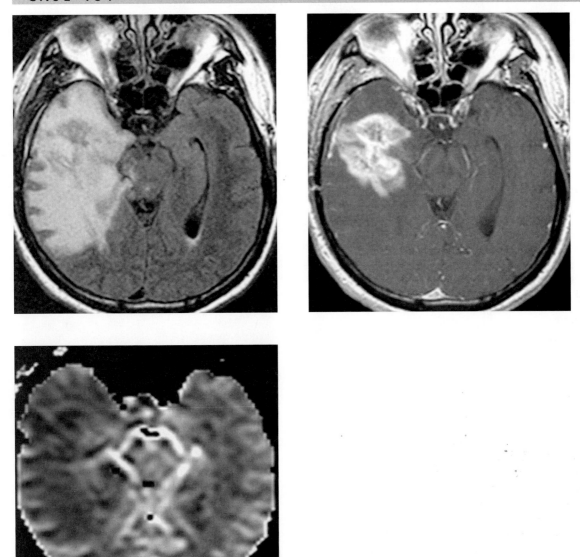

1. When is the best time to image a patient after resection of a brain tumor to assess for residual neoplasm?

2. Is hemorrhage most commonly present in early, early delayed, or late delayed radiation injury?

3. What diagnosis is favored in this patient treated previously for glioblastoma multiforme?

4. What would spectroscopy of the enhancing mass look like in this patient?

Radiation Necrosis after Treatment of High-Grade Glioma

1. Within 48 hours after surgery (before vascularized enhancing scar tissue develops).

2. Late delayed.

3. This case shows a very low relative cerebral blood volume (rCBV), consistent with radiation necrosis. Progressive neoplasm typically shows elevated rCBV in regions of enhancement.

4. Very low choline levels favoring radiation necrosis.

Reference

Mullins ME, Barest GD, Schaefer PW, Hochberg FH, Gonzalez RG, Lev MH: Radiation necrosis versus glioma recurrence: conventional MR imaging clues to diagnosis, *Am J Neuroradiol* 26:1967–1972, 2005.

Cross-Reference

Neuroradiology: THE REQUISITES, 2nd ed, pp 167–170, 584.

Comment

Magnetic resonance imaging is performed to assess for residual neoplasm in patients after brain tumor resection. Findings will determine the need for additional therapy (repeat surgery or the addition of radiation or chemotherapy). Because granulation tissue is often highly vascularized, it may enhance for months after surgery. Typically, granulation tissue develops within the first 3 days after surgery. Therefore, in patients with enhancing tumors before surgical resection, it is especially important to perform postoperative imaging within 48 hours after surgery because granulation tissue is just developing and frequently does not enhance. The finding of enhancing tissue on these initial postoperative scans should raise concern about residual neoplasm. Because T1W-hyperintense hemorrhage is usually present in the operative bed after tumor resection, it is important to compare enhanced images with unenhanced T1W images obtained in the same plane as the postcontrast images. Sequential imaging usually distinguishes residual tumor from surgical changes. Postoperative hematoma resolves, and granulation tissue typically decreases in size over time. In contrast, residual tumor grows.

In patients treated with radiation therapy after surgery, differentiation between radiation necrosis and recurrent high-grade glioma can be challenging. The conventional MR imaging characteristics of recurrent high-grade tumors and radiation necrosis overlap and include edema, mass effect, and contrast enhancement. Findings that tend to favor radiation effects over recurrent or progressive neoplasm include conversion from no enhancement to enhancement, new regions of enhancement in areas remote from the primary tumor site, and new periventricular deep white matter enhancement with poorly demarcated margins. Advanced MR imaging of enhancing regions typically shows low choline and low rCBV in the setting of radiation necrosis. When present together, findings that tend to favor progressive glioma include involvement of the corpus callosum, spread across the midline, and multiple regions of enhancement in the treated bed that have elevated choline and rCBV. In patients treated for high-grade gliomas or glioblastoma multiforme, it is important to recognize that, on a histologic level, microscopic glioma is usually present. In this case of predominant radiation necrosis with low rCBV, despite aggressive enhancement that was rapidly progressing over serial examinations, pathologic examination showed less than 5% neoplasm in the enhancing mass.

Notes

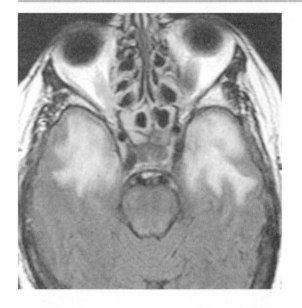
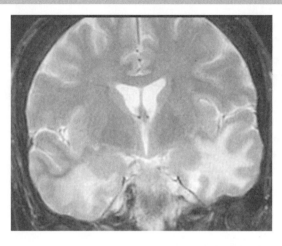
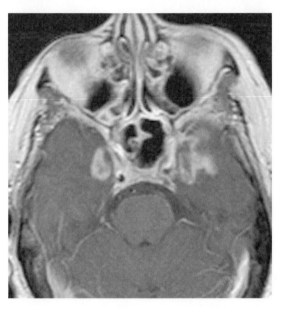
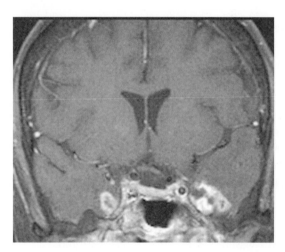

1. What is the differential diagnosis?

2. What is the diagnosis in this asymptomatic patient with a history of nasopharyngeal cancer?

3. What factors contribute to the development of this entity?

4. What is the incidence of radiation necrosis after radiosurgery for an arteriovenous malformation?

CASE 132

Radiation Necrosis after Radiation Therapy for Nasopharyngeal Cancer

1. Infection (encephalitis, abscess formation), demyelination, neoplasm, and radiation necrosis.

2. Radiation necrosis.

3. The total radiation dose, the interval over which it is given, the number and size of fractions per irradiation, patient age, and patient survival time.

4. Approximately 3% to 10%. Radiation necrosis is asymptomatic in more than 50% of these patients.

Reference

Chong VF-H, Rumpel H, Mukherji SK: Temporal lobe changes following radiation therapy: imaging and proton MR spectroscopic findings, *Eur Radiol* 11:317–324, 2001.

Cross-Reference

Neuroradiology: THE REQUISITES, 2nd ed, pp 167–169, 649–650.

Comment

This case shows the classic appearance of radiation necrosis after treatment for nasopharyngeal cancer. There is bilaterally symmetric T2W hyperintensity in the white matter of the inferior temporal lobes, with enhancement and necrosis. This patient completed radiation therapy 2 years ago. Brain changes due to radiation may be divided into those occurring early (during therapy) and those that are delayed. Delayed radiation changes may be further divided into early (within 3–4 months of therapy) and late (months to years after therapy). In early radiation injury, as well as early delayed injury, MR imaging typically shows T2W hyperintensity (edema) in the white matter that is frequently reversible. Late delayed injury is usually related to vascular injury and demyelination and appears as focal or diffuse abnormal T2W signal intensity, with mass effect and enhancement.

In the setting of arteriovenous malformations and head and neck cancers managed with radiation therapy, the diagnosis of radiation necrosis usually is not difficult to make (as long as you think of it!). However, in patients treated with radiation for primary brain tumors, the distinction between recurrent tumor and radiation necrosis may be difficult because both present as enhancing necrotic masses. Recurrent tumor often has increased activity relative to normal brain tissue on positron emission tomography, whereas radiation necrosis typically shows reduced activity. MR perfusion imaging typically shows elevated regional cerebral blood volume in tumor compared with reduced regional cerebral blood volume in necrosis. When the mass is remote from the primary tumor site, the diagnosis of radiation necrosis may be easier to establish.

Notes

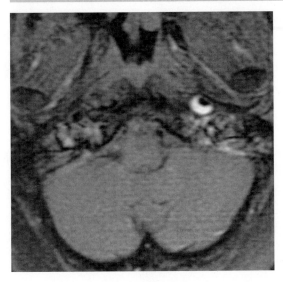 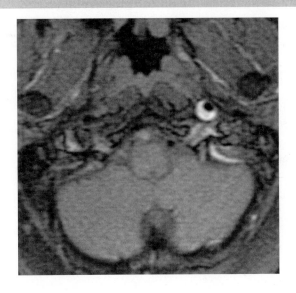

1. What structure is abnormal?

2. What is the cause of the high signal intensity around the vessel?

3. What is the advantage of acquiring noncontrast fat-suppressed T1W images?

4. How did this patient present clinically?

Internal Carotid Artery Dissection

1. The left internal carotid artery.

2. Intramural hematoma (methemoglobin).

3. With fat suppression, vascular mural blood products (which remain hyperintense) can be distinguished from perivascular fat (which saturates out).

4. With neck pain, Horner's syndrome, or transient ischemic attack or stroke.

Reference

Ozdoba C, Sturzenegger M, Schroth G: Internal carotid artery dissection: MR imaging features and clinical-radiologic correlation, *Radiology* 199:191–198, 1996.

Cross-Reference

Neuroradiology: THE REQUISITES, 2nd ed, pp 221–224.

Comment

This case illustrates the characteristic appearance of a dissection of the internal carotid artery. MR imaging shows overall enlargement of the left internal carotid artery when compared with the right due to extensive intramural hematoma (methemoglobin) that is hyperintense on unenhanced T1W images. Narrowing of the arterial lumen that is still patent as signal void (black blood), consistent with flow, is clearly present. MR imaging combined with MR angiography is sensitive for detecting vascular dissections because they allow evaluation of both the vascular lumen (like angiography) and the vessel wall and the tissues around the vascular structures. An occluded vessel can usually be differentiated from one that is narrowed but patent using a combination of conventional spin-echo MR imaging and MR angiography. It is important to acquire phase-contrast MR angiography because, with this sequence, the mural hematoma, which has high signal intensity, is nulled. The clinician may be "burned" if only time-of-flight MR angiography is used in which mural hematoma may be mistaken for flow because it remains hyperintense on this sequence.

Vascular dissections (tears in the intima that allow blood to travel in the arterial wall) may result from trauma or neck manipulation (eg, as provided by chiropractors) and are more common in patients with underlying vascular dysplasias (fibromuscular dysplasia, Marfan syndrome, Ehlers-Danlos syndrome, and cystic medial necrosis). Treatment in uncomplicated cases usually includes anticoagulation therapy and aspirin. It is important to obtain follow-up MR imaging in these patients to assess for recanalization of the vascular lumen or progressive stenosis. In addition, these patients are at increased risk for the development of pseudoaneurysms, which can be catastrophic if they go undetected and rupture. The most common complication of vascular dissection is thromboembolic disease (transient ischemic attack and stroke) that may occur days to weeks after the dissection.

Notes

* Horner syndrom

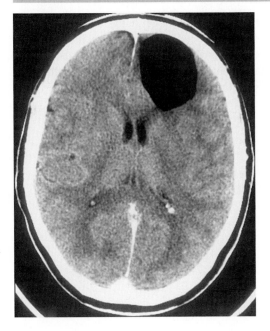 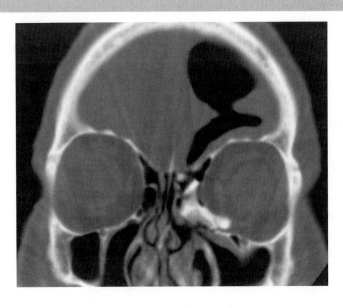

1. What underlying defects allow this condition to develop?

2. What is the most common cause of this entity?

3. This entity is most commonly described in association with what paranasal sinus tumor?

4. Intracranial air is designated as "tension pneumocephalus" under what clinical circumstance?

Tension Pneumocephalus

1. Tension pneumocephalus can develop when there is communication between the extracranial and intracranial compartments (usually there is a bone defect accompanied by a dural defect).

2. Trauma resulting in fractures of the paranasal sinuses.

3. Osteoma of the frontal sinuses or ethmoid air cells.

4. Tension pneumocephalus implies the presence of neurologic symptoms due to intracranial air that results in increased intracranial pressure.

References

Sprague A, Poulgrain P: Tension pneumocephalus: a case report and literature review, *J Clin Neurosci* 6:418–424, 1999.

Tobey JD, Loevner LA, Yousem DM, Lanza DC: Tension pneumocephalus: a complication of invasive ossifying fibroma of the paranasal sinuses, *AJR Am J Roentgenol* 166:711–713, 1996.

Cross-Reference

Neuroradiology: THE REQUISITES, 2nd ed, pp 631–632.

Comment

The term tension pneumocephalus describes the situation in which there are neurologic symptoms due to intracranial air that results in increased intracranial pressure. Symptoms are similar to those of other space-occupying lesions. Tension pneumocephalus can develop when there is communication between the extracranial and intracranial compartments (usually through a bone defect that is accompanied by a dural defect). When the intracranial pressure is lower such that the ingress of air into the intracranial compartment is favored, tension pneumocephalus may result. The most common cause of tension pneumocephalus is trauma resulting in fractures of the frontal sinuses and ethmoid air cells. It may also occur as a result of craniofacial surgery or tumors of the paranasal sinuses (most commonly described with osteomas). The pathogenesis of tension pneumocephalus is ascribed to a ball-valve mechanism. In the presence of a bony defect resulting in communication between the paranasal sinuses and anterior cranial fossa, pressure within the sinuses may transiently be increased with coughing or sneezing. In this situation, air flows from the sinuses into the lower-pressure intracranial compartment until there is equilibration of pressure. Less commonly, a negative intracranial pressure gradient, such as might be seen with a large CSF leak, may draw air into the cranial compartment.

The diagnosis of pneumocephalus is readily established with CT, which can detect very small volumes of air (reportedly as small as 0.5 mL). CT also establishes the presence of mass effect and is useful in identifying osseous defects in the cranium.

Notes

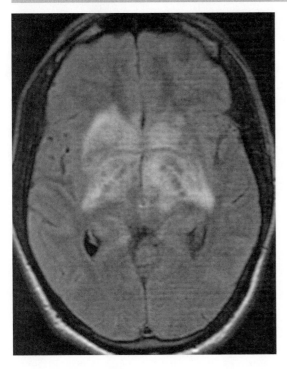 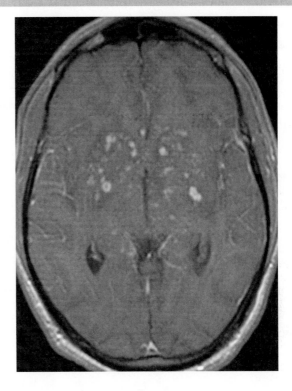

1. What fungal infections predominantly infect immunocompromised patients?

2. What fungal infections may occur in both immunocompetent and immunocompromised patients?

3. Why is there a lower incidence of both hydrocephalus and enhancement of parenchymal lesions in immunocompromised patients with CNS infections compared with immunocompetent patients with the same infections?

4. What laboratory studies may be performed to diagnose cryptococcosis?

Cryptococcosis

1. *Candida, Aspergillus,* and *Mucor.*

2. *Cryptococcus, Coccidioides,* and *Histoplasma.*

3. This likely reflects the inability of these patients to mount significant inflammatory and cell-mediated immune responses.

4. The diagnosis of cryptococcosis may be established by analysis of the CSF with India ink, detection of cryptococcal antigen, or positive findings on fungal cultures.

Reference

Kovoor JM, Mahadevan A, Narayan JP, Govindappa SS, Satishchandra P, Taly AV: Cryptococcal choroid plexitis as a mass lesion: MR imaging and histopathologic correlation, *AJNR Am J Neuroradiol* 23:273–276, 2002.

Cross-Reference

Neuroradiology: THE REQUISITES, 2nd ed, pp 311–312.

Comment

This case shows high signal intensity in the bilateral basal ganglia and thalami which is somewhat bilaterally symmetric. Buried within the flair hyperintensity are small focal regions of hypointensity within the deep gray matter with associated enhancement on the gadolinium enhanced T1-weighted image. In addition, to a lesser degree regions of parenchymal abnormality with enhancement at the gray-white matter interface in the cerebrum were also present as was mild communicating hydrocephalus [images not shown].

In this case enhancement is present. However, in patients with human immunodeficiency virus (HIV) infection, there can be a paucity of enhancement related to the inability to mount an inflammatory reaction which is related to the severity of the immunodeficient state of the patient. The CT and MR imaging findings are often nonspecific and one may not be able to distinguish among the various fungal infections, as well as toxoplasmosis and tuberculosis. Lymphoma in the setting of AIDS must also be considered.

Fungal infection in the CNS results in granulomatous changes that may affect the intracranial vasculature, meninges, and/or brain parenchyma. In patients with cryptococcosis, CT and MR imaging may be normal. Alternatively, a spectrum of imaging findings may occur, including dilated perivascular spaces; parenchymal cryptococcomas (more common in the deep gray matter of the basal ganglia and thalami than in the cerebral cortex); and, less commonly, miliary disease with parenchymal, leptomeningeal, and intraventricular nodules.

When infection spreads along the perivascular (Virchow-Robin) spaces that accompany perforating arteries, these perivascular spaces may become distended with mucoid, gelatinous material that is made by the organism's capsule.

Large accumulations of organisms and gelatinous material have been referred to as *gelatinous pseudocysts.* The diagnosis of CNS cryptococcosis may be established by analysis of the CSF with Indian ink, detection of cryptococcal antigen, and/or positive fungal cultures.

Notes

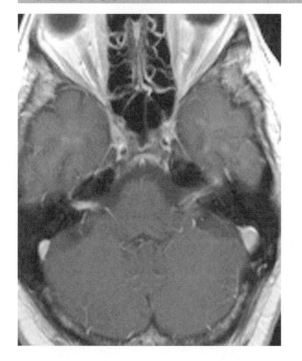 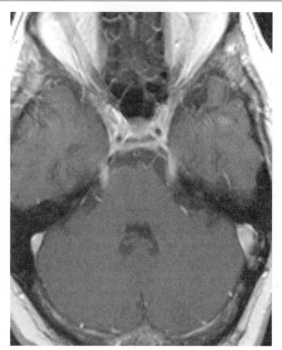

1. What are the major imaging findings?

2. What is the differential diagnosis?

3. What are the most common extracranial malignancies to involve the leptomeninges?

4. Blockage of the basal cisterns and arachnoid villi may result in what condition?

Subarachnoid Seeding—Leptomeningeal Carcinomatosis

1. Leptomeningeal enhancement bilaterally along cranial nerve V (trigeminal nerves) in the pontine cistern, and in the bilateral internal auditory canals.

2. Carcinomatous meningitis, CSF subarachnoid seeding from a primary CNS malignancy, inflammatory or granulomatous disease (sarcoidosis, tuberculosis), and infectious meningitis.

3. Leukemia, lymphoma, adenocarcinomas (particularly of the breast and lung), and melanoma.

4. Obstructive communicating hydrocephalus.

Reference

Tsuchiya K, Katase S, Yoshino A, Hachiya J: FLAIR MR imaging for diagnosing intracranial meningeal carcinomatosis, *AJR Am J Roentgenol* 176:1585–1588, 2001.

Cross-Reference

Neuroradiology: THE REQUISITES, 2nd ed, pp 109–111.

Comment

Leptomeningeal carcinomatosis is a relatively uncommon presentation of metastatic disease to the CNS in patients with extracranial malignancies. Carcinomatous meningitis is reported in approximately 2% to 3% of patients with such malignancies; however, as treatment for cancer improves and patients live longer, it is likely that the incidence of subarachnoid seeding from systemic malignancies will increase. Patients may present with nonspecific symptoms, including headache and meningeal signs; however, they may also present with cranial neuropathies and symptoms related to obstructive communicating hydrocephalus. Histologic examination of leptomeningeal spread typically shows metastatic cellular infiltrates within the subarachnoid space.

Contrast-enhanced CT is insensitive for the detection of leptomeningeal spread. Contrast-enhanced MR imaging is currently the imaging modality of choice for detecting subarachnoid seeding; however, it is not always sensitive either. Lumbar puncture to obtain CSF for cytologic evaluation for malignant cells remains the gold standard for diagnosing carcinomatous meningitis (serial punctures may be necessary).

In this case of multiple myeloma, enhancement can be seen within the internal auditory canals bilaterally, particularly on the right. In addition, there is bilateral enhancement of the cisternal portions of cranial nerve V. In hematologic malignancies, such as leukemia and lymphoma, spread is usually directly to the leptomeninges. In systemic cancers, such as lung and breast carcinoma, although spread may occur directly to the meninges, frequently, subarachnoid seeding may be the result of rupture of superficial cerebral metastasis into the subarachnoid space. In patients with carcinomatous meningitis, enhancement may be seen along the perivascular spaces within the brain parenchyma and along the ependymal surface of the ventricles.

Notes

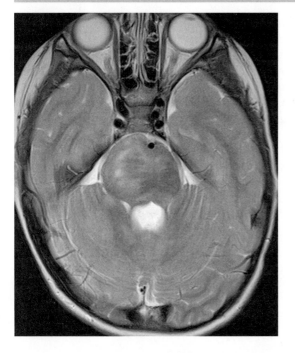 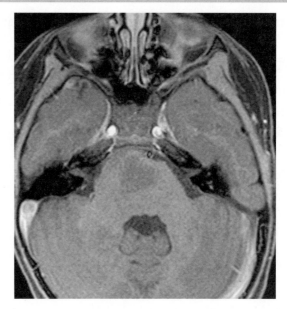

1. What part of the brainstem is most commonly affected with this entity?

2. What is the most common histologic subtype?

3. What is the typical location of a posterior fossa ependymoma?

4. What is the differential diagnosis of a brainstem mass in a child?

Brainstem Astrocytoma

1. The pons.

2. Diffuse fibrillary subtype.

3. The fourth ventricle.

4. The differential diagnosis includes astrocytoma; non-neoplastic diseases, such as demyelinating disease (acute disseminated encephalomyelitis), rhomboencephalitis, and tuberculosis (more common outside the United States); and lymphoma. Exophytic and enhancing masses can mimic medulloblastoma or ependymoma.

Reference

Young Poussaint T, Yousuf N, Barnes PD, Anthony DC, Zurakowski D, Scott RM: Cervicomedullary astrocytomas of childhood: clinical and imaging follow-up, *Pediatr Radiol* 29:662–668, 1999.

Cross-Reference

Neuroradiology: THE REQUISITES, 2nd ed, pp 121–122.

Comment

This case shows the characteristic appearance of a low-grade brainstem astrocytoma, including high signal intensity within the pons on T2W images. It also shows marked expansion of the brainstem, most notably the pons, but also extending exophytically into the prepontine cistern and around the basilar artery (note effacement of the prepontine cistern and invagination [encasement] of the basilar artery). The enhancement pattern of brainstem gliomas is quite variable, ranging from regions of avid nodular enhancement to minimal or no enhancement (as in this case).

Approximately 80% of brainstem gliomas occur during childhood. Brainstem neoplasms are uncommon, accounting for 10% to 15% of CNS tumors in children, with a peak age at presentation of less than 14 years. Most are gliomas, including slow-growing fibrillary or pilocytic astrocytoma, malignant astrocytoma, and glioblastoma multiforme. Most tumors are of the diffuse fibrillary subtype; however, more than half of them eventually show regions of anaplastic transformation and have a poor long-term prognosis. These tumors may initially infiltrate the brainstem without tissue destruction, and few deficits may be present, despite extensive disease. Presenting symptoms include cranial nerve deficits, motor or sensory deficits, ataxia, abnormal eye movements, somnolence, and hyperactivity. Hydrocephalus is a late finding, with the exception of tumors arising in immediate proximity to the aqueduct.

Magnetic resonance imaging is the imaging modality of choice for evaluation of brainstem abnormalities. Its multiplanar capabilities, improved resolution, and relative absence of scanning artifacts frequently present on CT scans, have resulted in improved detection of abnormalities in the posterior fossa. In addition, MR imaging is useful for planning radiation therapy. Because of the infiltrative nature and characteristic location of brainstem astrocytomas, radiation therapy remains the main therapeutic option. In cases in which tumor is exophytic, the exophytic portion can often be resected.

Notes

- glioma
- lymphoma
- infection, TB
- inflammation ADEM

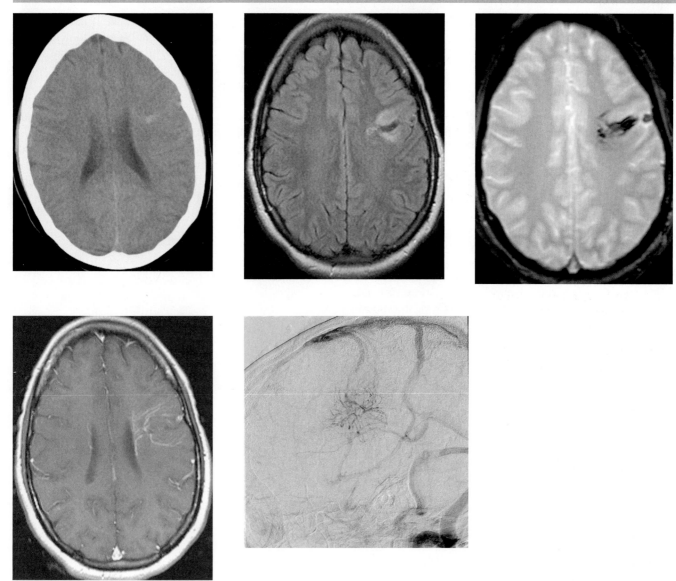

1. What is the best diagnosis in this postpartum patient with seizure?

2. What systemic disorders are associated with a hypercoagulable state and venous thrombosis?

3. What is the most serious complication associated with venous thrombosis?

4. Developmental venous anomalies (DVAs) in what part of the intracranial compartment are associated with a slightly higher incidence of hemorrhage?

CASE 138

Thrombosis of a Developmental Venous Anomaly—Postpartum

1. Thrombosis of the main vein of a developmental venous anomaly.

2. Dehydration, deficiency of antithrombin-III or protein C or S, nephrotic syndrome, use of oral contraceptives, circulating antiphospholipid antibodies, homocystinuria, L-asparaginase, underlying malignancy, pregnancy, postpartum state, and infections (meningitis, sinusitis, otomastoiditis).

3. Hemorrhagic venous infarction.

4. The posterior fossa.

Reference

Masson C, Godefroy O, Leclerc X, Colombani JM, Leys D: Cerebral venous infarction following thrombosis of the draining vein of a venous angioma (developmental abnormality), *Cerebrovasc Dis* 10:235–238, 2000.

Cross-Reference

Neuroradiology: THE REQUISITES, 2nd ed, pp 131–132, 219–220.

Comment

This case shows acute thrombosis of the main draining vein of a large left frontal lobe developmental venous anomaly (venous angioma) in a 27-year-old postpartum woman who presented with new-onset seizure shortly after childbirth. The CT scan shows serpentine high density within the main trunk of the DVA that extends down to the margin of the left lateral ventricle. The appearance of the area of high density is not that of acute subarachnoid hemorrhage or primary parenchymal hemorrhage. The FLAIR images show high signal intensity in the adjacent left frontal lobe that did not show restricted diffusion, consistent with edema around a small amount of parenchymal hemorrhage. The enhanced MR images show the characteristic appearance of a DVA, as does the delayed venous phase of the patient's conventional cerebral angiogram.

Venous thrombosis is underdiagnosed because of lack of consideration. It has many clinical presentations, including headache and papilledema related to increased intracranial pressure, as well as focal neurologic deficits and seizures in cases complicated by intraparenchymal hemorrhage, edema, or venous infarction. In the differential diagnosis of intracerebral hemorrhage, in the absence of known risk factors (eg, trauma or hypertension), it is important to consider venous thrombosis complicated by venous infarction.

Developmental venous anomalies are usually incidental lesions that are clinically silent because they are low-flow, low-pressure vascular malformations that drain normal brain. The annual bleeding risk associated with a venous angioma is approximately 0.20% per year. The bleeding risk is slightly higher with DVAs located in the posterior fossa, and in relation to pregnancy. Even when they occasionally bleed, management is usually conservative. Rarely reported is thrombosis of the main trunk of these malformations, with management in some cases being observation, whereas in other cases, anticoagulation therapy is administered.

Notes

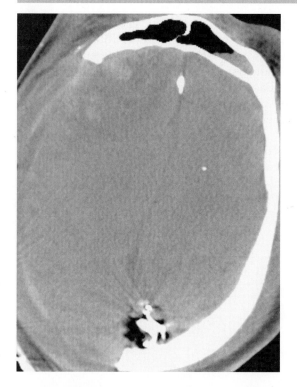

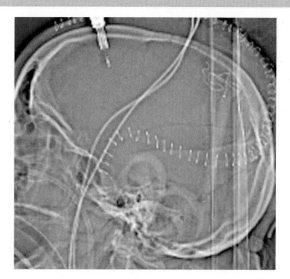

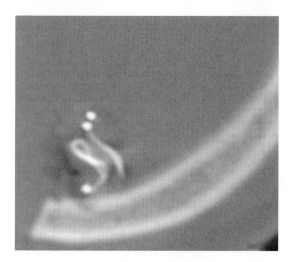

1. What is the surgical mishap here?

2. For significant brownie points, what are the official medical terms for this entity (truly Greek to me!)?

3. What kind of foreign body reactions can occur?

4. What may these foreign body reactions be mistaken for on CT or MR imaging?

Textiloma or Gossypiboma—Retained Surgical Sponge

1. Retained surgical sponge.

2. Textilomas or gossypibomas.

3. An aseptic fibrous reaction that results in granuloma formation, or an exudative reaction that leads to abscess formation.

4. Brain tumors.

References

Okten AL, Adam M, Gezercan Y: Textiloma: a case of foreign body mimicking a spinal mass, *Eur Spine J* 15:626–629, 2006.

Ribalta T, McCutcheon IE, Neto AG, et al: Textiloma (gossypiboma) mimicking recurrent intracranial tumor, *Arch Pathol Lab Med* 128:749–758, 2004.

Cross-Reference

Neuroradiology: THE REQUISITES, 2nd ed, pp 282–287.

Comment

A variety of hemostatic agents are routinely used to control intraoperative bleeding in many surgical subspecialties, including neurosurgery. Nonresorbable materials include various forms of cotton pledgets and cloth (such as muslin) and synthetic rayon hemostats (cottonoids and kites). These agents are removed before surgical closure, except in the case of muslin, which may be used to repair or reinforce intracranial aneurysms. Hemostatic agents can be mistakenly left behind during operations. Such foreign materials cause foreign body reaction in the surrounding tissue (called textilomas or gossypibomas).

Cottonoids and kites are synthetic strips and pledgets composed of rayon fibers that contain a filament or strip impregnated with radio-opaque barium sulfate that is visible on plain film radiographs and CT scans, as in this case. Complications caused by these foreign bodies are well known, but cases are rarely published because of medicolegal implications. Some textilomas cause infection or abscess formation in the early stage, whereas others remain clinically silent for many years. Such foreign bodies can often mimic tumors or abscesses clinically or radiologically. There are reports of other hemostatic materials (Gelfoam [Pfizer, New York, NY], Surgicel [Johnson & Johnson, New Brunswick, NJ) causing foreign body reactions that cannot be distinguished from recurrent tumors on MR imaging. The MR imaging appearance of foreign materials left behind during surgery can differ, depending on the type of material left behind, the time elapsed since surgery, and the type of foreign body reaction that occurs. There are two types of foreign body reactions: (1) aseptic fibrous reaction, which involves adhesion formation, or encapsulation; and (2) granuloma formation, or an exudative reaction, which leads to abscess formation.

It is possible to overlook cotton and gauze pads in the surgical field. Such materials should always have a tag that allows them to be easily located and removed, and all materials that are placed in the wound temporarily must be counted with meticulous care. Once hemostasis is achieved, the operative site should be flushed with saline and carefully examined for foreign materials.

Notes

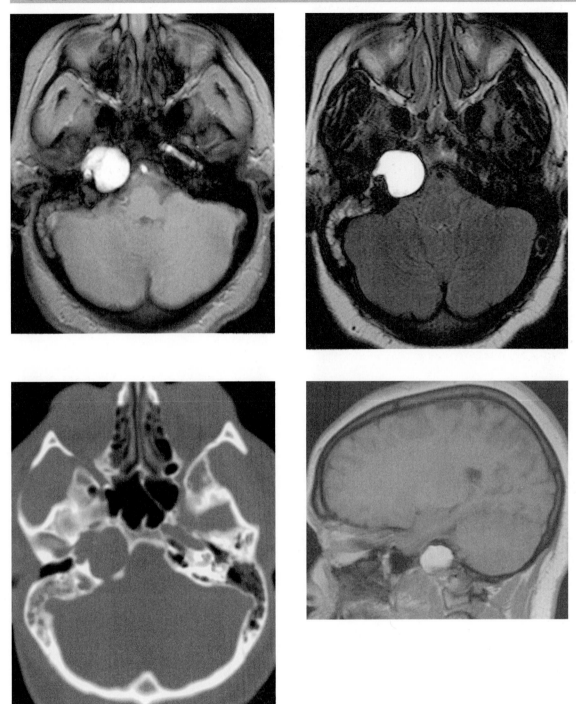

1. The presence of calcification is often indicative of what type of lesions?

2. What portion of the temporal bone is located directly behind the horizontal petrous internal carotid artery?

3. What is the etiology of this lesion?

4. The presence of fluid–fluid levels, especially on T2W images, is usually indicative of what lesion?

CASE 140

Petrous Apex Cholesterol Granuloma

1. Chondroid lesions, such as chondrosarcomas or chondromas.

2. The petrous apex.

3. Recurrent microhemorrhages due to rupture of small blood vessels within the petrous air cells as a result of negative pressure gradients.

4. Cholesterol granuloma.

References

Chang P, Fagan PA, Atlas MD, Roche J: Imaging destructive lesions of the petrous apex, *Laryngoscope* 108: 599–604, 1998.

Palacios E, Valvassori G: Petrous apex lesions: cholesterol granuloma, *Ear Nose Throat J* 78:234, 1999.

Cross-Reference

Neuroradiology: THE REQUISITES, 2nd ed, pp 600–602.

Comment

Cholesterol granulomas, also known as blue-domed or chocolate cysts, typically arise in the petrous apex. They are believed to be due to chronic obstruction of previously pneumatized petrous air cells, resulting in negative pressure within them. As a result of these negative pressure gradients, there are recurrent microhemorrhages caused by rupture of small blood vessels. A foreign body reaction involving the mucosal lining of the petrous air cells occurs, with giant cell proliferation and a fibroblastic reaction, as well as deposition of cholesterol crystals within the cyst. These are reportedly more common in the setting of chronic otomastoiditis, although this has not necessarily been my experience or observation. On CT, these lesions typically have a benign appearance that manifests as an expansile mass lesion with demarcated margins, as in this case involving the right petrous apex. Cholesterol granulomas, when large enough, may be multilobular. There is usually thinning of the cortex with large lesions; however, there is no bony destruction. On MR imaging, cholesterol granulomas are hyperintense on all pulse sequences. In particular, the marked hyperintensity on unenhanced T1W images is classic, distinguishing it from many other lesions, and the presence of hemorrhage–fluid levels within these lesions is highly characteristic. Normal fat may occur in the petrous apex and, because it is hyperintense on both T1W and fast spin-echo T2W imaging, may be mistaken for a cholesterol granuloma. This error can be avoided by obtaining fat-saturated T1W images in which fat will lose signal, but the cholesterol granuloma will continue to glow!

The differential diagnosis of a benign-appearing expansile petrous apex mass includes cholesterol granuloma, mucocele, and epidermoid cyst. Mucoceles are frequently unilocular and show peripheral enhancement. The signal characteristics of mucoceles will vary, depending on the protein concentration and viscosity within them, as well as the cross-linking of glycoproteins. Epidermoid cysts may have a benign appearance, but can have more concerning radiologic findings, such as bone erosion or destruction. They are typically similar to CSF on T1W and T2W images, are hyperintense on FLAIR imaging, and show restricted diffusion. Less common and more aggressive "cystic-appearing" masses that may involve the petrous apex include hemorrhagic metastases and plasmacytoma and multiple myeloma.

Notes

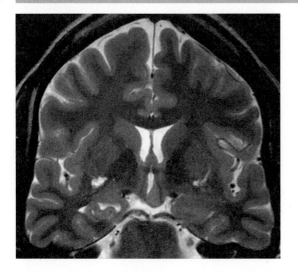 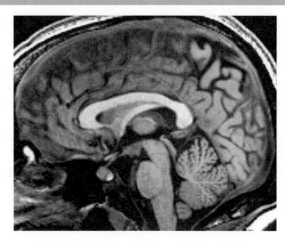

1. Where anatomically is the lesion located?

2. What is the typical clinical presentation of this lesion?

3. What is the typical imaging appearance of this entity?

4. What is the differential diagnosis?

Hamartoma of the Hypothalamus

1. At the tuber cinereum (floor of the third ventricle), anterior to the mammillary bodies.

2. Precocious puberty and gelastic seizures.

3. These lesions usually follow the signal characteristics of gray matter on T1W imaging, but may be isointense or hyperintense on FLAIR and T2W imaging. They typically do not enhance.

4. Hypothalamic glioma; however, the anatomic location of a tuber cinereum hamartoma, its imaging appearance, and the clinical history usually allow correct diagnosis.

References

Freeman JL, Coleman LT, Wellard RM, et al: MR imaging and spectroscopic study of epileptogenic hypothalamic hamartomas: analysis of 72 cases, *AJNR Am J Neuroradiol* 25:450–462, 2004.

Saleem SN, Said AHM, Lee DH: Lesions of the hypothalamus: MR imaging diagnostic features, *RadioGraphics* 27:1087–1108, 2007.

Cross-Reference

Neuroradiology: THE REQUISITES, 2nd ed, pp 548, 550.

Comment

The hypothalamus may be affected by a spectrum of pathology, including developmental lesions, primary tumors, systemic tumors that involve the CNS (such as lymphoma), vascular malformations, and inflammatory processes, including granulomatous disease. MR imaging findings, combined with the patient's clinical presentation and age, are usually able to distinguish among the differential possibilities.

This case illustrates a characteristic appearance of a hypothalamic hamartoma at the tuber cinereum. The mass is mildly hypointense relative to gray matter on T1W imaging, is isointense to gray matter on T2W imaging, and sits just anterior to the mammary bodies at the level of the floor of the third ventricle. Mild T2W hyperintensity relative to gray matter, absence of contrast enhancement, and stability in lesion size are the classic MR imaging findings of these hamartomas. MR imaging and spectroscopy (reduced *N*-acetylaspartate and increased myoinositol) suggest decreased neuronal density and gliosis in these lesions compared with normal gray matter. Hamartomas are benign nonneoplastic lesions that are likely congenital. Many are asymptomatic, but symptoms may be more common in children and with larger lesions, and typically include gelastic seizures ("fits of laughter") and central precocious puberty. Knowledge of this lesion and its radiologic and clinical presentations allows the diagnosis to be established in most cases. Occasionally, atypical imaging findings (marked hyperintensity on T2W imaging or lesions larger than 2.5 cm) raise the possibility of a hypothalamic glioma. In such cases, follow-up imaging at several-month intervals can be obtained (hamartomas should not grow).

Notes

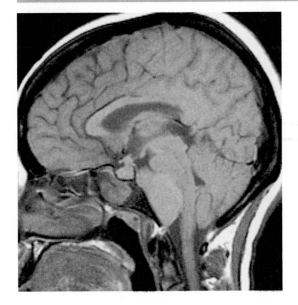

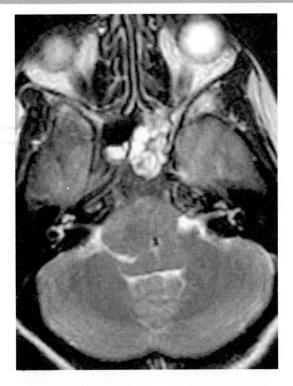

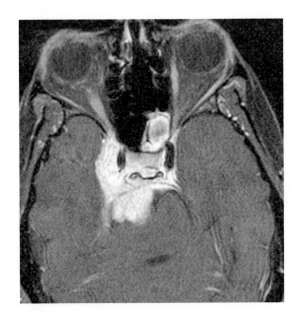

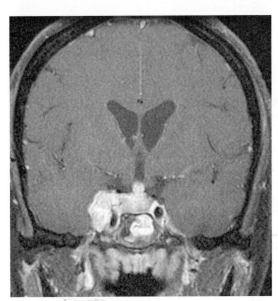

1. What are the main diagnostic considerations in this 24-year-old patient?

2. What imaging finding makes meningioma less likely?

3. CNS involvement is found in what percentage of patients?

4. What cranial nerves course through the cavernous sinus?

Hodgkin's Disease—Dural Based

1. Neoplasms, including meningioma, lymphoma, and much less commonly, metastatic disease. Inflammatory conditions, such as sarcoidosis, are also strong considerations.

2. There is a mass along the pituitary stalk or infundibulum.

3. Approximately 5% to 15%.

4. Cranial nerves III, IV, V (first and second divisions), and VI.

References

Ghofrani M, Tantiwongkosi B, Smith AS, Wasdahl DA: Richter transformation of chronic lymphocytic leukemia presenting as a dural-based non-Hodgkin lymphoma, *AJNR Am J Neuroradiol* 28:318–320, 2007.

Roman-Goldstein S, Jones A, Delashaw JB, McMenomey S, Neuwelt EA: Atypical central nervous system lymphoma at the cranial base: report of four cases, *Neurosurgery* 43:613–615, 1998.

Cross-Reference

Neuroradiology: THE REQUISITES, 2nd ed, pp 109–110, 153–157.

Comment

These images show an extra-axial mass in the prepontine cistern that is isointense to brain parenchyma on T2W imaging. Neoplastic processes that may be hypointense on T2W imaging include meningioma, lymphoma, and less commonly, plasmacytoma and metastases. Sarcoid may also be hypointense on T2W imaging. The mass enhances intensely and homogeneously, and it extends into the right cavernous sinus. Another important imaging finding is diffuse hypointensity of the clivus, which may be seen with meningioma, lymphoma (corresponding sclerosis on CT scan is more common with Hodgkin's disease), sarcoid, and metastatic disease. A salient finding is that there is a mass along the pituitary stalk or infundibulum that makes granulomatous diseases, such as sarcoid and lymphoma, more suspect in this 24-year-old patient. In this case, a steroid trial resulted in significant reduction in the size of the mass, and surgical biopsy showed Hodgkin's disease.

Dural-based metastases usually spread along the dura as a result of hematogenous dissemination. Dural involvement may also occur secondary to extraosseous spread of bone metastases. Much less commonly, a brain metastasis may spread to the dura. Common causes of dural metastases include lung, breast, and prostate carcinoma as well as melanoma. Breast carcinoma is the most common neoplasm associated with dural metastases, followed by lymphoma, which is unique in that dural lymphoma may be the primary source of neoplasm. This case is unusual in that the vast majority of dural-based lymphoma is non-Hodgkin's lymphoma, but this case represents a rare instance of Hodgkin's disease. In children, the most common causes of dural metastases are adrenal neuroblastoma and leukemia. Inflammatory lesions that can mimic dural metastases include sarcoidosis, Langerhans' cell histiocytosis, and Erdheim-Chester disease. Dural-based disease may be the predominant imaging finding and may be mistaken for a meningioma, as in this case!

Notes

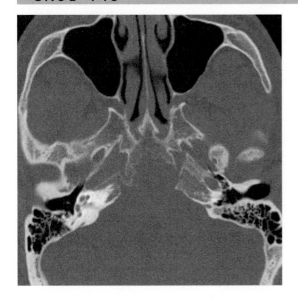

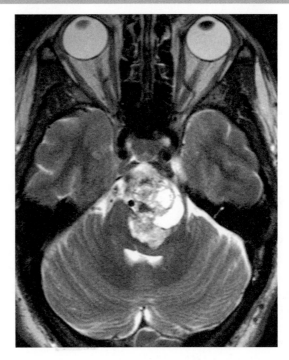

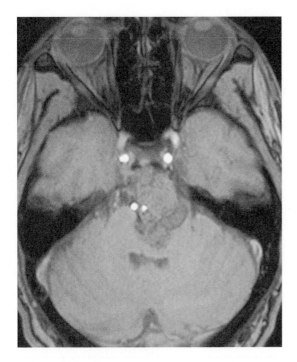

1. What was this patient's clinical presentation?

2. Notochordal remnants give rise to what type of tumor?

3. Chordomas are most frequently found in what location?

4. Although histologically benign, what two tumors may have distant metastases?

Clival Chordoma

1. Palsy of cranial nerve VI.

2. Chordoma.

3. The sacrum (50%).

4. Giant cell tumors and chordomas.

Reference

Erdem E, Angtuaco EC, Van Henert R, Park JS, Al-Mefty O: Comprehensive review of intracranial chordoma, *Radio-Graphics* 23:995–1009, 2003.

Cross-Reference

Neuroradiology: THE REQUISITES, 2nd ed, pp 560, 603, 734, 828–829.

Comment

Chordomas arise in locations where notochordal remnants are found. They occur most commonly in the sacrum (50%), followed by the clivus (35%) and the spine, especially the upper cervical spine (C1–2) [15%]. Although chordomas are considered benign neoplasms, based on their histologic appearance, they grow quite invasively, particularly at the skull base, where they can invade foramina or the cavernous sinus or extend into the posterior and middle cranial fossa. Like giant cell tumors, chordomas may metastasize in a small percentage of patients. CT and MR imaging play complimentary roles in assessing tumors of the base of the skull. On CT, calcification is seen in 50% of cases, and regions of bone erosion or destruction are clearly delineated. Multiplanar MR imaging allows complete evaluation of the extent of the lesion. On MR imaging, the signal characteristics of chordomas are variable. These tumors are typically hypointense to isointense to brain on T1W imaging and are normally hyperintense on T2W imaging. There may be marked heterogeneity due to cellularity, vascularity, or calcification. Most chordomas enhance, although some predominantly cystic tumors have minimal enhancement. In my experience, tumors arising at the C1–2 region have been associated with less enhancement and more cystic-type changes.

The differential diagnosis includes chondroid lesions (chondrosarcoma), metastatic disease, multiple myeloma, and lymphoma. The presence of a calcified matrix usually limits the differential diagnosis to chordoma versus chondrosarcoma. In my experience and as the literature indicates, it may be difficult to distinguish these two entities. Chordomas tend to be midline lesions, whereas chondrosarcomas tend to be more lateral. Clinical symptoms of chordomas and chondrosarcomas may be quite similar at the skull base, including headache and cranial neuropathies (frequently affecting cranial nerve VI).

Clinical presentation is usually in the second through fourth decades of life.

Notes

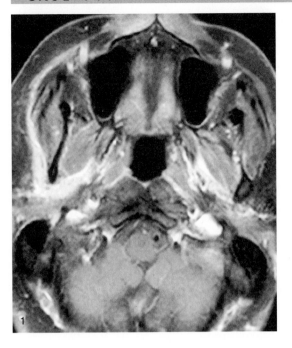

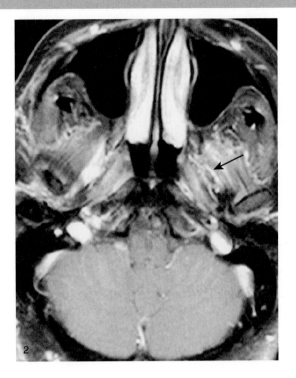

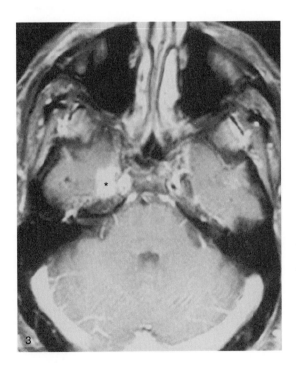

1. What is the diagnosis?

2. What cranial nerves is tumor tracking along?

3. What primary tumor of the salivary glands is notorious for its propensity for perineural spread?

4. What branch of cranial nerve V transmits tumor to Meckel's cave through the foramen ovale?

Perineural Spread of Skin Cancer—Basal Cell Carcinoma

1. Perineural spread of tumor, in this case, skin cancer.

2. Cranial nerves V (trigeminal) and VII (facial).

3. Adenoid cystic carcinoma, which has perineural spread in 50% of cases.

4. The auriculotemporal branch.

Reference

Ginsberg LE, Eicher SA: Great auricular nerve: anatomy and imaging in a case of perineural tumor spread, *Am J Neuroradiol* 21:568–571, 2000.

Cross-Reference

Neuroradiology: THE REQUISITES, 2nd ed, pp 698–699, 710–711.

Comment

This case illustrates a classic appearance of perineural spread of skin carcinoma (basal cell carcinoma in this patient). The patient, who had previously had a skin cancer removed from his right cheek, presented with new facial numbness, fasciculations, and mild facial weakness. The first image shows prominent enhancement of right cranial nerve VII tracking from superficial fibers along the cheek into the parotid gland. In addition to cranial nerve VII, the parotid gland may also contain branches of the auriculotemporal rami of the third division of cranial nerve V. As seen in this case, tumor may spread along branches of the auriculotemporal nerve, through the foramen ovale (*arrow* on the normal left side), and into Meckel's cave (*). In the third image, note the enhancement of the right facial nerve in the temporal bone, including the labyrinthine portion that takes tumor to the fundus of the internal auditory canal.

Perineural spread of tumor represents tracking of tumor along nerve sheaths, frequently discontinuous and remote from the site of the primary neoplasm. It occurs with a spectrum of tumors, including skin cancer (basal cell and desmoplastic melanoma are notorious for this tendency, but squamous cell carcinoma is common and may also have perineural spread); squamous cell carcinoma of the head and neck (in particular, nasopharyngeal cancer); primary salivary neoplasms (most notably, adenoid cystic carcinoma); lymphoma in the periorbital region; and other skull base neoplasms. Because perineural spread of tumor may not be symptomatic, the radiologist must always be on the hunt for this in appropriate clinical scenarios. Perineural spread is a poor prognostic indicator. Lesions believed to be resectable for cure may be deemed unresectable. Radiation fields may need to be expanded.

Notes

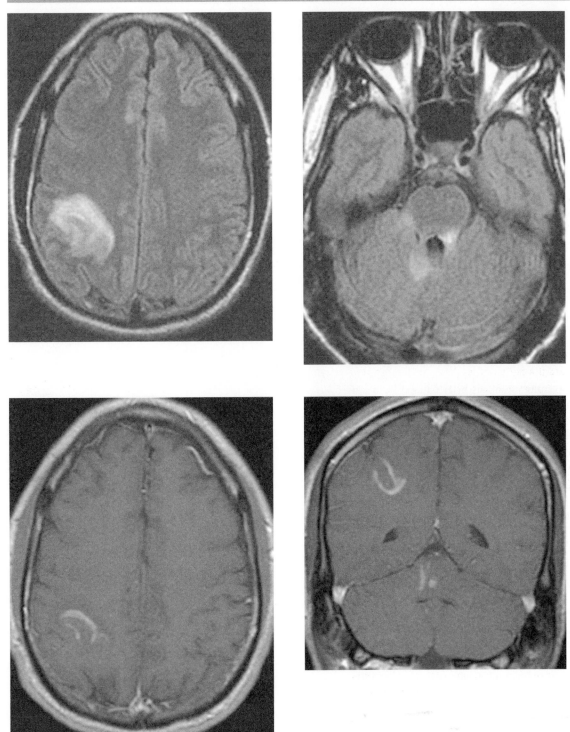

1. What is the differential diagnosis?

2. What is the most common presenting cranial nerve palsy in multiple sclerosis?

3. What is the most common presenting cranial neuropathy in Lyme disease?

4. What is the most common MR imaging finding in patients with Lyme disease?

Central Nervous System Lyme Disease

1. Demyelinating disease, vasculitis, infectious disease (Lyme disease, syphilis [*Treponema pallidum*]), and other inflammatory processes, such as neurosarcoid.

2. Optic neuritis.

3. Bell's palsy (cranial nerve VII, the facial nerve).

4. Normal findings.

Reference

Charles V, Duprez TP, Kabamba B, Ivanolu A, Sindic CJ: Poliomyelitis-like syndrome with matching magnetic resonance features in a case of Lyme neuroborreliosis, *J Neurol Neurosurg Psychiatry* 78:1160–1161, 2007.

Cross-Reference

Neuroradiology: THE REQUISITES, 2nd ed, pp 309–311, 344.

Comment

Lyme disease is a multisystem disorder caused by a spirochetal (*Borrelia burgdorferi*) infection that is transmitted most commonly by the deer tick (*Ixodes dammini*). The characteristic initial bull's-eye skin lesion (erythema chronicum migrans) is pathognomonic of this infection and is the typical presentation of the first of the three recorded clinical stages. In this clinical stage, the rash is usually accompanied by constitutional symptoms, including myalgia, headache, and low-grade fevers. Stage II disease is characterized by disseminated infection and is normally manifest by neurologic and cardiac abnormalities. Stage II typically occurs weeks to months after the initial infection. In stage III (persistent infection), patients usually present with neurologic (meningitic) or rheumatologic symptoms months to years after infection. Neurologic manifestations may develop in up to 15% of patients with Lyme disease and include cranial neuropathies (especially Bell's palsy), meningitis, cerebellar findings, ophthalmic involvement (conjunctivitis, keratitis, and ocular inflammation), or encephalopathy, with memory loss and cognitive disorders. The diagnosis of Lyme disease is made based on clinical presentation and serologic findings. Treatment is with antibiotics.

The findings on MR imaging may include multiple periventricular and subcortical white matter–hyperintense lesions on T2W images. The subcortical white matter of the frontal and parietal lobes may be preferentially affected. Contrast enhancement of the white matter lesions, meninges, or cranial nerves may be seen. Focal lesions in the deep gray matter (basal ganglia, thalami), brainstem (pons), and hydrocephalus have also been reported.

Notes

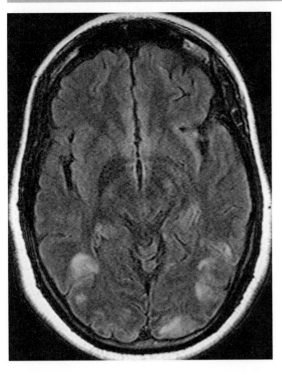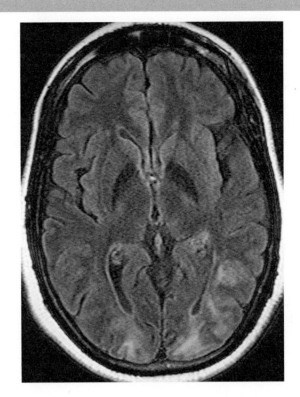

1. What is the most common cause of this entity in women?

2. What areas of the brain are particularly susceptible to the changes of hypertension?

3. What are the most common imaging findings in hypertensive encephalopathy?

4. What was this patient's clinical presentation?

Reversible Posterior Leukoencephalopathy

1. Pregnancy-related hypertension (toxemia or eclampsia).

2. The cerebellum and occipital lobes (posterior circulation).

3. CT shows low attenuation in areas of involvement, whereas T2W images show increased signal intensity within the cortex and subcortical white matter that is frequently bilateral and symmetric. The occipital and parietal lobes are most often affected.

4. Seizures and headaches.

Reference

Casey SO, Sampaio RC, Michel E, Truwit CL: Posterior reversible encephalopathy syndrome: utility of fluid-attenuated inversion recovery MR imaging in the detection of cortical and subcortical lesions, *AJNR Am J Neuroradiol* 21:1199–1206, 2000.

Cross-Reference

Neuroradiology: THE REQUISITES, 2nd ed, pp 206, 354–356.

Comment

The images show foci of increased signal intensity within the subcortical white matter (and cortex) that is predominantly in the occipital lobes; however, regions of signal alteration are also present in the parietal lobes. This case shows many of the typical imaging manifestations of reversible posterior leukoencephalopathy. The posterior circulation is more sensitive to the changes of accelerated hypertension. This may be related to a difference in sympathetic innervation (sparse innervation by sympathetic nerves). One theory is that the normal autoregulatory control of the cerebral vasculature that allows continuous perfusion over a range of blood pressures is exceeded. This may result in engorgement of the distal cerebral vessels, with hyperperfusion and breakdown of the blood–brain barrier. Signal abnormalities may represent reversible vasogenic edema. The imaging findings, in combination with the patient's clinical presentation (elevated blood pressure associated with progressive neurologic symptoms, including change in mental status, headache, blurred vision, seizures, and focal neurologic deficits), allow the correct diagnosis. Both the symptoms and the radiologic findings may be reversible with treatment of the elevated blood pressure.

In addition to foci of abnormal signal intensity at the gray–white matter interface in the occipital and parietal lobes, the frontal and temporal lobes may be affected, as may the cerebellum and pons. Enhancement in regions of signal abnormality may be observed. Acute hemorrhage may be present, although this is less common.

Similar, potentially reversible changes may occur with the use of intravenous drugs, such as cocaine; in patients treated with chemotherapeutic agents (cytosine arabinoside, methotrexate, cisplatin); in those undergoing radiation therapy; and in patients with eclampsia.

Notes

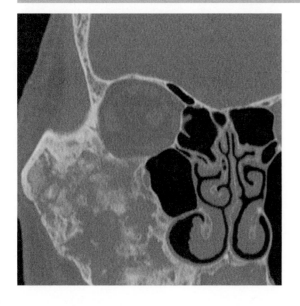
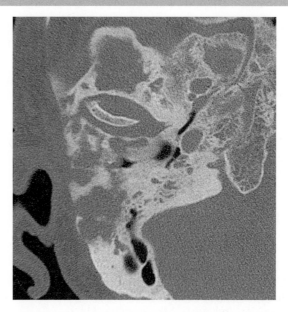
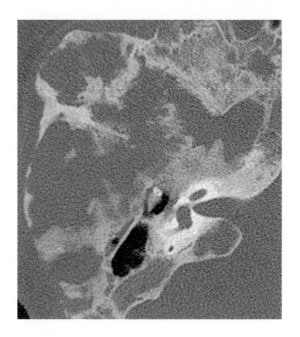
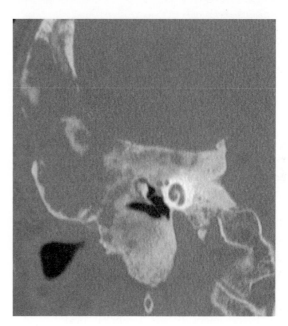

1. What is this patient's underlying diagnosis?

2. Does this patient have predominantly conductive or sensorineural hearing loss?

3. What is the cause of the patient's hearing loss?

4. In the craniofacial form of fibrous dysplasia, what bones are least affected?

Fibrous Dysplasia of the Temporal Bone

1. Fibrous dysplasia.

2. Conductive hearing loss.

3. Acquired narrowing of the external auditory canal and involvement of the ossicles, which have fibrous adhesion to the scutum or lateral wall of the ear cavity.

4. The temporal and occipital bones.

References

Güngör A, Cincik H, Çolak A, Poyrazoğlu E: Fibrous dysplasia involving the temporal bone: report of four cases, *Internet Journal of Otorhinolaryngology* 2, 2003.

Lustig LR, Holliday MJ, McCarthy EF, Nager GT: Fibrous dysplasia involving the skull base and temporal bone, *Arch Otolaryngol Head Neck Surg* 127:1239–1247, 2001.

Cross-Reference

Neuroradiology: THE REQUISITES, 2nd ed, pp 513, 662, 864.

Comment

Fibrous dysplasia represents a disturbance of normal bone development in which there is a defect in osteoblastic differentiation and maturation that originates in the mesenchymal precursor of the bone. It is characterized as a slow, progressive replacement of bone by proliferative isomorphic fibrous tissue, intermixed with poorly formed and irregularly arranged trabeculae of woven bone. Fibrous dysplasia has a predilection for the facial and cranial bones, where it causes deformity and a spectrum of dysfunction, depending on the specific cranial bones involved.

The temporal bone occasionally may be involved by fibrous dysplasia. Involvement of the temporal bone results in painless progressive enlargement of the squamosa, mastoid, or external canal. The male:female ratio is 2:1. The left and right ears are affected equally. The craniofacial form of fibrous dysplasia occurs in 10% to 25% of patients with the monostotic form of the disease and in 50% with the polyostotic form. The most common sites of involvement include the frontal, sphenoid, maxillary, and ethmoidal bones. The occipital and temporal bones are less commonly affected. Temporal bone involvement occurs in fewer than 15% of cases. Involvement of the sphenoid wing and temporal bones may result in vestibular dysfunction, tinnitus, and hearing loss. The secondary complications of fibrous dysplasia seen in this case may include external cholesteatoma behind external auditory canal stenosis, or obliteration or erosion of the middle ear ossicles, inner ear capsule, and fallopian canal, leading to labyrinthitis and facial nerve palsy.

Notes

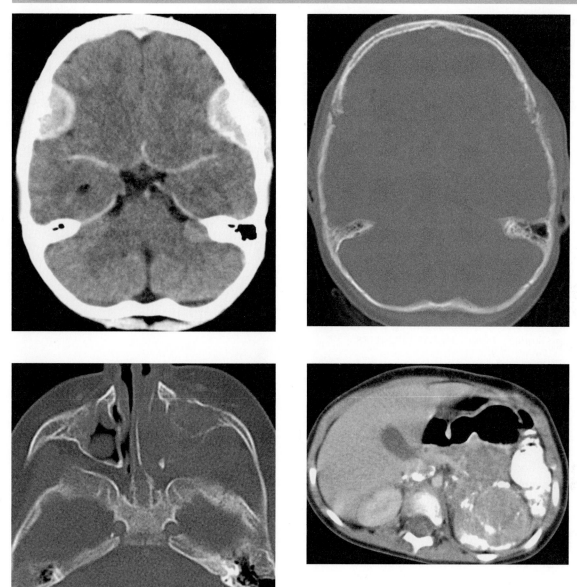

1. What are the findings on imaging?

2. What is the best diagnosis in this 1-year-old child?

3. What type of nuclear medicine scan is used in the routine staging of this entity?

4. What are causes of false-negative findings on metaiodobenzylguanidine (MIBG) scans?

Neuroblastoma—Metastases to the Cranium

1. There are bilaterally symmetric destructive masses with laminated periosteal reaction of the cranium along the coronal sutures. There are associated extracranial soft tissue masses with extension also to the intracranial extra-axial compartment. Lesions are also noted in the facial bones. These represent metastatic disease.

2. Metastatic neuroblastoma. The primary lesion is located in the left adrenal gland.

3. Iodine 131- or iodine 123-labeled MIBG scan.

4. Lack of tumor cell MIBG avidity; nonvisualization of lesions because of marked radiotracer uptake in normal liver, myocardium, salivary glands, intestines, and thyroid.

Reference

Kushner BH: Neuroblastoma: a disease requiring a multitude of imaging studies, *J Nucl Med* 45:1172–1188, 2004.

Cross-Reference

Neuroradiology: THE REQUISITES, 2nd ed, pp 512, 720, 827.

Comments

Neuroblastoma is the most common extracranial pediatric solid tumor and the most common neoplasm in infancy. The majority of cases present in children by the age of 5 years. These neoplasms arise from precursors of the sympathetic nervous plexus. The primary site is usually the adrenal gland, but these tumors may arise in paraspinal locations anywhere from the neck through the pelvis. High urinary catecholamine levels are present in more than 90% of cases. The embryonal type of this neoplasm often encases vascular structures and usually presents with metastatic disease (bone, lymph nodes, liver). Defining the extent of disease requires CT or MR imaging, bone scan, MIBG scan, bone marrow tests, and urine catecholamine measurements. The natural history is variable, but is largely predictable from the clinical and biologic features. The biologic features distinguish low-risk (90% survival) from high-risk (30% survival) cases. Some patients with a favorable clinical profile (localized tumor) are likely to have fatal metastatic disease because of the biologic features of the tumor, whereas other patients with widespread disease are likely to survive because of good biologic markers of the tumor.

Patients usually present with symptoms attributable to the local effects of the primary or metastatic tumor. Ecchymotic orbital proptosis ("raccoon eyes") results from metastatic involvement of the periorbital bones and soft tissue (spread to the skull is common). This 1-year-old boy was brought to the emergency room because his parents felt "bumps" on his head. A small subset of patients, approximately 2%, present with a paraneoplastic syndrome that may include watery diarrhea or opsoclonus-myoclonus-ataxia syndrome. The diarrhea mimics intestinal malabsorption and results from vasoactive intestinal peptide production by tumor cells that resolves after tumor resection.

Notes

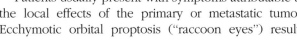

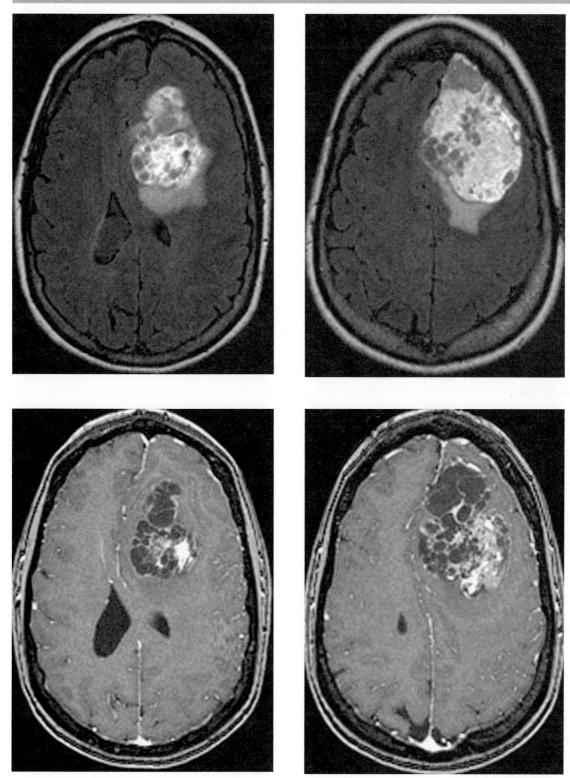

1. What is the differential diagnosis?

2. What percentage of intracranial meningiomas are cystic?

3. What is the most common site of cystic meningiomas?

4. What histologic cell type most commonly causes cystic intracranial metastases?

Cystic Meningioma—with Cellular Atypia

1. Meningioma, glial neoplasm, and metastatic disease.

2. Approximately 5%.

3. Along the cerebral convexity.

4. Adenocarcinoma.

Reference

Wasenko JJ, Hochhauser L, Stopa EG, Winfield JA: Cystic meningiomas: MR characteristics and surgical correlations, *Am J Neuroradiol* 15:1959–1965, 1994.

Cross-Reference

Neuroradiology: THE REQUISITES, 2nd ed, pp 98–105.

Comment

Cystic meningiomas are uncommon tumors, representing approximately 2% to 5% of meningiomas (some series report up to 10%), and they can be confused with metastatic or glial tumors with cystic components. Cystic meningiomas typically occur at the cerebral convexity or along the greater wing of the sphenoid, and rarely have been described in the ventricles and suprasellar cistern. Cystic meningiomas may be morphologically divided into three major types: cystic areas contained within the tumor; cystic areas at the periphery of the tumor, but within the tumor margins (as in this case); and cystic areas peripheral to the tumor, lying on or occasionally within the adjacent brain. The majority of cystic meningiomas are histopathologically meningothelial. Cellular atypia and sometimes malignant features are seen in a higher percentage of these cystic variants (compared with the garden variety meningioma); therefore, multiple intraoperative biopsies and frozen sections are recommended. There is still debate about the etiology of the cyst wall.

Magnetic resonance imaging shows the extra-axial location of these tumors and their cystic components. MR imaging with contrast enhancement may distinguish cyst walls containing tumor cells (these cyst walls enhance) from cyst walls containing gliotic tissue without tumor invasion (these cyst walls typically do not enhance). There is no clear correlation between cyst signal intensity and cyst content. MR imaging findings correlate well with the surgical appearance and pathologic results, and these findings allow the preoperative diagnosis of cystic meningioma. Division of this entity into three types of cysts aids the neurosurgeon, who must decide whether total resection is feasible. To obtain total resection and reduce the risk of recurrence, the surgeon must ensure that the plane of resection is between the thin enhancing membrane of the tumor cyst and the adjacent arachnoid. In cases in which the cyst is intra-axial or trapped CSF, the cyst wall adjacent to or within the brain parenchyma usually is not included in the resection.

Notes

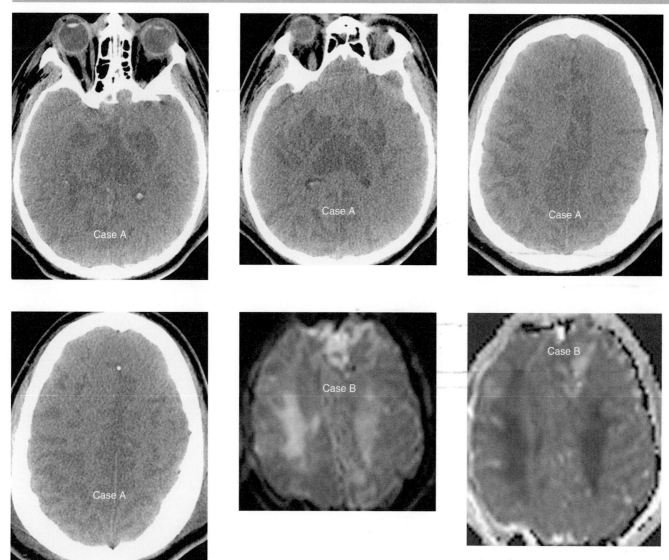

1. What are the major imaging findings in Case A?

2. What are common causes of anoxic-ischemic encephalopathy?

3. What is the watershed territory in fetuses and newborns?

4. What are the pathologic findings in adults with global hypoxic-ischemic encephalopathy?

Global Anoxic Brain Injury

1. Diffuse hypodensity in the gray matter, including the cerebral cortex globally, as well as the deep gray matter (bilateral basal ganglia, thalami) and hippocampi. The brainstem is also hypodense and there is early sulcal or cisternal effacement.

2. Global perfusional abnormalities (cardiac arrest, prolonged severe hypotension) and disturbances resulting in decreased blood oxygenation may result in the same picture (including respiratory arrest, asphyxia, and carbon monoxide inhalation).

3. The deep periventricular white matter. As a result, radiologic and pathologic manifestations of global hypoxic-ischemic injury are present within the deep white matter and result in periventricular leukomalacia.

4. In severe cases, generalized cortical laminar necrosis. Involvement of the globus pallidus, putamen, and caudate nuclei is common, as in this case. The other common pattern of abnormality is infarcts in the watershed territories at the confluence between the anterior, middle, and posterior cerebral artery territories.

Reference

Dettmers C, Solymosi L, Hartmann A, Buermann J, Hagendorff A: Confirmation of CT criteria to distinguish pathophysiologic subtypes of cerebral infarction, *AJNR Am J Neuroradiol* 18:335–342, 1997.

Cross-Reference

Neuroradiology: THE REQUISITES, 2nd ed, pp 206, 353–355.

Comment

Global hypoxic-ischemic injury is typically related to decreased perfusion; less commonly, it may be related to a disturbance in blood oxygenation. Postanoxic encephalopathy typically occurs after a period in which a diffuse episode of cerebral hypoperfusion has occurred. The patient may have a lucid interval, but over a 1- to 2-week period, undergo a precipitous decline that may even result in death. In this scenario, the pathologic changes are most pronounced in the white matter, where there is demyelination and sometimes necrosis (as in Case B, a patient who had prolonged hypotension after a motor vehicle collision). Carbon monoxide poisoning may produce a similar clinical course and radiologic appearance.

In the acute setting of global hypoxic-ischemic injury, unenhanced CT may show global loss of gray–white matter differentiation, diffuse gray matter hypodensity, and sulcal effacement, as in Case A. On MR imaging, T2W hyperintensity may be seen in the watershed territories (acute watershed ischemia may show contrast enhancement in the early stages). In laminar necrosis, T2W hyperintensity may be seen globally throughout the cortex. Imaging in the subacute phase may demonstrate cortical hemorrhage in the setting of laminar necrosis, which is commonly of high signal intensity on unenhanced T1W images. In the subacute to chronic stages, hypointensity in the cortex and on gradient echo images may be noted.

Notes

Challenge

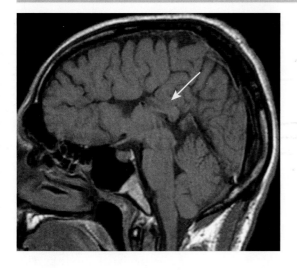
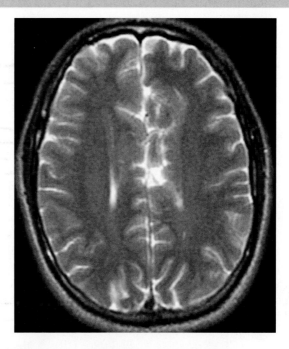
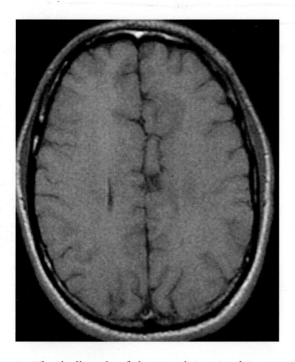
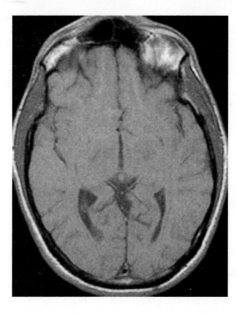

1. The hallmark of the condition in this case is absence of what structure?

2. What is the triad of lesions seen in septo-optic dysplasia (deMorsier's syndrome)?

3. How can maximal pressure hydrocephalus be distinguished from alobar holoprosencephaly (HPE)?

4. What subtype of HPE is associated with anterior dysgenesis of the corpus callosum?

CASE 151

Lobar Holoprosencephaly

1. The hallmark of all holoprosencephalies (alobar, semilobar, and lobar) is the absence of the septum pellucidum.

2. (1) Complete or partial absence of the septum pellucidum; (2) optic nerve hypoplasia; and (3) hypothalamic-pituitary dysfunction, which typically manifests as growth retardation and short stature. There may be an ectopic posterior pituitary gland.

3. In maximal-pressure hydrocephalus the midline structures are present (although chronic ventricular enlargement may result in failure to visualize the septum pellucidum). In alobar holoprosencephaly the interhemispheric fissure and midline structures are absent with failure of separation of the right and left cerebral hemispheres.

4. Lobar HPE.

References

Albayram S, Melham E, Mori S, et al: Holoprosencephaly in children: diffusion tensor MR imaging of white matter tracts of the brainstem. Initial experience, *Radiology* 223:645–651, 2002.

Barkovich A, Simon E, Clegg N, Kinsman S, Hahn J: Analysis of the cerebral cortex in holoprosencephaly with attention to the sylvian fissures, *AJNR Am J Neuroradiol* 23:143–150, 2002.

Cross-Reference

Neuroradiology: THE REQUISITES, 2nd ed, pp 421–423.

Comment

The HPEs are a spectrum of disorders characterized by hypoplasia of the rostral end of the neural tube and the premaxillary segment of the face (lack of forebrain induction). HPE is characterized by failure of cleavage of the embryonic prosencephalon, which is normally complete by embryonic day 35. With this comes partial to complete failure of separation of the telencephalon and diencephalon into the right and left cerebral hemispheres and basal ganglia or thalami, respectively. Because the optic vesicles and olfactory bulbs evaginate from the prosencephalon, visual disturbances and incomplete formation of the olfactory system are frequently present. Hypoplasia of the premaxillary segment results in facial anomalies, including cleft lip and palate; abnormalities of the orbit (cyclopia, hypotelorism); and forehead proboscis.

Holoprosencephaly may be divided into subtypes: alobar (the most severe form), semilobar, lobar (the mildest form of the major subtypes), and middle interhemispheric variant. There is no clear distinction between subtypes. In alobar HPE, the falx, interhemispheric fissure, and septum pellucidum are absent. There is failure of separation of the cerebrum and the ventricular system, resulting in a mono-ventricle contiguous with a dorsal cyst. In semilobar HPE, the interhemispheric fissure and falx cerebri are usually formed posteriorly and absent anteriorly. In lobar HPE, the interhemispheric fissure and falx anteriorly are hypoplastic. Often the posterior corpus callosum or splenium is formed, as in this case (*arrow*). The third ventricle is usually well formed. In semilobar and lobar HPE, the ventricular system shows variable degrees of development. The middle interhemispheric variant differs from classic HPE in that the posterior frontal and parietal lobes are most significantly affected rather than the basal forebrain. The anterior frontal lobes and occipital lobes are separated, and the genu and splenium of the corpus callosum are formed, but the callosal body is absent. The hypothalamus and lentiform nuclei appear separated, but the caudate nuclei and thalami are incompletely separated in many cases. Heterotopias and cortical dysplasia are common associated anomalies of HPE, as seen in this case, in the left greater than right medial frontal lobes.

Notes

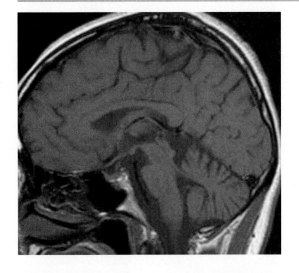

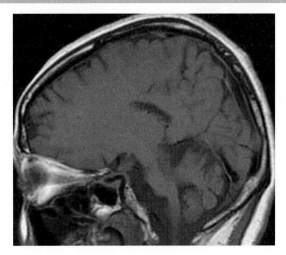

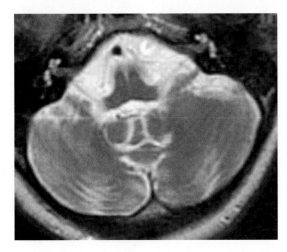

1. What is the most common clinical presentation of patients with degenerative processes of the cerebellum?

2. In olivopontocerebellar degeneration (OPCD), myelin loss and gliosis usually begin in what structure?

3. What are common causes of acquired cerebellar degeneration?

4. Regarding Friedreich ataxia, what is the inheritance pattern and what chromosome is implicated?

Olivopontocerebellar Degeneration

1. Ataxia.

2. The pons. Degeneration begins in the pontine nuclei and progresses along the pontocerebellar tracts through the middle cerebellar peduncles and into the cerebellum.

3. Substance abuse (alcohol), medications (anticonvulsants, such as phenytoin), paraneoplastic syndromes, and some chemotherapeutic agents, to name a few.

4. Autosomal (dominant and recessive forms) and chromosome 9, respectively.

Reference
Nakagawa N, Katayama T, Makita Y, et al: A case of spinocerebellar ataxia type 6 mimicking olivopontocerebellar atrophy, *Neuroradiology* 41:501–503, 1999.

Cross-Reference
Neuroradiology: THE REQUISITES, 2nd ed, pp 397–398.

Comment
Olivopontocerebellar degeneration may be transmitted through autosomal dominant inheritance or may occur sporadically. Although the onset of symptoms in OPCD may span several decades, two peaks of presentation are noted. Sporadic cases are more common and tend to affect people in midlife, whereas familial cases usually present earlier in young adulthood. The cause of sporadic olivopontocerebellar atrophy is not known, but the disease is progressive. The main clinical presentation is truncal ataxia, first involving the legs and then the arms. Patients may also have nystagmus, dysarthria, and tremors. Parkinsonian features may develop, accompanied by mild dementia and ophthalmoplegia, pyramidal tract signs, and autonomic disturbance. It is characterized by atrophy of the cerebellum, pons, medullary olives, and other brainstem structures.

Pathologically, in OPCD, there is loss of myelin and gliosis of the pontocerebellar pathways, beginning in the pontine nuclei and progressing into the cerebellum (the hemispheres and, to a lesser degree, the vermis), with neuronal loss of the cerebellar cortex. The development of MR imaging has greatly enhanced the ability to evaluate the degenerative processes of the cerebellum, brainstem, and spinal cord. On MR imaging, atrophy of the involved structures (pons, middle cerebellar peduncles, inferior olives, and cerebellum) is evident. In addition, there may be mild hyperintensity on T2W images in the involved structures in OPCD.

Notes

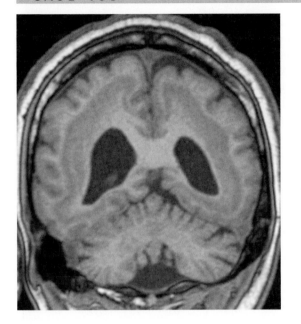 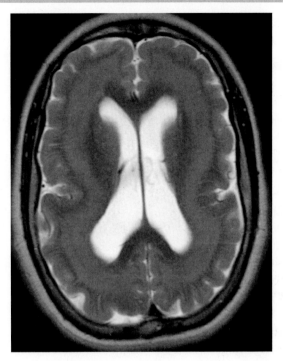

1. What are three major types of heterotopia?

2. What is hemimegalencephaly?

3. What is the definition of cortical dysplasia?

4. Along what structures do neurons migrate from the germinal zone to the cortex region?

Band Heterotopia—Pachygyria

1. Subependymal, focal, and diffuse (band, laminar).

2. Hamartomatous overgrowth of a cerebral hemisphere.

3. After migration from the germinal zone to the cortical region, there is failure in the development of a normal six-layered cortex.

4. The radial glial fibers.

References

Barkovich AJ: Morphologic characteristics of subcortical heterotopia: MR imaging study, *AJNR Am J Neuroradiol* 21:290–295, 2000.

Iannetti P, Spalice A, Raucci U, Perla FM: Functional neuroradiologic investigations in band heterotopia, *Pediatr Neurol* 24:159–163, 2001.

Cross-Reference

Neuroradiology: THE REQUISITES, 2nd ed, pp 427–429.

Comment

Heterotopias are migrational abnormalities in which normal neurons occur in abnormal locations as a result of failure of migration along the radial glial fibers from the germinal region to the cortex. Three well-recognized types of heterotopia include focal, subependymal, and diffuse (laminar, band). Subcortical heterotopia is a newer term that refers to a specific entity in which neurons are abnormally located predominantly in the subcortical white matter. The cortical dysplasias are different from the heterotopias in that they do not represent a failure of normal migration, but rather a failure in the development of a normal six-layered cortex after migration from the germinal matrix to the cortical region.

Diffuse or band heterotopia refers to a layer of gray matter whose migration has arrested such that it is localized between the subcortical white matter laterally and the deep white matter medially. The inner and outer margins of the heterotopic neurons are well demarcated. Therefore, the band of gray matter is separated from the overlying cortex by a mantle of subcortical white matter. Band heterotopias are frequently associated with overlying cortical dysplasias (pachygyria, polymicrogyria), as in this case. The severity of the cortical dysplasia is directly related to the severity of the band heterotopia: the thicker the band, the more severe the overlying dysplasia will be. Similarly, patients with band heterotopia tend to have more pronounced clinical symptoms. In addition to seizures, which may have an age of onset ranging from infancy to young adulthood, many children have moderate to severe developmental delay.

Hemimegalencephaly refers to hamartomatous overgrowth of a cerebral hemisphere. Migrational abnormalities are usually present within the affected hemisphere, but they may also be present on the contralateral side. On imaging, there is usually enlargement of the affected cerebral hemisphere and the ipsilateral lateral ventricle, as well as associated cortical dysplasias.

Notes

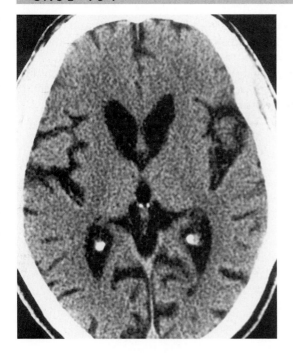 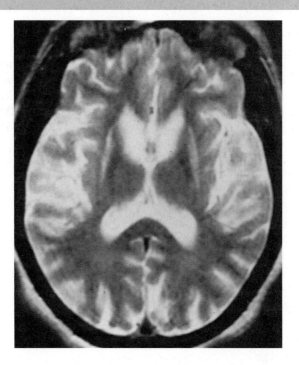

1. What is the imaging finding?

2. Lesions involving the extrapyramidal nuclei (deep gray matter) typically result in what type of neurologic disorders?

3. Hallervorden-Spatz syndrome is an autosomal recessive disorder that results in accumulation of iron products in which structures of the deep gray matter?

4. In Wilson's disease (hepatolenticular degeneration), abnormal copper deposition is caused by a deficiency of what serum transport protein?

Huntington's Disease

1. Bilateral caudate atrophy.

2. Motor dysfunction or movement disorders.

3. The globus pallidus or substantia nigra.

4. Ceruloplasmin.

References

Krausz Y, Bonne O, Marciano R, Yaffe S, Lerer B, Chisin R: Brain SPECT imaging of neuropsychiatric disorders, *Eur J Radiol* 21:183–187, 1996.

Montoya A, Price BH, Menear M, Lepage M: Brain imaging and cognitive dysfunctions in Huntington's disease, *J Psychiatry Neurosci* 31:21–29, 2006.

Cross-Reference

Neuroradiology: THE REQUISITES, 2nd ed, p 391.

Comment

A variety of disease processes affect the extrapyramidal nuclei (basal ganglia, thalami) as well as the nuclei in the brainstem. These conditions are most commonly degenerative or metabolic, and many are inherited. Among the neurodegenerative processes that can affect the deep gray matter are Huntington's disease, Wilson's disease, and Hallervorden-Spatz syndrome. Toxic exposures may also result in abnormalities of the deep gray matter. Lesions in these structures typically result in movement disorders that can occur in isolation or in combination and include the following subtypes: abnormalities in muscle tone, involuntary movements, abnormal postural reflexes, and the inability to carry out voluntary movements. Toxic exposures that affect the basal ganglia include carbon monoxide, cyanide, hydrogen sulfide, ethylene glycol, and toluene. Although there is wide variation in the deep gray matter structures involved, many diseases have characteristic involvement of specific structures.

Huntington's disease is inherited in an autosomal dominant manner that results in progressive degeneration of brain cells. The gene responsible for the disease is located on chromosome 4. Clinical manifestations typically include involuntary movement (choreoathetosis), rigidity, dementia, and emotional instability. Cognitive deficits are believed to be due to abnormal connectivity between the deep gray matter and the cortex. The disease typically presents in the fourth or fifth decade of life. The disease is progressive, with death occurring 15 to 20 years after its onset. On imaging, as in this case, Huntington's disease is characterized by atrophy of the caudate nuclei, which results in ballooning of the frontal horns of the lateral ventricles ("boxcar" ventricles). There may also be involvement of the putamen, which can

atrophy. MR imaging shows signal changes in these nuclei. These changes may be hyperintense on T2W images, as in this case, which is believed to be related to gliosis; other cases show T2W hypointensity, which is likely related to iron deposition. Other major imaging findings include cortical atrophy.

Notes

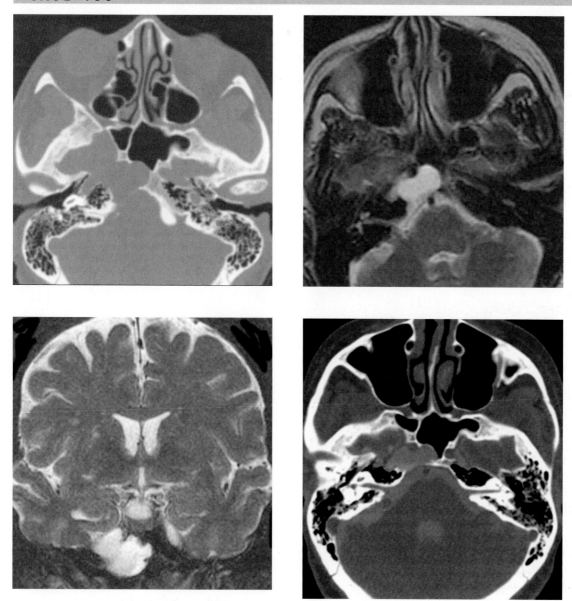

1. What anatomic part of the skull base does this lesion arise from?

2. What lesion arising in this area has bone destruction and restricted diffusion?

3. What is the diagnosis in this case?

4. What condition is associated with a partially empty sella, arachnoid pits, CSF leaks, and meningoceles at the skull base?

Meningocele and Pseudomeningocele of the Skull Base (Petrous Apex)

1. The petrous apex.

2. An epidermoid.

3. Meningocele (or possibly a pseudomeningocele from Meckel's cave).

4. Benign intracranial hypertension.

Reference

Silver RI, Moonis G, Schlosser RJ, Bolger WE, Loevner LA: Radiographic signs of elevated intracranial pressure in idiopathic CSF leaks: a possible presentation of idiopathic intracranial hypertension, *Am J Rhinol* 21:257–261, 2007.

Cross-Reference

Neuroradiology: THE REQUISITES, 2nd ed, pp 418–419, 600–602, 616–617, 628–629, 643.

Comment

This case shows a well-demarcated, chronic-appearing lesion of the right petrous apex. There is expansion, smooth cortical bone thinning without bone destruction, and cortication medially, suggesting a long-standing process. The lesion is isointense to CSF on T2W images, and on the coronal T2W image, it is difficult to determine whether this lesion is separate from or an extension of Meckel's cave into the osseous base of the skull. CT cisternography (instillation of contrast material into the thecal sac by lumbar puncture, followed by CT imaging after graceful tilting of the patient so that the contrast agent spreads through the subarachnoid spaces in the head) confirms that the petrous apex lesion communicates with the CSF spaces.

The differential diagnosis of a benign-appearing, expansile petrous apex mass includes cholesterol granuloma, mucocele, epidermoid, meningocele, and occasionally, an aneurysm of the internal carotid artery. Mucoceles are frequently unilocular and show peripheral enhancement. The signal characteristics of mucoceles will vary, depending on the protein concentration and viscosity. Epidermoid cysts may have a benign appearance, or they can have more concerning radiologic findings, such as bone erosion or destruction. They typically appear similar to CSF on T1W and T2W images and hyperintense on FLAIR imaging, and demonstrate restricted diffusion. Cholesterol granulomas, when large, may be multilocular. There is usually thinning of the cortex with large lesions without bone destruction. Cholesterol granulomas are often hyperintense on all pulse sequences. In particular, the marked hyperintensity on unenhanced T1W images distinguishes these from many other lesions, and the presence of hemorrhage–fluid levels within these lesions is highly characteristic.

Notes

Petrous aped:
chloestral granuloma
muc

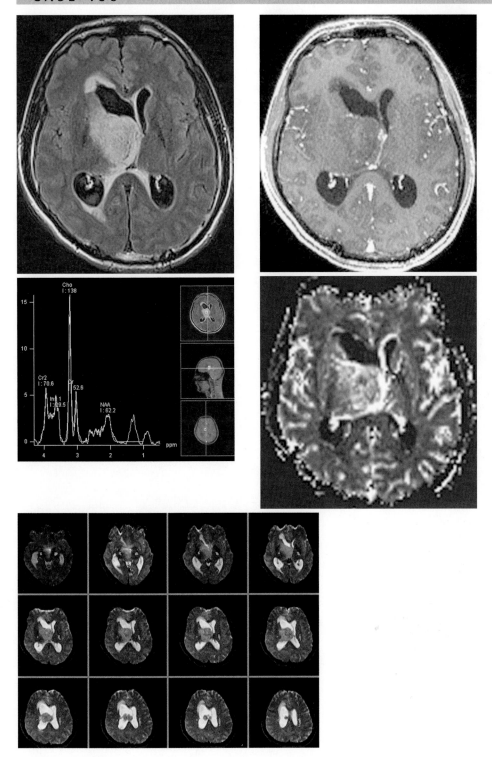

1. What glial neoplasm is most commonly associated with hemorrhage?

2. What are the pathologic criteria for grading gliomas?

3. What features seen on conventional MR imaging are associated with higher-grade gliomas?

4. What functional in vivo MR imaging techniques may be used to provide supplemental information about glioma grade?

CASE 156

Right Thalamic Glioblastoma

1. Glioblastoma multiforme (GBM).

2. The presence of necrosis, number of mitoses, vascular endothelial proliferation, cellular density, and nuclear pleomorphism.

3. The presence of necrosis, enhancement, hemorrhage, and marked mass effect.

4. MR spectroscopy and perfusion imaging. An elevated choline : *N*-acetylaspartate ratio has been a reliable predictor of higher-grade neoplasms, and the presence of lactic acid has been indicative of higher-grade neoplasms. Elevated regional cerebral blood volume (rCBV) correlates with higher histologic grade (the higher the rCBV, the greater the likelihood that the mass is a GBM).

References

Earnest F IV, Kelly PJ, Scheithauer BW, et al: Cerebral astrocytomas: histopathologic correlation of MR and CT contrast enhancement with stereotactic biopsy, *Radiology* 166:823–827, 1988.

Lupo JM, Cha S, Chang SM, Nelson SJ: Analysis of metabolic indices in regions of abnormal perfusion in patients with high grade glioma, *AJNR Am J Neuroradiol* 28:1455–1461, 2007.

Cross-Reference

Neuroradiology: THE REQUISITES, 2nd ed, pp 139–143.

Comment

This case illustrates a solid mass centered in the right thalamus, with an exophytic component extending into the ventricle. There is mass effect, with partial obstruction of the foramen of Monroe resulting in hydrocephalus and transependymal flow of CSF along the margin of the right lateral ventricle. Most GBMs enhance and usually demonstrate heterogeneity because of the presence of necrosis or hemorrhage. Margins of the enhancing component are usually ill defined, and there is irregular thick peripheral enhancement due to central necrosis. Enhancement may extend into the adjacent white matter. In a newly identified brain tumor in which biopsy is anticipated, regions of enhancement correlate with regions of solid tumor on pathologic examination. Therefore, contrast is useful in identifying areas for stereotactic biopsy. In addition, enhanced images may identify tumor spread to regions that otherwise would not be noticed on unenhanced images, such as the leptomeninges, subarachnoid space, or subependymal region along the ventricular margins.

In this less typical case, the GBM is centered in the deep gray matter (most GBMs occur in the cerebral lobes), has no significant central necrosis, and shows only mild central enhancement. The functional in vivo techniques of MR spectroscopy and MR perfusion imaging allow correlation of metabolic activity with the vascular properties, respectively, and provide further insight into the grade of the primary glial neoplasm. In this case, these techniques were helpful in characterizing the high-grade nature of this neoplasm. Specifically, proton spectroscopy shows an elevated choline:NAA ratio (>2), and perfusion imaging shows markedly elevated rCBV, indicative of a high-grade neoplasm. For the neurosurgeon planning stereotactic biopsy, location of eloquent areas of brain relative to the tumor is critical to reduce potential neurologic deficits. Diffusion tensor imaging tractography in this case clearly identifies the corticospinal tracts (*green*).

Notes

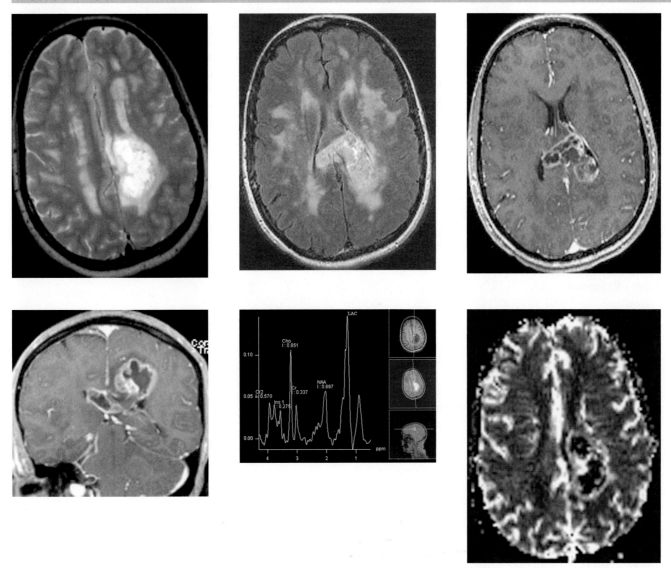

1. The patient has a diagnosis of multiple sclerosis. What are the two main diagnostic considerations for the corpus callosum mass in this case?

2. What is the histologic correlate of a decrease in *N*-acetylaspartate levels?

3. Elevated glutamate or glutamine peaks have been described in which of the following: glioblastoma multiforme (GBM), tumefactive multiple sclerosis, or anaplastic astrocytoma?

4. The foci of elevated regional cerebral blood volume on perfusion imaging favors what diagnosis?

Multiple Sclerosis and Glioblastoma

1. High-grade glioma (GBM) and demyelinating disease (tumefactive multiple sclerosis).

2. Loss of normal neurons due to replacement by abnormal cells or neuronal destruction.

3. Tumefactive multiple sclerosis. ↑ glutamate

4. GBM.

Reference

Cianfoni A, Niku S, Imbesi SG: Metabolite findings in tumefactive demyelinating lesions utilizing short echo time proton magnetic resonance spectroscopy, *AJNR Am J Neuroradiol* 28:272–277, 2007.

Cross-Reference

Neuroradiology: THE REQUISITES, 2nd ed, pp 332–336.

Comment

"Tumefactive" multiple sclerosis, high-grade glioma (GBM), and occasionally an abscess can appear similar on imaging, particularly in the absence of a clinical history. Multiple sclerosis typically occurs in younger patients, and there are often additional clinical or imaging findings to suggest this diagnosis. On close questioning, patients often have neurologic symptoms that are spaced both in time and in location. Furthermore, MR imaging may demonstrate white matter lesions separate from the mass that are suggestive of multiple sclerosis.

Advanced MR imaging sequences may be of value. Perfusion imaging in this case shows markedly elevated regional cerebral blood volume in the enhancing rim of the necrotic mass, suggesting a high-grade glioma or GBM rather than demyelination. GBM was confirmed at surgical biopsy. Nonspecific spectroscopic findings in tumefactive multiple sclerosis include elevation of choline, lactate, and lipid peaks, and a decrease in the *N*-acetylaspartate peak. These spectroscopic characteristics reflect the histologic correlate of marked demyelination in the absence of significant inflammation. Gliomas also consistently show reductions in *N*-acetylaspartate and increases in phospholipids, reflecting the replacement of normal neuronal tissue with a proliferating cellular process. Increases in lactate are not uncommon as a result of tissue ischemia and necrosis, as in this case. Variable increases in lipid levels may be seen.

Elevation of glutamate or glutamine peaks favors tumefactive demyelination and is typically not seen in aggressive neoplasms (not present in this case). Serial proton MR spectroscopy can be a useful, noninvasive method of overcoming the diagnostic dilemma of differentiating glioma from acute tumefactive demyelination.

Persistent elevation of choline and lactate levels favors a glioma. Normalization of the initial increases in phospholipids, lipid, and lactate peaks within 3 to 4 weeks, followed by persistent, marked reductions of the neuronal marker *N*-acetylaspartate, has been described over time in tumefactive demyelination.

Notes

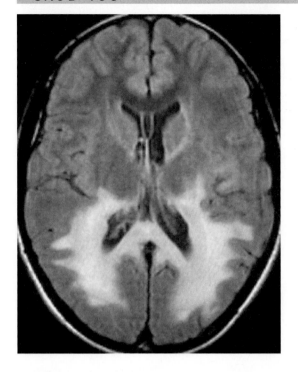 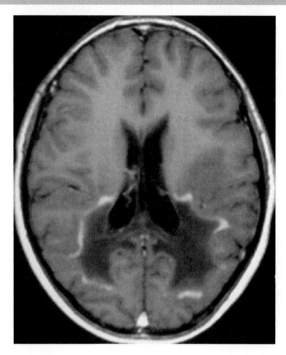

1. What is the characteristic MR imaging appearance of metachromatic leukodystrophy?

2. What do the areas of enhancement represent in this case?

3. How is adrenoleukodystrophy genetically transmitted?

4. What leukodystrophy results from a deficiency in the enzyme *N*-acetylaspartoacylase?

Adrenoleukodystrophy

1. There is a confluent, symmetric white matter abnormality that begins in the frontal lobes and progresses posteriorly. There is usually relative sparing of the subcortical U-fibers and the white matter within the basal ganglia.

2. Active demyelination and perivascular inflammation.

3. X-linked or autosomal recessive.

4. Canavan disease.

Reference

Rajanayagam V, Balthazor M, Shapiro EG, Krivit W, Lockman L, Stillman AE: Proton MR spectroscopy and neuropsychological testing in adrenoleukodystrophy, *AJNR Am J Neuroradiol* 18:1909–1914, 1997.

Cross-Reference

Neuroradiology: THE REQUISITES, 2nd ed, pp 361, 363.

Comment

Adrenoleukodystrophy is an X-linked or autosomal recessive disorder that is related to a single enzyme deficiency (acyl coenzyme A synthetase) within intracellular peroxisomes. This enzyme is necessary for β oxidation in the breakdown of very long-chain fatty acids that accumulate in erythrocytes, plasma, and fibroblasts, as well as the CNS white matter and adrenal cortex. Boys typically present between the ages of 4 and 10 years. The clinical presentation may include behavioral disturbance, visual symptoms, hearing loss, seizures, and eventually spastic quadriparesis. Patients often present with adrenal insufficiency (Addison's disease), which may occur before or after the development of neurologic symptoms.

As in other demyelinating and dysmyelinating disorders, MR is the imaging modality of choice for the detection of white matter disease, being far superior to CT. In adrenoleukodystrophy, the most common pattern of white matter disease is bilaterally symmetric abnormalities within the parietal and occipital white matter, extending across the splenium of the corpus callosum. The disease may continue to progress anteriorly to involve the frontal and temporal lobes. The region of active demyelination, usually along the anterior margin, may show contrast enhancement. Less typical presentations include predominantly frontal lobe involvement or holohemispheric involvement. Adrenoleukodystrophy also involves the cerebellum, spinal cord, and peripheral nervous system. Findings on MR imaging correlate well with neuropsychological measures.

Notes

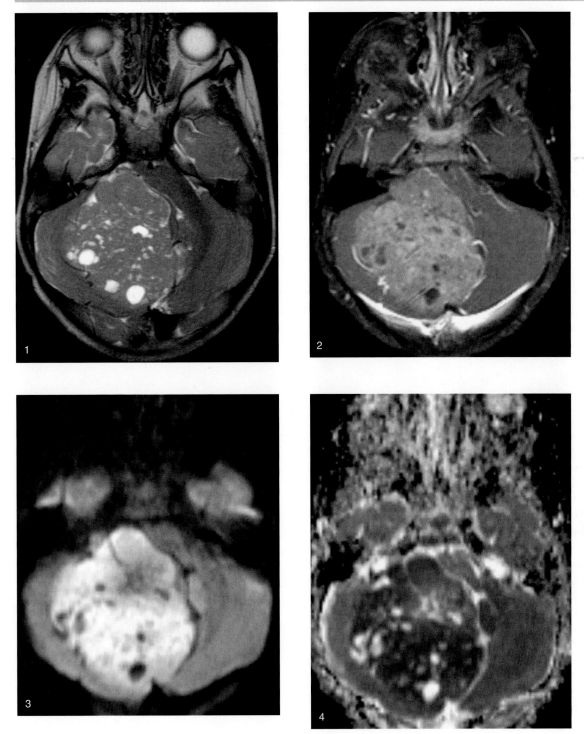

1. What is the differential diagnosis of a midline posterior fossa mass in a child?

2. What primitive neuroectodermal tumor occurs in the pineal gland?

3. Where in the posterior fossa do medulloblastomas characteristically present in adults?

4. What percentage of patients with medulloblastomas present with subarachnoid seeding of tumor?

Medulloblastoma

1. The major diagnostic considerations are medulloblastoma and fourth ventricular ependymoma. Ependymomas typically arise in the fourth ventricle and expand it, whereas medulloblastomas typically compress it. Unlike medulloblastomas, ependymomas characteristically grow through the foramina of Magendie and Luschka. Less commonly, cerebellar astrocytomas may occur in the midline; however, they usually are hemispheric.

2. Pineoblastoma.

3. The lateral cerebellar hemisphere. They are usually desmoplastic.

4. Approximately 30%.

Reference

Rumboldt Z, Camacho DLA, Lake D, Welsh CT, Castillo M: Apparent diffusion coefficients for differentiation of cerebellar tumors in children, *Am J Neuroradiol* 27:1362–1369, 2006.

Cross-Reference

Neuroradiology: THE REQUISITES, 2nd ed, pp 122–126.

Comment

Medulloblastomas account for up to one third of all pediatric posterior fossa tumors. They occur more commonly in boys than in girls (approximately 3:1) and arise from the superior medullary velum of the fourth ventricle from primitive neuroectoderm. In children, they are typically midline masses associated with the inferior vermis, but occasionally may present as a lateral cerebellar hemispheric mass, as in this case. Importantly, subarachnoid seeding of the leptomeninges is very common at presentation (reported in up to 30% of cases in some series); therefore, patients should have a screening contrast enhanced MR imaging study of the spine to exclude this type of spread.

On unenhanced CT, medulloblastomas are typically hyperdense relative to brain parenchyma because of their dense cellularity. They are demarcated masses, and calcification, cystic change, or hemorrhage may be present in up to 10% to 20% of lesions. On MR imaging, the signal characteristics of medulloblastomas vary considerably on T2W imaging, depending on the presence of hemorrhage and the degree of cellularity. Most medulloblastomas show avid but heterogeneous contrast enhancement. Typically, they efface the fourth ventricle and present with hydrocephalus.

Accurate preoperative diagnosis is important in pediatric cerebellar tumors because this may affect the surgical approach. Diffusion MR imaging allows assessment of microscopic water diffusion within tissues, and with neoplasms, this diffusion seems to be primarily based on cellularity. Increasing cellularity leads to increased signal intensity on diffusion imaging and hypointensity on corresponding apparent diffusion coefficient (ADC) maps. Studies have suggested that diffusion imaging and ADC values may be useful in helping to distinguish among histologic types of pediatric brain tumors. Juvenile pilocytic astrocytomas have shown high ADC values and ratios. In contrast, medulloblastomas that characteristically are cellular have shown restricted diffusion, as in this case, with high signal intensity on diffusion images (image 3) and hypointensity on ADC maps (image 4). The cellularity of ependymomas is between that of astrocytomas and that of medulloblastomas. Hence, pilocytic astrocytomas are most often hyperintense on ADC maps, medulloblastomas are hypointense, and ependymomas fall somewhere in between.

Notes

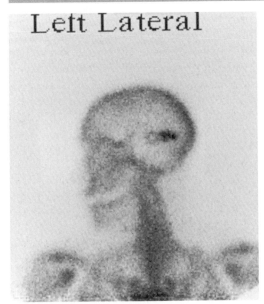

Left Lateral

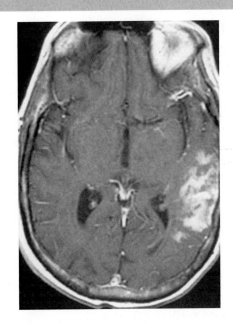

1. Using only the bone scan, what are the diagnostic considerations?

2. What radiopharmaceuticals are most commonly used for bone scanning?

3. What factors affect the accumulation of technetium-labeled radiopharmaceuticals in bone?

4. Using the bone scan and enhanced MR images, what is the best diagnosis?

Middle Cerebral Artery Territory Stroke Mimicking a Bone Metastasis

1. Metastatic disease, primary bone neoplasm, bone dysplasia (eg, Paget's disease), or an intracranial lesion.

2. Technetium-labeled phosphate analogs.

3. Blood supply, the amount of mineralized bone, bone turnover, and systemic factors (medications, such as hormones or vitamins).

4. A subacute to chronic stroke in the left middle cerebral artery territory mimicking a bone lesion.

References

Hoggard N, Wilkinson ID, Paley MN, Griffiths PD: Imaging of haemorrhagic stroke, *Clin Radiol* 57: 957–968, 2002.

Rappaport AH, Hoffer PB, Genant HK: Unifocal bone findings by scintigraphy: clinical significance in patients with known primary cancer, *West J Med* 129: 188–192, 1978.

Cross-Reference

Neuroradiology: THE REQUISITES, 2nd ed, pp 174–196.

Comment

The left lateral projection from the patient's delayed bone scan shows increased radiotracer activity projecting over the temporal bone region (it is important to remember that an anteroposterior view is necessary to accurately localize the abnormality). This was the only abnormality on the patient's bone scan. Corresponding enhanced MR imaging shows mild local mass effect in the superficial portion of the posterior left temporal lobe with cortical enhancement; the imaging findings are consistent with a stroke. In this patient with renal cell carcinoma, the bone scan was initially interpreted as showing metastatic disease. It is important to remember that any process that stimulates deposition of calcium within soft tissues, the solid organs, or areas of infarction may result in increased uptake of technetium-labeled radiopharmaceuticals. Similarly, in circumstances in which there is increased blood flow or luxury perfusion, there will also be increased radiotracer uptake. Infarctions in the brain may take up radionuclide, as can brain metastases from systemic cancers, which have a predilection to calcify (mucinous adenocarcinomas, including breast and gastrointestinal carcinomas; sarcomas; and in children, neuroblastomas). In a patient with a known systemic malignancy, an isolated region of increased radiotracer uptake in the cranium should be further assessed with additional imaging (plain films, CT, or MR imaging as needed) before it is assumed to represent metastatic disease. In this patient, MR imaging was obtained 1 week after the bone scan because of new-onset left upper extremity weakness. Images showed an acute infarct in the distal right middle cerebral artery territory (not shown) and, at the same time, confirmed a subacute to chronic infarct in the left middle cerebral artery territory. In addition, no calvarial lesion was identified on MR imaging.

Notes

infarct enhancement 2-3w Max (Acute)

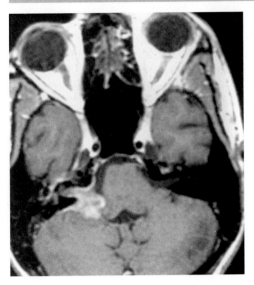 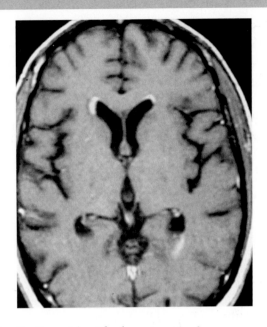

1. What is the differential diagnosis for the findings identified on imaging?

2. What imaging findings are typical of CNS involvement in patients infected with cytomegalovirus (CMV) in utero?

3. What is the most neoplastic common cause of ependymal enhancement in the setting of AIDs infection?

4. What were the patient's acute symptoms at clinical presentation?

Cytomegalovirus Meningitis and Ependymitis in a Patient with AIDS

1. Infection (ventriculitis, ependymitis) and neoplasm (lymphoma or seeding from a systemic or primary brain neoplasm).

2. Bilateral ventricular subependymal calcification, ventricular enlargement, periventricular hypodensity on CT or hyperintensity on T2W MR imaging, atrophy, and migrational anomalies (pachygyria or polymicrogyria).

3. Lymphoma.

4. Sensorineural hearing loss and vertigo.

References

Boska MD, Mosley RL, Nawab M, et al: Advances in neuroimaging for HIV-1 associated neurological dysfunction: clues to diagnosis, pathogenesis and therapeutic monitoring, *Curr HIV Res* 2:61–68, 2004.

Vinters HV, Kwok MK, Ho HW, et al: Cytomegalovirus in the nervous system of patients with the acquired immune deficiency syndrome, *Brain* 112:245–268, 1989.

Cross-Reference

Neuroradiology: THE REQUISITES, 2nd ed, pp 300–301, 304.

Comment

Cytomegalovirus is present in the latent form in the majority of the American population. Reactivation usually results in a subclinical or mild flu-like syndrome. In immunocompromised patients, reactivation can result in disseminated infection, usually involving the respiratory and gastrointestinal tracts; however, rarely, it can infect the nervous system. In the CNS, CMV may cause meningoencephalitis and ependymitis. Symptoms may be acute or chronic, developing over months. Patients may have fever, altered mental status, and progressive cognitive decline. Patients may also present with cranial neuropathies (as in this case). CMV polymerase chain reaction in the CSF is sensitive and specific for the diagnosis of AIDS-related CMV infection of the CNS. However, conventional CSF findings and neuroimaging may not adequately assess the severity of CNS CMV disease, as demonstrated at autopsy.

Magnetic resonance imaging is the diagnostic study of choice in assessing immunocompromised patients suspected of having CNS infection. Imaging may show atrophy; high signal intensity in the periventricular white matter, typically not associated with significant mass effect; and retinitis (frequently seen in the AIDS population) in patients with CMV infection. Although patients with CNS infection may also have ependymal and subependymal involvement, associated imaging findings often are not present. When present, T2W signal abnormality and enhancement along the ependyma are valuable in establishing this diagnosis. Currently, the most common cause of ependymal enhancement in the setting of AIDS is lymphoma.

Notes

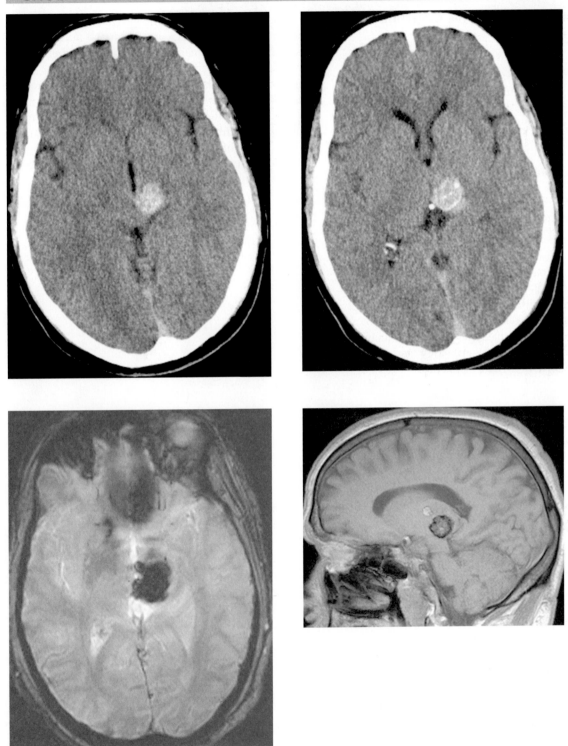

1. What is the differential diagnosis in this patient with traumatic injury?

2. What is the best diagnosis?

3. What imaging findings favor an uncomplicated cavernous malformation?

4. What is the most common location for a cavernous malformation in the brainstem?

Upper Brainstem and Thalamic Cavernous Malformation

1. Hemorrhage, hemorrhage into an underlying lesion, and cavernous malformation.

2. Occult vascular malformation (cavernous malformation).

3. The mass is demarcated or circumscribed, it has calcification, and there is no surrounding hypodensity to suggest edema.

4. The pons.

References

Porter RW, Detwiler PW, Spetzler RF, et al: Cavernous malformations of the brainstem: experience with 100 patients, *J Neurosurg* 90:50–58, 1999.

Zausinger S, Yousry I, Brueckmann H, Schmid-Elsaesser R, Tonn JC: Cavernous malformations of the brainstem: three-dimensional-constructive interference in steady-state magnetic resonance imaging for improvement of surgical approach and clinical results, *Neurosurgery* 58:322–330, 2006.

Cross-Reference

Neuroradiology: THE REQUISITES, 2nd ed, pp 231–234, 551.

Comment

This case shows the typical appearance of an uncomplicated cavernous malformation involving the upper brainstem or cerebral peduncle and left thalamus. In the absence of edema, hemorrhage within the cavernous malformation is unlikely. The differentiation of a cavernous malformation from a hemorrhagic neoplasm on MR imaging occasionally can be difficult in the face of acute hemorrhage, particularly in the presence of edema and mass effect. Several imaging features may help to distinguish these two lesions. Findings favoring a cavernous malformation include focal heterogeneous high signal intensity, representing methemoglobin; a complete hypointense peripheral ring, representing hemosiderin, as in this case; and the absence of enhancing solid tissue. When all else fails, follow-up imaging in 4 to 6 weeks may be performed to assess for the expected temporal evolution of hemorrhage when secondary to a cavernous malformation.

Cavernous malformations may be present in up to 5% of the population. Most are located superficially in the cerebrum and are often closely associated with the adjacent subarachnoid space. They may occur deep within the cerebral hemispheres, although this is less common. Cavernous malformations occur less frequently in the infratentorial compartment. The most common brainstem location is the pons. Many are incidental asymptomatic lesions detected on imaging performed for other indications, as in this patient with traumatic injury. When lesions are symptomatic, symptoms may be related to lesion location or acute hemorrhage. In the cerebrum, the most common presentation is seizures. In the infratentorial compartment, neurologic deficits may occur on the basis of acute hemorrhage, thrombosis, or progressive enlargement of a cavernous malformation related to recurrent hemorrhages.

Notes

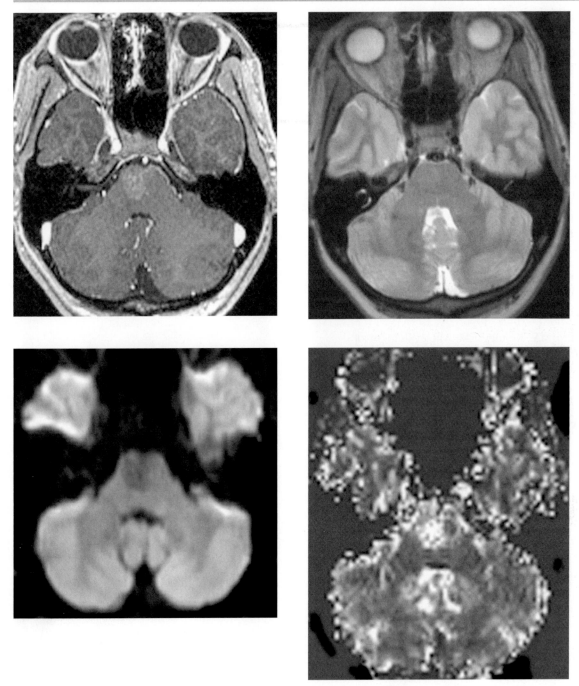

1. What is the most common clinical presentation of these abnormalities?

2. On MR imaging, what are useful findings that distinguish capillary telangiectasias from other lesions (such as inflammatory disease or neoplasm)?

3. What other occult vascular malformations can capillary telangiectasias be associated with?

4. What would a conventional angiogram of a developmental venous anomaly (DVA) show?

Capillary Telangiectasia and Developmental Venous Anomaly of the Brainstem

1. Capillary telangiectasias and DVAs are usually clinically silent, incidental lesions detected on MR imaging performed for other indications.

2. On T2W imaging, most of these lesions have very mild or no associated signal abnormality. Gradient echo imaging frequently shows hypointensity consistent with blood products.

3. DVAs (venous angiomas) and cavernomas.

4. Angiographically, the arterial and capillary phases are normal, and there may be opacification of the DVA during the venous phase.

References

Barr RM, Dillon WP, Wilson CB: Slow-flow vascular malformations of the pons: capillary telangiectasias?, *Am J Neuroradiol* 17:71–78, 1996.

Lee C, Pennington MA, Kenney CM: MR evaluation of developmental venous anomalies: medullary venous anatomy of venous angiomas, *Am J Neuroradiol* 17: 61–70, 1996.

Cross-Reference

Neuroradiology: THE REQUISITES, pp 231, 234.

Comment

Capillary telangiectasias represent a cluster of abnormally dilated capillaries with intervening normal brain tissue. They usually represent clinically silent lesions that are detected on imaging studies acquired for unrelated reasons. Angiographically, they are most often occult. This case nicely illustrates the typical appearance of a capillary telangiectasia on MR imaging: a poorly demarcated region of "feathery" contrast enhancement, corresponding T2W images that show no significant associated signal abnormality, and gradient echo susceptibility images that show hypointensity in the lesion. It has been postulated that T2W shortening on gradient echo imaging may be related to intravascular deoxyhemoglobin from stagnant blood flow. In this case, regional cerebral blood volume shows increased flow that is believed to reflect pooling of blood in dilated capillaries and venules. Capillary telangiectasias may coexist with other vascular malformations, including cavernomas and DVAs.

DVAs are typically incidental vascular malformations representing an aberration in venous drainage. Within the venous network is intervening normal brain tissue, and no arterial elements are associated with these lesions. The angiomas are composed of a tuft of enlarged venous channels that drain into a common venous trunk, which then subsequently drains into the deep or superficial venous system. Typically, the lesions are clinically silent, although they may be associated with intracranial hemorrhage. These lesions have a characteristic MR imaging appearance, representing a cluster of veins oriented in a "radial" pattern that drain into a large central vein. There is usually no significant signal abnormality in the adjacent brain parenchyma. Angiographically, the arterial and capillary phases are normal, and there may be opacification of the DVA during the venous phase.

Notes

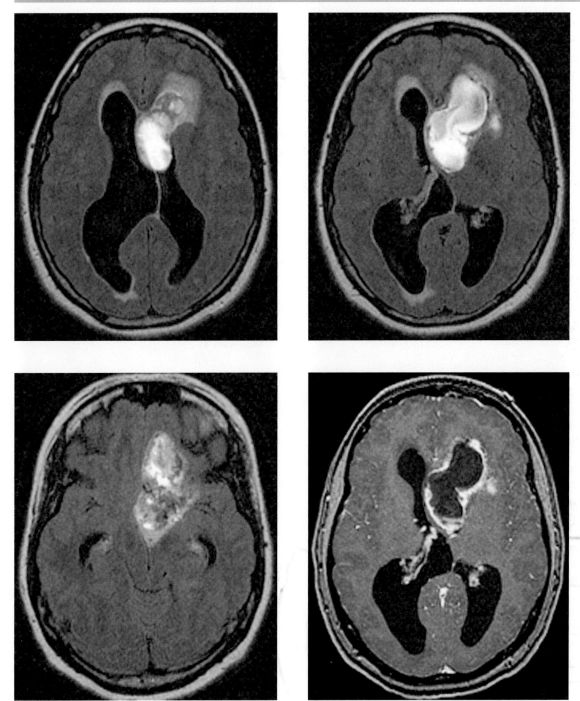

1. What are the most common locations for choroid plexus papillomas in children and adults, respectively?

2. On imaging and conventional pathologic examination, central neurocytomas are frequently indistinguishable from what primary glial neoplasm?

3. What is the most common site for intraventricular meningiomas?

4. Craniopharyngiomas occasionally arise within what ventricle?

Central Neurocytoma

1. In children, the atria of the lateral ventricles. In adults, the fourth ventricle.

2. Oligodendroglioma. Electron microscopy and immuno-histochemistry show neurosecretory granules and the neuronal marker synaptophysin, respectively, which are characteristic of central neurocytoma.

3. The atria of the lateral ventricles.

4. The third ventricle.

References

Cooper JA: Central neurocytoma, *RadioGraphics* 22:1472, 2002.

Shin JH, Lee HK, Khang SK, et al: Neuronal tumors of the central nervous system: radiologic findings and pathologic correlation, *RadioGraphics* 22:1177–1189, 2002.

Cross-Reference

Neuroradiology: THE REQUISITES, 2nd ed, p 145.

Comment

Central neurocytomas typically have a homogeneous cell population with neuronal differentiation. These benign neuroepithelial neoplasms occur in young and middle-aged adults. Patients may be asymptomatic, or may present with headache and signs of increased intracranial pressure, frequently due to hydrocephalus, as in this case. Central neurocytomas arise most commonly within the body of the lateral ventricle (less frequently, the third ventricle), adjacent to the septum pellucidum and foramen of Monroe. They have a characteristic attachment to the superolateral ventricular wall. Most are confined to the ventricles, although occasionally parenchymal extension may occur, as in this case, where there is growth into the frontal lobe. These features may help to distinguish neurocytomas from other intraventricular tumors, such as astrocytoma, giant cell astrocytoma, ependymoma, intraventricular oligodendroglioma, and meningioma. Preoperative diagnosis of central neurocytoma may help in planning therapy, because this tumor has a better prognosis than other intraventricular tumors arising in this area.

On CT and MR imaging, neurocytomas typically are heterogeneous masses that contain multiple cysts. They are well demarcated, with smooth, lobulated margins and moderate vascularity. Most neurocytomas have calcifications. On MR imaging, the more solid component of these tumors tends to follow the signal characteristics of gray matter. Signal voids may be related to calcification or tumor vascularity. Contrast enhancement is variable, ranging from none to moderate. On imaging and conventional pathologic evaluation (light microscopy), these tumors are frequently indistinguishable from oligodendrogliomas. The distinction between these two neoplasms is important because central neurocytomas have a more benign course and treatment may differ. Although neurocytomas have a favorable prognosis, malignant variants and recurrences may rarely occur.

Notes

- Central neurocytoma
- ependymoma
- Astrocytoma
- intra vent oligodendroglione
- menangioma / mets

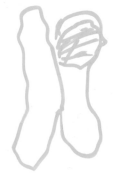

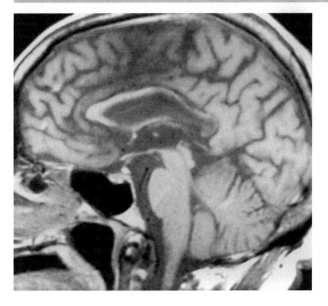

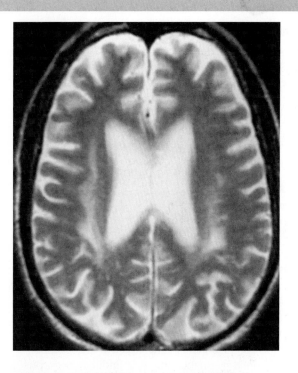

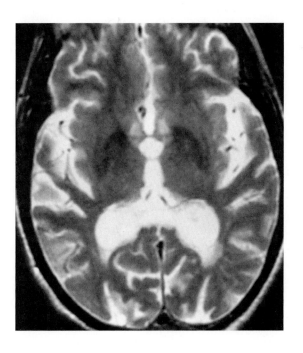

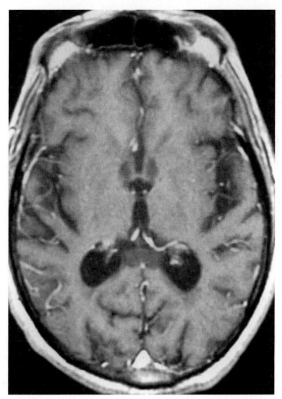

1. What are the imaging findings in this case?

2. What is the characteristic location for osmotic demyelination?

3. What was this patient's clinical presentation?

4. This entity is considered to be in what category of demyelinating disease?

Marchiafava-Bignami Disease

1. Abnormal T2W image hyperintensity, with corresponding hypointensity on unenhanced T1W images of the splenium of the corpus callosum. There is also atrophy of the splenium. In addition, in this 48-year-old patient, there is global cerebral atrophy and multiple additional foci of T2W hyperintensity are seen in the periventricular white matter.

2. The pons.

3. Progressive dementia.

4. Extrapontine myelinolysis.

References

Arbelaez A, Pajon A, Castillo M: Acute Marchiafava-Bignami disease: MR findings in two patients, *AJNR Am J Neuroradiol* 24:1955–1957, 2003.

Kawarabuki K, Sakakibara T, Hirai M, Yoshioko Y, Yamamoto Y, Yamaki T: Marchiafava-Bignami disease: magnetic resonance imaging findings in corpus callosum and subcortical white matter, *Eur J Radiol* 48:175–177, 2003.

Cross-Reference

Neuroradiology: THE REQUISITES, 2nd ed, pp 356–358.

Comment

Marchiafava-Bignami disease is a toxic demyelinating disorder initially described by two Italian pathologists. They identified it at autopsy in three patients with chronic alcoholism who presented in status epilepticus that subsequently progressed to coma. All three patients consumed large quantities of red wine. This has also been described in patients with significant nutritional deficiencies, and it has been described in other populations and with other alcoholic beverages. This diagnosis should be considered in patients with acute encephalopathy or progressive dementia and alcoholism. The disease may present acutely, with rapid deterioration, or may exist in a chronic form over a period of years. It is most commonly seen in men, and usually occurs in the third to fifth decade.

On pathologic evaluation, Marchiafava-Bignami disease is typified by demyelination and necrosis, and it occurs most commonly in the corpus callosum; however, there may be extensive demyelination involving multiple areas of the brain, as in this case, including the deep and periventricular white matter, as well as other commissural fibers. Occasionally, this may involve the subcortical white matter, but typically, the subcortical U-fibers are spared. Sagittal T1W images are valuable in assessing these patients because these images show the extensive callosal atrophy and the associated focal necrosis as demarcated regions of signal abnormality that are hypointense on T1W imaging and hyperintense on T2W imaging. This case nicely demonstrates all of these findings. The acute form of this disease presents with seizures, muscular hypertonia, dysphagia, and coma, and it is often fatal. In the acute form, diffusion-weighted images show hyperintensity (restricted diffusion), and there may be enhancement in affected regions of white matter. In the absence of a patient history, it would be difficult to distinguish this diagnosis from the other demyelinating processes that are more common, such as multiple sclerosis. However, Marchiafava-Bignami disease should be considered in patients with encephalopathy and a history of chronic alcoholism.

Notes

DWI restricted

Demyelinating D: MS
ADEM
Alcoholic   Marchiafava
encephalopathy   bignami

Corpus callosum

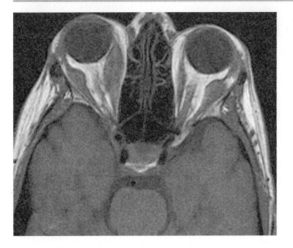
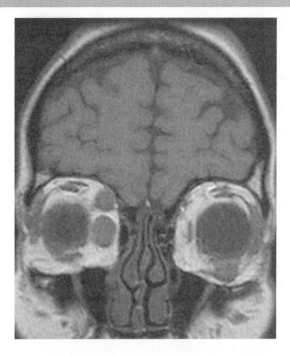
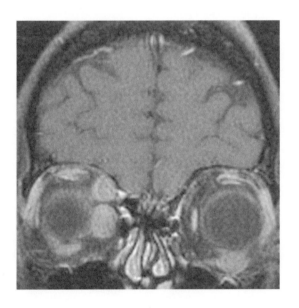
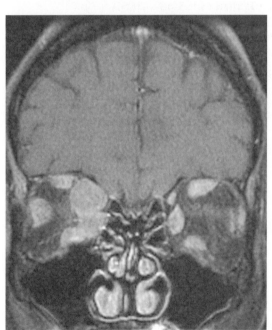

1. Why is thyroid ophthalmopathy an unlikely diagnosis in this case?

2. What is the classic presentation of orbital pseudotumor?

3. What bone comprising the orbit is most commonly affected with metastatic disease?

4. What characteristic imaging finding, when present, is highly suggestive of metastatic breast carcinoma to the orbit?

Metastatic Carcinoid to the Orbital Extraocular Muscles

1. In thyroid ophthalmopathy, the tendinous insertions on the globe are typically spared (involvement is seen in this case); and in this case, there are discrete masses along the muscle bellies, rather than fusiform enlargement that is typical of thyroid disease.

2. Pain! Patients may also have unilateral exophthalmos, lid swelling, chemosis, and restricted ocular motility.

3. The greater wing of the sphenoid bone.

4. Enophthalmos. Inward retraction of the globe (just like the skin of the affected breast) is characteristic of metastatic scirrhous breast carcinoma.

References

Borota OC, Kloster R, Lindal S: Carcinoid tumour metastatic to the orbit with infiltration to the extraocular orbital muscle, *APMIS* 113:135–139, 2005.

Hanson MW, Schneider AM, Enterline DS, Feldman JM, Gockerman JP: Iodine-131-mataiodobenzylguanidine uptake in metastatic carcinoid tumor to the orbit, *J Nucl Med* 39:647–650, 1998.

Cross-Reference

Neuroradiology: THE REQUISITES, 2nd ed, pp 501, 503, 512–513, 638.

Comment

Carcinoid tumors arise from Kulchitsky cells that originate in the neural crest. Most carcinoids arise in the gastrointestinal tract or the lung. This case represents metastatic carcinoid to the orbit, specifically, to the extraocular muscles. With rare exception, the reported metastatic carcinoid tumors to the uvea all developed from primary bronchial carcinoids. In contrast, the vast majority of reported orbital metastases arose from ileal carcinoids. The metastatic potential of carcinoid tumors is related to the site of origin and to tumor size, with histologic features playing a lesser role. In symptomatic patients with intestinal carcinoid, more than 90% have metastatic disease, which is most common to the lymph nodes and liver. Tumors larger than 1 cm are more likely to metastasize.

Metastatic disease to the orbits is common. The imaging diagnosis of orbital metastases as the first manifestation of metastatic disease is not uncommon. For every case of clinically evident orbital metastases, there are several asymptomatic cases that go unrecognized. The most common location for orbital metastases is the globe, usually involving the region of the choroid and retina. Ocular metastases characteristically involve the uveoscleral region. The most common tumors to metastasize to the globe are breast and lung carcinoma in adults. Outside of the globe, orbital metastases most often are extraconal and are often related to bone metastases. Intraconal metastatic disease is usually related to direct extension of an ocular metastasis. Clinical manifestations of ocular metastases are variable. Some patients may be asymptomatic, whereas others may have proptosis, blurred vision, pain, or ophthalmoplegia, depending on the site of involvement.

Notes

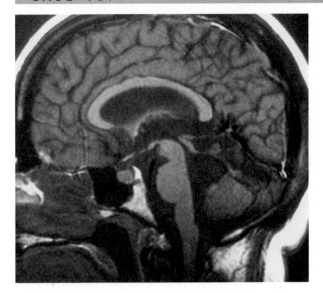

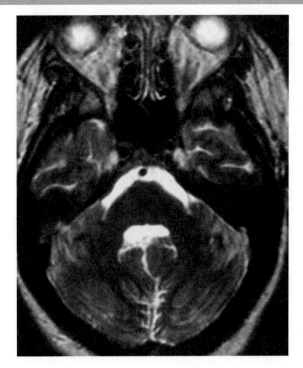

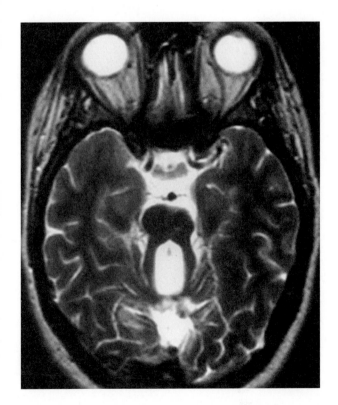

1. How can Dandy-Walker malformation be distinguished from cerebellar hypoplasia or dysplasia?

2. What are common causes of acquired cerebellar volume loss or atrophy?

3. Which type of Chiari malformation is not associated with lumbosacral myelomeningocele?

4. What is the hallmark finding in Joubert's syndrome?

Joubert's Syndrome *AR*

1. Dandy-Walker malformations are characterized by a retrocerebellar cyst that communicates with the fourth ventricle. In true Dandy-Walker malformations, the posterior fossa is usually enlarged. In addition, up to 75% of patients with these malformations have associated hydrocephalus or supratentorial anomalies that are not typical of most cerebellar hypoplasias.

2. Alcohol, phenytoin, malnutrition, a spectrum of neurodegenerative disorders, and certain paraneoplastic syndromes.

3. Chiari I and Chiari III malformations.

4. The hallmark of Joubert's syndrome is separation or disconnection of the cerebellar hemispheres, which are apposed but not fused in the midline.

References

Friede RL, Boltshauser E: Uncommon syndromes of cerebellar vermis aplasia. I: Joubert syndrome, *Dev Med Child Neurol* 20:758–763, 1978.

Sener RN: MR imaging of Joubert's syndrome, *Comput Med Imaging Graph* 19:481–486, 1995.

Cross-Reference

Neuroradiology: THE REQUISITES, 2nd ed, pp 433–434.

Comment

Cerebellar developmental anomalies have been loosely categorized into complete or incomplete cerebellar agenesis, median aplasia or hypoplasia, and lateral aplasia or hypoplasia. These aberrations in cerebellar development may result in prominent CSF spaces or CSF collections or cystic dilation of the fourth ventricle (giant cisterna magna, Dandy-Walker malformations) in the posterior fossa. Other rarer entities are associated with enlargement or an abnormal configuration of the fourth ventricle. Such entities include aplasia or a spectrum of hypoplasias involving the cerebellar hemispheres, vermis, or brainstem. Unlike Dandy-Walker malformations, these cerebellar hypoplasias are not associated with posterior fossa cysts and less commonly have associated hydrocephalus or associated supratentorial anomalies.

The predominant abnormality in Joubert's syndrome is aplasia or hypoplasia of the vermis, particularly the superior portion. In addition, these patients have dysplastic cerebellar tissue, including heterotopic and dysplastic cerebellar nuclei; abnormal development of the inferior olivary nuclei; and incomplete formation of the pyramidal decussation. It is an autosomal recessive disorder.

Magnetic resonance images in these patients show a characteristic appearance. Specifically, sagittal T1W images demonstrate a diminutive vermis. Axial images in particular show an enlarged fourth ventricle with a "bat-wing" shape. The superior cerebellar peduncles are vertically oriented and elongated in the anteroposterior direction. Because of the dysgenesis of the vermis, the hallmark of Joubert's syndrome is separation or disconnection of the cerebellar hemispheres, which are apposed but not fused in the midline.

Notes

- Alcohol
- phenytoin
- malnutrition
- neurodegenerative
- paraneoplastic (med Tem lobe pone)

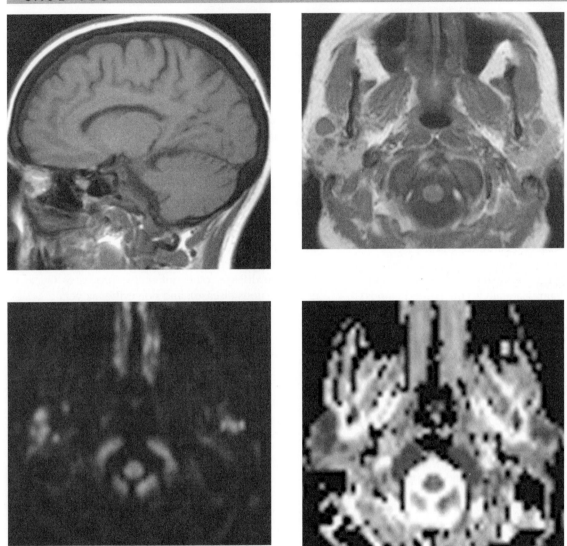

1. What are the major imaging findings?

2. What is the differential diagnosis of diffuse marrow abnormality in this 64-year-old patient?

3. What is the differential diagnosis of solid bilateral parotid nodules?

4. What is the best diagnosis in this case?

Systemic Non-Hodgkin's Lymphoma

1. Diffuse replacement of the calvarial, clival and skull base marrow with tissue hypointense to white matter; and multiple bilateral parotid nodules.

2. Infiltrative marrow disorders, including hematologic malignancies (leukemia, lymphoma, multiple myeloma), metastatic disease (breast and lung), and chronic anemia. In isolation, this finding can occasionally represent a normal variation.

3. Usually, purely solid bilateral nodules represent lymph nodes. The differential diagnosis includes lymphoma (almost always non-Hodgkin's), sarcoid, Sjögren's syndrome (with or without superimposed lymphoma), rheumatoid arthritis, and rarely, metastatic disease (usually unilateral and most often from skin cancer; occasionally, midline scalp skin cancers may drain bilaterally to the parotid glands).

4. Non-Hodgkin's lymphoma.

Reference

Loevner LA, Tobey JD, Yousem DM, Sonners AI, Hsu WC: MR characteristics of cranial marrow in adults with systemic disorders compared to normal controls, *AJNR Am J Neuroradiol* 23:248–254, 2002.

Cross-Reference

Neuroradiology: THE REQUISITES, 2nd ed, pp 708–709.

Comment

This case illustrates diffuse calvarial and skull base marrow replacement, in addition to solid bilateral parotid masses consistent with lymph nodes. The best diagnosis, based on all of the imaging findings, is non-Hodgkin's lymphoma. In this case, lymph node and bone marrow biopsy both showed small B-cell lymphoma. Did you notice that the bilateral parotid masses show restricted diffusion (very suggestive of lymphoma)?

Magnetic resonance imaging is well suited to the evaluation of bone marrow because it can differentiate fat from other tissues. Signal intensity is directly related to relative amounts of fat, water, and cells in the marrow. Hematopoietic (red) marrow is composed of approximately 40% fat, 40% water, and 20% protein, compared with inactive fatty (yellow) marrow, which contains approximately 80% fat, 10% to 15% water, and 5% protein. On unenhanced T1W images, yellow marrow is hyperintense relative to muscle; it approaches the intensity of subcutaneous fat. Cellular red marrow has intermediate signal intensity, which may be isointense or slightly hyperintense relative to muscle, depending on the cell:fat ratio. Marrow conversion is a normal process

in which yellow marrow gradually replaces red marrow. At birth, marrow is predominantly red in both the appendicular and axial skeletons. In the appendicular skeleton, most of the marrow has undergone conversion by the time an individual is 25 years of age. Residual red marrow is found in the proximal metaphyses of the femurs and humeri. In the axial skeleton, a larger portion of the marrow in adults remains hematopoietic compared with the appendicular skeleton.

A spectrum of processes may affect bone marrow. When demand for hematopoeisis is increased in response to systemic stresses, such as chronic anemia, heart failure, or heavy smoking, reconversion of fatty marrow to cellular marrow may occur in an anatomic pattern opposite to that of conversion. In addition, cellular replacement of bone marrow may occur in hematologic malignancies, metastatic disease, other infiltrative processes (such as granulomatous disease), and polycythemia vera.

Notes

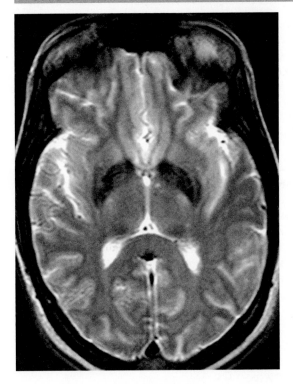 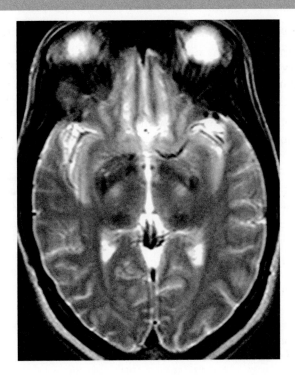

1. What is the pertinent imaging finding?

2. Positive findings on Perls' staining indicate the presence of what type of product?

3. What deep gray nucleus shows increasing amounts of iron deposition with age?

4. What deep gray matter structures typically do not show hypointensity on T2W images in normal patients, regardless of age?

5. For double brownie points, what underlying neurodegenerative disease does this patient have?

Abnormal Iron Deposition in Deep Gray Matter Nuclei

1. T2W hypointensity in the deep gray matter of the basal ganglia (bilateral lentiform nuclei) and pulvinar of the thalami.

2. Iron (ferric)-containing compounds.

3. The lentiform nucleus, especially the globus pallidus.

4. The caudate nucleus and thalamus.

5. Amyotrophic lateral sclerosis (did you note the bilaterally symmetric T2W hyperintensity in the corticospinal tracts)?

References

Loevner LA, Shapiro RM, Grossman RI, Overhauser J, Kamholz J: White matter changes associated with partial deletion of the long-arm of chromosome 18 (18q-syndrome): a dysmyelinating disorder?, *AJNR Am J Neuroradiol* 17:1843–1848, 1996.

Milton WJ, Atlas SW, Lexa FJ, Mozley PD, Gur RE: Deep gray matter hypointensity patterns with aging in healthy adults: MR imaging at 1.5 T, *Radiology* 181:715–719, 1991.

Cross-Reference

Neuroradiology: THE REQUISITES, 2nd ed, pp 53–55, 336, 388–389, 391–392.

Comment

Detection of iron deposition within the deep gray matter of the brain (globus pallidus, putamen, caudate nucleus, thalamus), as well as the dentate nuclei, substantia nigra, and red nuclei, manifests as hypointensity on T2W images and may serve as an indirect marker of cerebral neurodegenerative processes. Axial T2W gradient echo susceptibility imaging shows striking hypointensity in involved structures due to paramagnetic effects. Although there is a spectrum of normal iron deposition within the basal ganglia and brainstem nuclei noted on pathologic examination and to some extent confirmed on MR imaging, certain trends are clear. Specifically, in healthy young adults, hypointensity within the substantia nigra, red nucleus, and dentate nucleus is seen on T2W images. Both evaluation of pathologic specimens and MR imaging suggest that the volume of iron products in these structures does not significantly increase with age. Although hypointensity in the globus pallidus is often present in young adults, the amount of hypointensity (reflective of iron deposition) increases with age. In addition, whereas hypointensity may be seen in the putamen, in normal subjects, this typically is not seen before the sixth decade. Of note, hypointensity in the thalamus or caudate nucleus generally is not present in normal subjects, regardless of age, and hypointensity in these locations is indicative of CNS disease.

A variety of CNS disorders may be suggested by the detection of hypointensity within the deep gray matter and nuclei that is different from the expected normal patterns. Increased brain iron levels may be seen in a variety of pathologic states, including demyelinating or dysmyelinating diseases (multiple sclerosis), the leukodystrophies, brain anoxia and infarction, movement disorders (Wilson's disease, Hallervorden-Spatz disease), endocrinologic or metabolic disorders (hyperparathyroidism, hypoparathyroidism, pseudohypoparathyroidism), and significant closed head trauma. The patient in this case has underlying amyotrophic lateral sclerosis (Lou Gehrig's disease).

Notes

anoxia co
infarction
wilson
Hallervorden spatz
metabolic hyperpara
hypopara
pseudohypopara

ALS

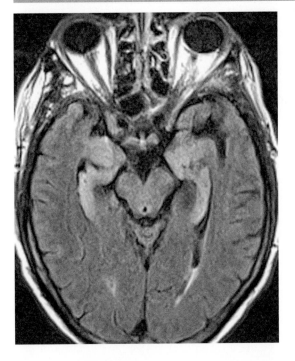

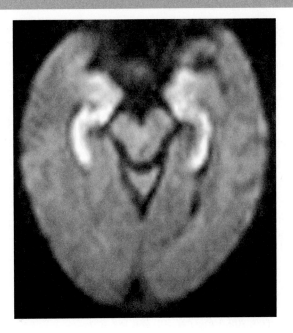

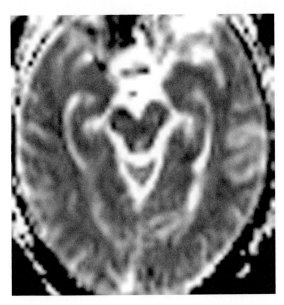

1. What structures are involved in this patient?

2. What is the differential diagnosis in an immunocompromised patient?

3. What was this patient's clinical presentation?

4. What group of patients is at increased risk for herpes zoster infection?

Herpes Encephalopathy—Human Herpesvirus-6 Infection after Organ Transplantation

1. The hippocampi and amygdala.

2. Herpes simplex type 1 encephalitis, other viral encephalopathies (influenza), paraneoplastic syndrome, and drug-induced encephalopathy.

3. Altered mental status, including disorientation.

4. Immunosuppressed patients.

Reference

Noguchi T, Mihara F, Yoshiura T, et al: MR imaging of human herpesvirus-6 encephalopathy after hematopoietic stem cell transplantation in adults, *AJNR Am J Neuroradiol* 27:2191–2195, 2006.

Cross-Reference

Neuroradiology: THE REQUISITES, 2nd ed, pp 288–290.

Comment

Human herpesvirus-6 (HHV-6) is a double-stranded DNA virus. More than 90% of the general population is seropositive for HHV-6. It is excreted by the salivary glands and may be passed to infants from their mothers. HHV-6 has a strong affinity for the CNS, and has been detected by polymerase chain reaction in up to one third of normal brain specimens, suggesting that the brain might be a latent viral site. Recently, HHV-6 encephalopathy has been reported in immunocompromised patients, especially patients who have undergone hematopoietic stem cell or solid-organ transplantation (lung and liver). Infection has typically been identified within 4 weeks of the transplantation. The pathogenesis is considered to be reactivation of the recipient's latent HHV-6 infection, and not infection from the donor. Immunocompromised patients are at risk for a spectrum of disease processes that may affect the CNS, and their symptoms are frequently nonspecific. Common neurologic symptoms in HHV-6 infection include disorientation, confusion, and short-term memory loss. Coma, hypopnea, and seizures have been reported.

Early MR imaging findings, as in this case, include high signal intensity on FLAIR, T2W and diffusion-weighted images of the mesial temporal lobe structures (hippocampus and amygdala). The diffusion-weighted abnormality is accompanied by hypointensity on apparent diffusion coefficient maps. Enhancement usually is not present. In transplantation, acyclovir is routinely administered to prevent reactivation of herpes viruses. However, acyclovir is not effective against HHV-6 because it lacks virus-specific thymidine kinase. Gancyclovir and foscarnet can be effective against HHV-6, but serious side effects, including myelosuppression and nephrotoxicity, may occur. Therefore, these drugs are not usually given prophylactically. Early diagnosis is critical to prevent serious neurologic sequelae. Mesial temporal involvement seen on MR images in a transplant recipient receiving preventive treatment with acyclovir is highly suggestive of HHV-6–associated encephalopathy.

Notes

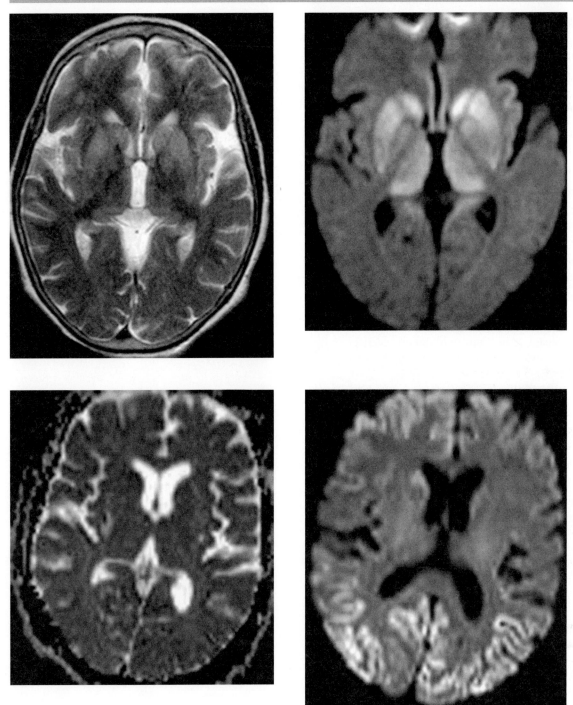

1. What are the imaging findings in this 48-year-old patient?

2. What was the clinical presentation of this patient?

3. What is the most common abnormality on CT in patients with this entity?

4. In addition to eating meat from infected animals (cows, sheep), what other modes of transmission have been associated with this infection?

Jakob-Creutzfeldt Disease

1. Increased signal intensity that is bilaterally symmetric in the deep gray matter of the basal ganglia and thalami that shows restricted diffusion. There is also involvement of the cortex, with greater cortical volume loss than expected for the patient's age.

2. Rapidly progressive dementia.

3. Cortical atrophy.

4. Corneal transplantation, cerebral electrode implantation, and cannibalism.

References

Hori M, Ishigame K, Aoki S, Araki T: Creutzfeldt-Jacob disease shown by line scan diffusion-weighted imaging, *Am J Roentgenol* 180:1481–1482, 2003.

Mao-Drayer Y, Braff SP, Nagle KJ, Pendlebury W, Penar PL, Shapiro RE: Emerging patterns of diffusion-weighted MR imaging in Creutzfeldt-Jakob disease: case report and review of the literature, *AJNR Am J Neuroradiol* 23:550–556, 2002.

Cross-Reference

Neuroradiology: THE REQUISITES, 2nd ed, pp 383–384.

Comment

Jakob-Creutzfeldt disease is rare and is caused by a prion agent composed of protease-resistant protein that affects the CNS and results in rapid, progressive neurodegeneration. Approximately 1 in every 1 million persons worldwide is infected. It is thought to be caused by a slow virus, an organism devoid of active nucleic acid. The most common clinical presentation is that of rapidly progressive dementia. Other neurologic symptoms include upper motor neuron signs, ataxia, myoclonus, and sensory deficits. The characteristic diagnostic triad of progressive dementia, myoclonic jerks, and periodic sharp-wave electroencephalographic activity is present in approximately 75% of cases. Prognosis is poor, with death usually occurring within 1 year from the onset of symptoms. Histologic evaluation shows neuronal degeneration and gliosis in the gray matter, especially the cortex, but also in the deep gray matter of the corpus striatum and thalami, as in this case. Spongiform changes are characteristic. Inflammatory changes are usually not present. The disease is best known in association with mad cow disease (bovine spongiform encephalopathy) in the United Kingdom; however, there have been scattered sporadic cases described with corneal transplantation as well as with implantation of cerebral electrodes.

Computed tomography may show no abnormality; however, atrophy (most commonly cortical) is the next most common presentation. On MR imaging, in addition to cortical atrophy, T2W hyperintensity in the deep gray matter, especially the caudate and putamen nuclei, but also the thalami, is observed. Lesions typically are bilateral and are not associated with enhancement or significant mass effect. In addition, abnormalities involving the gray and white matter have been noted within the cerebral hemispheres. Several reported cases of sporadic Creutzfeldt-Jakob disease have shown increased signal intensity in the basal ganglia or cerebral cortex on diffusion-weighted images (reduced diffusion), as in this case. Ribbon-like areas of hyperintensity in the cerebral cortex on diffusion-weighted images have also corresponded to the localization of periodic sharp-wave complexes on electroencephalogram.

Notes

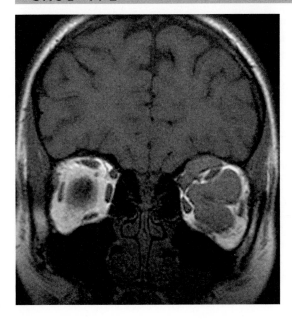
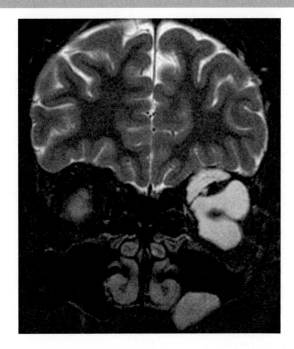

1. What structure runs between the superior extraocular muscle complex and the optic nerve?

2. What is the most common intraconal mass in adults?

3. Which vascular neoplasm is seen almost exclusively in infancy?

4. Where do lymphangiomas typically arise in the orbit?

Orbital Lymphangioma

1. Superior ophthalmic vein.

2. Cavernous hemangioma.

3. Capillary hemangioma.

4. The extraconal compartment.

References

Bilaniuk LT: Orbital vascular lesions: role of imaging, *Radiol Clin North Am* 37:169–183, 1999.

Kazim M, Kennerdell JS, Rothfus W, Marquardt M: Orbital lymphangioma: correlation of magnetic resonance images and intraoperative findings, *Ophthalmology* 99: 1588–1594, 1992.

Cross-Reference

Neuroradiology: THE REQUISITES, 2nd ed, pp 499–500.

Comment

The most common vascular neoplasms in the orbit include cavernous hemangioma, capillary hemangioma, and lymphangioma. They are usually distinguishable based on their location in the orbit, their imaging appearance, and the age of the patient.

Capillary hemangiomas are seen almost exclusively in children and usually present clinically within the first months of life. They usually peak in size within the first 18 months of life and then often undergo spontaneous regression. They are infiltrative lesions that may extend into the periorbita, eyelid, and conjunctiva. Because of their vascularity, they may increase in size during crying or coughing (Valsalva maneuvers). Capillary hemangiomas may involve any portion of the orbit and are frequently associated with vascular flow voids on MR imaging. Cavernous hemangiomas are the most common retrobulbar mass in adults. Their imaging appearance is distinctly different from that of capillary hemangiomas. These are demarcated lesions that appear hyperdense on unenhanced CT, hypointense on T1W imaging, and markedly hyperintense on T2W imaging. After contrast, they enhance avidly. Although phleboliths may be present, this finding is not as common as with hemangiomas in other parts of the body.

Lymphangiomas are poorly demarcated, infiltrating lesions that are less common than hemangiomas. They are usually extraconal in origin and may extend to involve the adjacent extraocular muscles, the soft tissues in the periorbital region, and the conjunctiva. Less commonly, they may extend to the intraconal compartment, as in this case. Small lesions may be asymptomatic; however, patients may become acutely symptomatic as a result of hemorrhage within the lesion. On MR imaging, lymphangiomas have a characteristic appearance. They are usually multilobular, with regions of cystic change and peripheral enhancement. Hemorrhage within cystic regions of the neoplasm is common and usually appears hyperintense on T1W imaging. When present, a key to the diagnosis is the finding of fluid–hemorrhage levels within the lesion. Because lymphangiomas are not encapsulated, surgical resection is difficult and recurrence common.

Notes

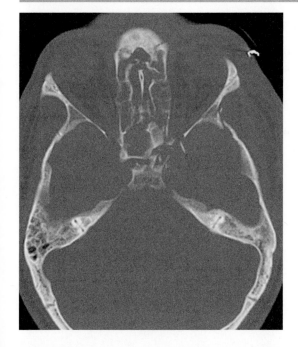

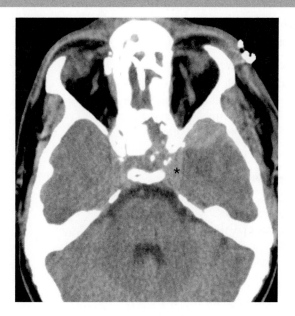

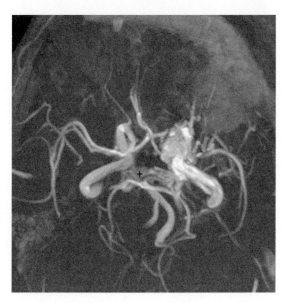

1. The * represents what anatomic structure?

2. What are the CT imaging findings in this case?

3. The compressed axial view of the MR angiography confirms what diagnosis?

4. The + represents what vascular structure?

Carotid–Cavernous Fistula—Part I

1. The * is the abnormally enlarged left cavernous sinus.

2. Multiple facial and skull base fractures, an enlarged left cavernous sinus, a mildly enlarged left superior ophthalmic vein, and a small left middle cranial fossa epidural hematoma.

3. A direct carotid–cavernous fistula.

4. The petrosal venous complex.

Reference

Barrow DL, Spector RH, Braun IF, et al: Classification and treatment of spontaneous carotid-cavernous sinus fistulas, *J Neurosurg* 62:248–256, 1985.

Cross-Reference

Neuroradiology: THE REQUISITES, 2nd ed, pp 263, 499, 500–501, 551.

Comment

There are two basic types of carotid–cavernous vascular malformations, direct (type A) and indirect (dural, types B–D), each of which has a different etiology. Carotid–cavernous fistulas represent a direct communication between the intracavernous portion of the internal carotid artery and the cavernous venous sinus. The typical clinical presentation of a carotid–cavernous fistula is ophthalmologic symptoms, including pulsatile proptosis, pain, chemosis, and orbital bruit. This is because the cavernous sinus directly communicates with the ophthalmic veins, and an abnormal shunt between the sinus and the internal carotid artery can transmit arterial pressure to these veins. In addition, arterial perfusion to the globe is decreased, leading to visual loss. Direct carotid–cavernous fistulas are most commonly the result of head trauma; however, spontaneous carotid–cavernous fistulas may be seen in a spectrum of disorders, including atherosclerosis in the elderly, rupture of a carotid–cavernous aneurysm, or in association with underlying vascular dysplasias. An indirect carotid–cavernous vascular malformation, otherwise known as a dural arteriovenous fistula, is a shunt between meningeal branches of the cavernous internal carotid artery (type B), meningeal branches of the external carotid artery (type C), or meningeal branches of both the intracavernous carotid artery and the external carotid artery (type D) with the cavernous venous sinus.

The clinical presentation and imaging findings are normally diagnostic of a direct carotid–cavernous fistula. CT and MR imaging often show enlargement of the superior ophthalmic vein, cavernous sinus, or petrosal venous plexus, as in this case. Proptosis, periorbital soft tissue swelling, and diffuse enlargement of the extraocular muscles are commonly present. MR angiography and catheter angiography show direct communication between the cavernous internal carotid artery and the cavernous venous sinus as well as early filling of the ipsilateral cavernous sinus, superior or inferior ophthalmic veins, and petrosal venous complex. In high-flow lesions, the contralateral venous system may opacify, as in this case, through both intercavernous veins and the petrosal venous complex.

Notes

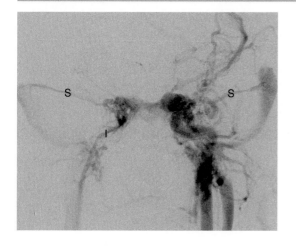

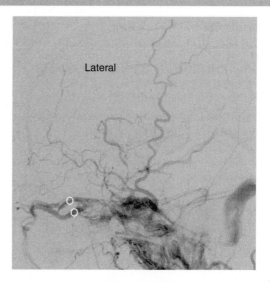

Lateral

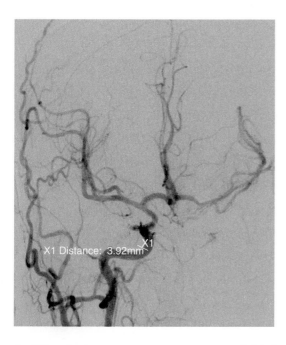

X1 Distance: 3.92mm

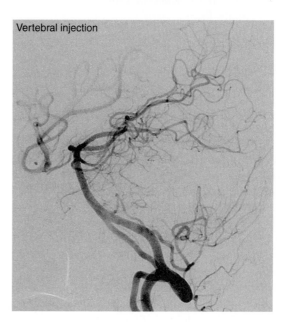

Vertebral injection

1. What is the most common cause of this lesion?

2. When there is cortical venous drainage with this entity, patients are at risk for what complication?

3. What is believed to be the cause of dural malformations involving the cavernous sinus?

4. In cases of high-flow direct carotid–cavernous fistulas, filling of the contralateral venous system may occur through what communicating veins?

Carotid–Cavernous Fistula—Part II

1. Trauma.

2. Intraparenchymal hemorrhage.

3. Venous thrombosis.

4. The petrosal venous plexus and intercavernous veins between the right and left cavernous sinuses. I = inferior petrosal vein; O = superior ophthalmic veins; S = superior petrosal vein.

References

Lewis AI, Tomsick TA, Tew JM Jr: Management of 100 consecutive direct carotid-cavernous fistulas: results of treatment with detachable balloons, *Neurosurgery* 36:239–244, 1995.

Wadlington VR, Terry JB: Endovascular therapy of traumatic carotid-cavernous fistulas, *Crit Care Clin* 15: 831–854, 1999.

Cross-Reference

Neuroradiology: THE REQUISITES, 2nd ed, pp 263, 499, 500–501, 551.

Comment

In this case, the left carotid injection shows the site of the fistula between the cavernous left internal carotid artery and the cavernous venous sinus. Contralateral injection of the right carotid artery and injection of the vertebral basilar arterial system are important in evaluating for collateral flow, particularly if the involved internal carotid artery must be sacrificed to close the fistula, as was necessary in this case. Right common carotid artery injection in this patient shows a patent anterior communicating artery with cross-filling of the left anterior and middle cerebral circulation. Left vertebral artery injection shows filling of the left supraclinoid internal carotid artery through a patent posterior communicating artery.

Management of these lesions in the majority of cases is usually with interventional neuroradiologic procedures. Symptomatic direct carotid–cavernous fistulas (type A) spontaneously resolve only in rare cases. The goal of treatment is to eliminate flow through the fistula as well as to maintain internal carotid patency when possible. Treatment of direct and indirect fistulas may differ. Direct carotid–cavernous fistulas are usually treated transarterially with detachable coils or balloon embolization, with flow directed through the fistula into the cavernous sinus, tamponading the hole in the internal carotid artery. In the event that a transarterial route is not possible or is ineffective, a transvenous approach using platinum coils may be warranted. This can be achieved either via the femoral route or surgically via the superior ophthalmic vein. Complicated carotid–cavernous fistulas, residual carotid–cavernous fistulas after embolization with an arterial approach, and dural arteriovenous fistulas of the cavernous sinus may sometimes need to be treated transvenously. Gamma knife radiosurgery has also been shown to be effective in treating indirect dural arteriovenous fistulas.

Notes

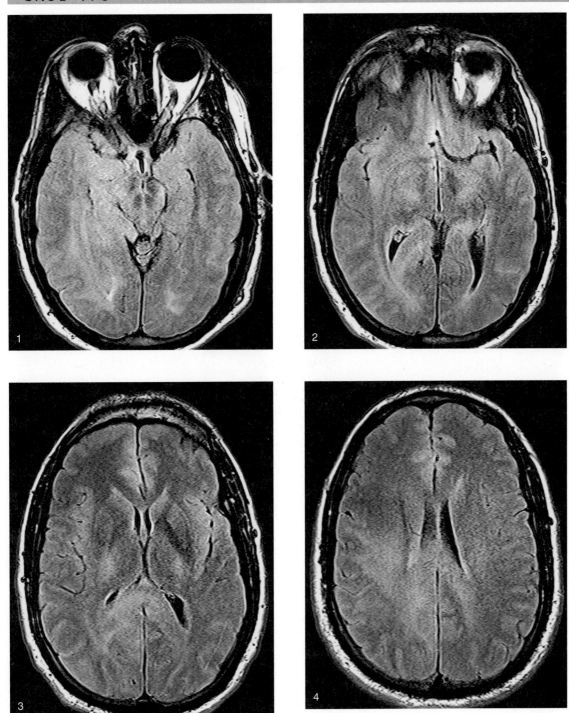

1. What are the three major types of noninfiltrating astrocytic tumors?

2. What is the histologic correlate of gliomatosis cerebri?

3. How often is the corpus callosum involved in gliomatosis cerebri?

4. What might MR perfusion imaging show in this patient?

Gliomatosis Cerebri

1. Subependymal giant cell astrocytoma, pilocytic astrocytoma, and pleomorphic xanthoastrocytoma.

2. Gliomatosis cerebri is composed of elongated glial cells that usually resemble astrocytes. The lesion is diffuse and infiltrates affected areas of brain while preserving the underlying histoarchitecture.

3. The corpus callosum is involved in approximately 50% of cases.

4. Low relative cerebral blood volume comparable to that of normal white matter.

Reference

Yip M, Fisch C, Lamarche FB: Gliomatosis cerebri affecting the entire neuraxis, *RadioGraphics* 23:247–253, 2003.

Cross-Reference

Neuroradiology: THE REQUISITES, 2nd ed, pp 147–148.

Comment

This case illustrates the typical radiologic appearance of gliomatosis cerebri. There is extensive abnormality within the brain that affects the white matter; however, the gray matter is also involved. This extensively infiltrative process affects large portions of the cerebrum, including the right temporal, occipital, and frontal lobes. There is mild gyral swelling and sulcal effacement. There is extension across the splenium of the corpus callosum that is mildly expanded, as well as the anterior commissure, with involvement of the left cerebrum to a lesser extent. There are no regions of necrosis, there is no circumscribed mass, and there is no enhancement (not shown). Also, on image 1, note the involvement of the optic chiasm and bilateral optic tracts.

Gliomatosis cerebri is characterized by an extensive infiltrative pattern throughout the involved portions of the brain disproportionate to the remainder of the histologic findings, including a relative paucity of cellularity, anaplasia, and necrosis. In addition to the disproportionate histologic findings relative to the degree of infiltration seen on MR imaging, clinical symptoms are characteristically mild relative to the degree of brain involvement. Patients often present only with altered mental status or a change in personality. Headaches and seizures may occur. Focal neurologic deficits occur late in the course of disease. Although this tumor may affect patients of any age, it most commonly presents between the third and fifth decades. In addition to the extensive parenchymal involvement and the signal alteration seen on MR imaging, other findings that may suggest the diagnosis include mild diffuse sulcal and ventricular effacement. Not uncommonly, a large resection or lobectomy is necessary to make the diagnosis pathologically because biopsy may provide insufficient material. Therefore, recognition of the imaging findings, in combination with the patient's history, is important in diagnosing this neoplasm. Radiologists play a critical role by suggesting the diagnosis, mapping the extent of disease, and guiding biopsy.

Notes

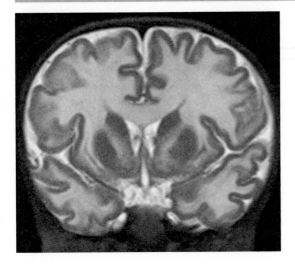

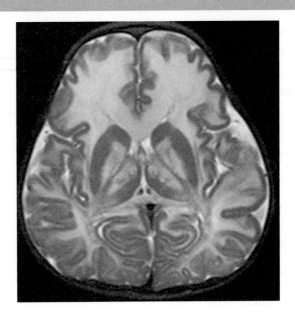

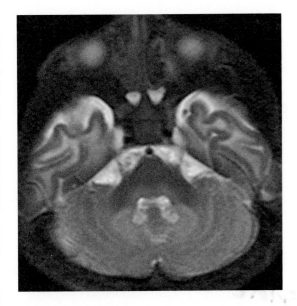

1. What leukodystrophies are associated with enlargement of the head?

2. What is the typical clinical presentation of the leukodystrophies?

3. What leukodystrophy is unusual in that it begins in the subcortical white matter rather than the deep white matter?

4. What enzyme deficiency is responsible for Canavan disease?

Canavan Disease

1. Alexander and Canavan diseases.

2. Progressive deterioration of motor function, cognitive decline, hypotonia, and spasticity.

3. Canavan disease.

4. Canavan disease is caused by mutations in the gene for an enzyme called N-acetylaspartoacylase.

Reference

Engelbrecht V, Scherer A, Rassek M, Witsack HJ, Modder U: Diffusion-weighted MR imaging in the brain in children: findings in the normal brain and in the brain with white matter diseases, *Radiology* 222: 410–418, 2002.

Cross-Reference

Neuroradiology: THE REQUISITES, 2nd ed, pp 361–362.

Comment

The leukodystrophies, or dysmyelinating disorders, represent a spectrum of inherited diseases that usually result in both abnormal formation and abnormal maintenance of myelin. Many of the more common of these rare disorders are inherited in an autosomal recessive pattern. In many of the leukodystrophies, specific enzyme deficiencies have been identified as the cause. These diseases cause abnormal growth or development of the myelin sheath, the fatty covering that acts as an insulator around nerve fibers in the brain. Myelin is made up of at least 10 different chemicals. Each of the leukodystrophies affects one (and only one) of these substances.

Canavan disease is transmitted as an autosomal recessive disorder usually identified in infants of Ashkenazi Jewish descent and in Saudi Arabians. It is the result of a deficiency of N-acetylaspartoacyclase. Infants may have macrocephaly due to enlargement of the brain. On histologic evaluation, there is diffuse demyelination and the white matter is replaced by microscopic cystic spaces, giving it a "spongy" appearance. In contrast to most of the other dysmyelinating syndromes, Canavan disease preferentially begins in the subcortical white matter and later spreads to diffusely involve the deep white matter. There may be sparing of the internal capsules. There may be bilaterally symmetric T2W signal abnormality in the deep gray matter, as in this case. The brainstem is involved in late disease. Usually, the ventricles remain normal or may be slightly small; however, in the late stages of disease, when cerebral atrophy occurs, there may be proportionate enlargement of the ventricles and cerebral sulci. Diffusion-weighted imaging shows diffuse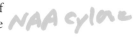

restriction, and spectroscopy shows high levels of N-acetylaspartoacyclase.

Alexander disease is different from many of the leukodystrophies in that no familial pattern has been recognized. Like Canavan disease, it presents with macrocephaly in addition to developmental delay and spasticity. The deep white matter is usually involved early, and the internal capsules are typically involved (in contrast to Canavan disease, in which they are often relatively spared).

Notes

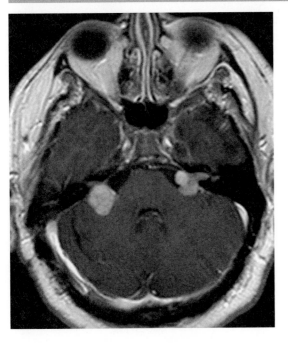 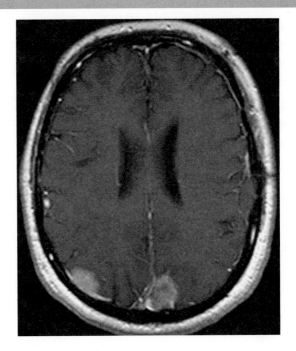

1. What are the imaging findings?

2. What syndrome does this patient have?

3. What primary glial neoplasm is this disorder associated with?

4. From what type of nerves do schwannomas typically arise?

Neurofibromatosis Type 2

1. Bilateral vestibular schwannomas and multiple dural-based, extra-axial masses, consistent with meningiomas.

2. Neurofibromatosis type 2.

3. Ependymoma.

4. Sensory nerves. Uncommonly, they may be associated with motor nerves, and this should prompt a workup for neurofibromatosis type 2.

References

Aoki S, Barkovich AJ, Nishimura K, et al: Neurofibromatosis types 1 and 2: cranial MR findings, *Radiology* 172:527–534, 1989.

Mautner V, Lindenau M, Baser ME, et al: The neuro-imaging and clinical spectrum of neurofibromatosis 2, *Neurosurgery* 38:880–885, 1996.

Cross-Reference

Neuroradiology: THE REQUISITES, 2nd ed, pp 452–453.

Comment

This case shows imaging findings characteristic of neurofibromatosis type 2, including bilateral vestibular schwannomas, as well as multiple dural-based, extra-axial, avidly enhancing masses, consistent with meningiomas.

Neurofibromatosis type 2 is an autosomal dominant disorder transmitted on chromosome 22. It typically presents in adolescence or young adulthood, and the most common clinical presentation is bilateral sensorineural hearing loss as a result of vestibular schwannomas. The radiologic hallmark of neurofibromatosis type 2 is the presence of bilateral vestibular schwannomas. Otherwise, the diagnosis of neurofibromatosis type 2 can be made if a patient has a unilateral vestibular schwannoma and a first-degree relative with neurofibromatosis type 2, or if patient has a first-degree relative with neurofibromatosis type 2 and at least two schwannomas, meningiomas, or ependymomas. Unlike neurofibromatosis type 1, cutaneous manifestations in neurofibromatosis type 2 are rare. CNS tumors are present in virtually 100% of patients with neurofibromatosis type 2. Schwannomas most commonly involve cranial nerve VIII. The trigeminal nerve is the next most common site for schwannomas. Although most of these tumors are sporadic, those arising from more than one cranial nerve or from cranial nerves III through VI should prompt a search for neurofibromatosis type 2. Other imaging findings that may be present in neurofibromatosis type 2 include prominent calcifications along the choroid plexus, or occasionally along the cerebral or cerebellar cortex. Lesions within the spinal canal are common and include schwannomas and meningiomas. Intramedullary tumors are typically ependymomas.

Notes

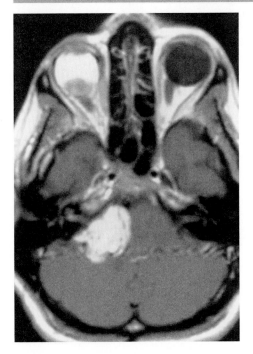 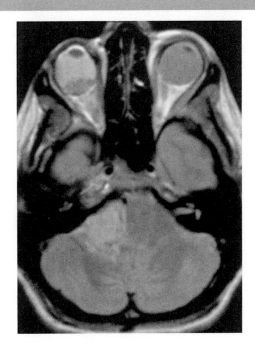

1. What is the most common primary intraocular malignancy in adults?

2. What is the most common site of metastases to the orbit?

3. What are the classic signal characteristics of ocular melanoma?

4. What metastatic tumor to the uveal tract may have signal characteristics similar to those of primary ocular melanoma?

Metastasis to the Cerebellopontine Angle—Ocular Melanoma

1. Melanoma.

2. The uveal tract.

3. Hyperintense on T1W imaging and hypointense on T2W imaging.

4. Metastatic mucin-secreting adenocarcinomas.

Reference

Feldman ED, Pingpank JF, Alexander HR: Regional treatment options for patients with ocular melanoma metastatic to the liver, *Ann Surg Oncol* 11:290–297, 2004.

Cross-Reference

Neuroradiology: THE REQUISITES, 2nd ed, pp 483–484.

Comment

This case shows a poorly demarcating enhancing mass in the right cerebellopontine angle, with extension into the internal auditory canal (IAC). The differential diagnosis includes schwannoma, meningioma, metastatic disease, and an inflammatory mass. The appearance of the mass is atypical for a meningioma, given the extension into the IAC and the poorly demarcated margins. Similarly, poorly defined boundaries, lack of cystic degeneration, and absence of expansion of the IAC, in conjunction with abnormality within it, are atypical features of vestibular schwannoma.

Malignant melanoma of the uveal tract represents the most common intraocular malignancy of adults. It is usually unilateral and commonly presents in the fifth and sixth decades. On CT, ocular melanomas are typically hyperdense relative to the vitreous and enhance after contrast. On MR imaging, melanotic melanomas are characteristically hyperintense on T1W and hypointense on T2W images. The signal characteristics are related to the paramagnetic effects of melanin. In the absence of intravenous contrast, melanoma could be mistaken for hemorrhage, such as that seen with retinal detachment. However, enhanced images typically show solid enhancing tissue with melanomas. Did you notice the primary melanoma of the right uveal tract?

The most common site of metastases to the orbit is also along the uveal tract, and for this reason, metastatic disease to the orbit may be confused with primary ocular melanoma. Metastatic mucin-secreting adenocarcinomas of the uveal tract have been noted to have signal characteristics similar to those of ocular melanoma.

The most important role of MR imaging is in detecting extraocular extension of primary ocular melanoma. Episcleral involvement, retrobulbar extension, and occasional perineural and intracranial subarachnoid spread may occur. Systemic metastases are most commonly noted in the liver and lungs, but may also be seen in the bone and brain. Therefore, a careful metastatic workup is required to prevent unnecessary enucleation. Two treatments for primary ocular melanoma include removal of the eye (enucleation) and irradiation. Recent studies suggest similar survival rates for these treatments.

Notes

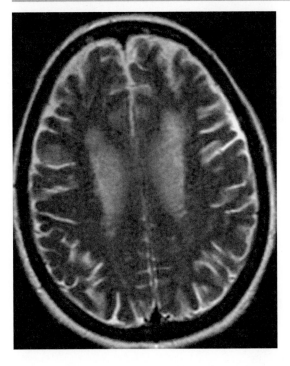

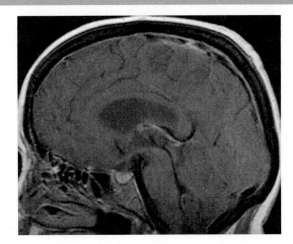

1. What is the finding on the axial FLAIR image?

2. What is the differential diagnosis?

3. What is the normal half-life of gadolinium chelates?

4. What skin condition has recently been reported as a complication of gadolinium administration in patients with renal failure?

Retained Gadolinium—Renal Failure

1. Diffuse hyperintensity in the CSF (subarachnoid spaces and ventricles).

2. Subarachnoid hemorrhage, meningitis, meningeal carcinomatosis, superior sagittal thrombosis, status epilepticus, renal failure, hyperoxygenation, and gadolinium given for a different MR imaging study 24 to 48 hours before brain MR imaging.

3. Approximately 1.6 hours.

4. Gadolinium-induced nephrogenic fibrosing dermopathy.

Reference

Morris JM, Miller GM: Increased signal intensity in the subarachnoid space on fluid-attenuated inversion recovery imaging associated with the clearance dynamics of gadolinium chelate: a potential diagnostic pitfall, *AJNR Am J Neuroradiol* 28:1964–1967, 2007.

Cross-Reference

Neuroradiology: THE REQUISITES, 2nd ed, pp 11–13, 20–21.

Comment

Fluid-attenuated inversion recovery is routinely used in brain imaging due to its high lesion-to-tissue contrast from T2 prolongation and nulling of the normal CSF background. Therefore, any alteration in the CSF results in increased signal intensity in the CSF. Flair imaging is particularly sensitive for pathologic entities that affect the CSF in the subarachnoid spaces. Hyperintense CSF in the subarachnoid spaces on FLAIR imaging has been reported in numerous conditions, including subarachnoid hemorrhage, meningitis, meningeal carcinomatosis, venous sinus thrombosis, status epilepticus, and stroke. Increased signal intensity in the subarachnoid spaces can be a diagnostic pitfall in patients receiving supplemental oxygen during MR imaging of the brain and in patients with renal insufficiency who have previously received gadolinium (as in this case).

Gadolinium has also been reported to diffuse across the choroid plexus and uveochoroid membrane in patients with impaired renal function, resulting in FLAIR hyperintensity in the ventricular system and in the vitreous and aqueous humor of the eye. The mechanism by which CSF diffuses into the CSF spaces is not clearly understood. It has been postulated that in patients with renal insufficiency, the gadolinium may move across an osmotic gradient at the circumventricular organs in the setting of prolonged elevation of plasma concentrations because it is primarily cleared through glomerular filtration.

Some patients will have undergone gadolinium-enhanced MR imaging 24 to 48 hours before MR imaging of the brain. The radiologist should be aware that delayed gadolinium chelate clearance can cause increased signal intensity in the CSF on FLAIR imaging in patients with or without renal failure and without abnormalities known to disrupt the blood–brain barrier.

Notes

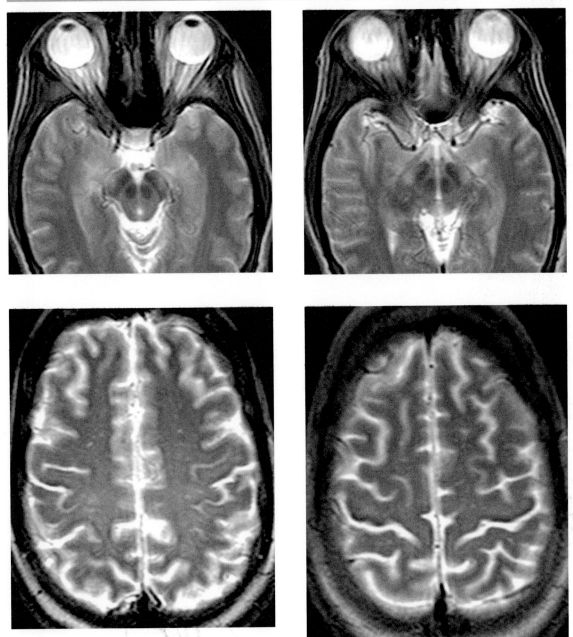

1. What anatomic structures are affected in this case on MR imaging?

2. This entity involves degeneration of what CNS structures?

3. In what part of the brainstem is the pyramidal decussation located?

4. What is the most common cause of death in these patients?

Amyotrophic Lateral Sclerosis—Lou Gehrig's Disease

1. There is bilaterally symmetric high signal intensity within the corticospinal tracts in the cerebral peduncles.

2. The motor neurons.

3. The medulla.

4. Death usually results from pulmonary causes (respiratory failure, infections).

Reference

Bowen BC, Pattany PM, Bradley WG, et al: MR imaging and localized proton spectroscopy of the precentral gyrus in amyotrophic lateral sclerosis, *AJNR Am J Neuroradiol* 21:647–658, 2000.

Cross-Reference

Neuroradiology: THE REQUISITES, 2nd ed, pp 388–389.

Comment

Amyotrophic lateral sclerosis (Lou Gehrig's disease) is the most common of the neurodegenerative disorders involving the motor neurons. It occurs in approximately 1 in every 100,000 people annually. Most cases are sporadic, although autosomal dominant transmission may occur. Amyotrophic lateral sclerosis typically presents in the sixth decade of life; clinical manifestations include hyperreflexia, weakness of the hands and forearms, spasticity, and cranial neuropathies. The hypoglossal nerve is most commonly affected, and its involvement may be detected on imaging as denervation atrophy with fatty replacement of the tongue.

Amyotrophic lateral sclerosis typically involves the corticospinal tracts and motor neurons. Progression is usually relentless, with death frequently occurring within 3 to 6 years of disease onset. The cause is unknown. In extreme cases, abnormal T2W signal intensity may extend from the cortex, along the precentral gyrus of the motor strip (pyramidal Betz's cells or upper motor neurons); through the corona radiata, the posterior part of the posterior limb of the internal capsule, the cerebral peduncles, and brainstem; and down to the ventral and lateral portions of the spinal cord. Abnormal T2W hypointensity, believed to be related to the deposition of iron or other minerals, may be present along the cerebral cortex in the motor strip, as in this case. SPECT with *N*-isopropyl-p-I123 iodoamphetamine may show decreased uptake in the cerebral cortex, including the motor cortex. Spectroscopy of the precentral gyrus region has shown a strong correlation between reduced *N*-acetylaspartate and glutamate levels and elevated choline and myoinositol levels and severity of disease. MR imaging of the spinal cord may show atrophy along the corticospinal tracts.

Notes

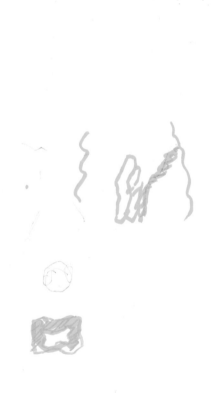

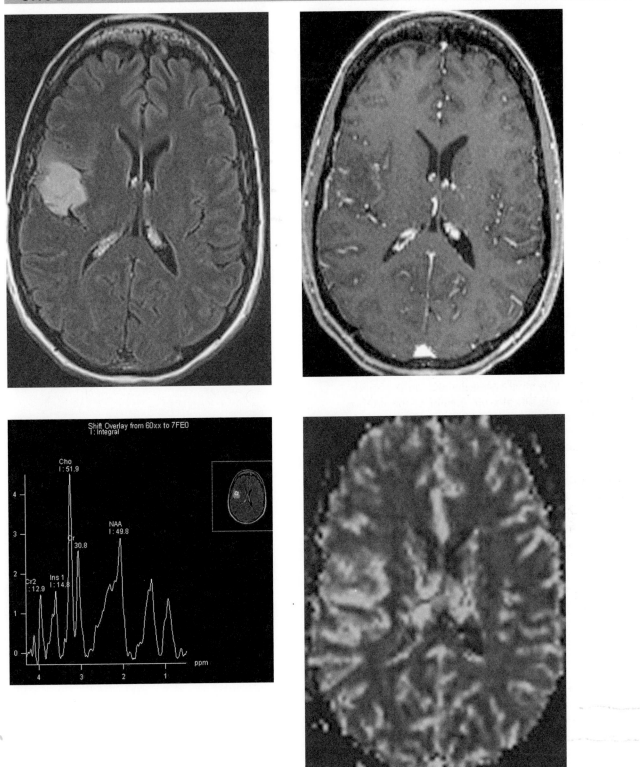

1. Based on the FLAIR and gadolinium-enhanced T1W images, what is the most likely diagnosis?

2. Taking into account the findings on perfusion scan and MR spectroscopy, what is the best diagnosis?

3. On pathologic examination, how is the histologic grade of a primary glial tumor determined?

4. What histologic features in particular favor a glioblastoma multiforme (GBM)?

High-Grade Anaplastic Astrocytoma

1. Infiltrating low-grade astrocytoma.

2. Infiltrating high-grade anaplastic astrocytoma.

3. The regions of a tumor showing the highest degree of anaplasia are used to determine the histologic grade.

4. The presence of necrosis and vascular endothelial proliferation.

Reference

Lupo JM, Cha S, Chang SM, Nelson SJ: Analysis of metabolic indices in regions of abnormal perfusion in patients with high grade glioma, *AJNR Am J Neuroradiol* 28:1455–1461, 2007.

Cross-Reference

Neuroradiology: THE REQUISITES, 2nd ed, pp 128–129, 139, 142–143.

Comment

This case shows abnormal signal intensity in the superficial cortex and subcortical white matter of the inferior right frontal lobe and superior right temporal lobe. There is mild local mass effect manifested by gyral expansion and sulcal effacement. No avid contrast enhancement is identified. These features on conventional FLAIR and gadolinium-enhanced images suggest a low-grade astrocytoma. On proton MR spectroscopy, an increased choline peak is highly suggestive of a malignant neoplasm. Importantly, perfusion imaging shows markedly elevated regional cerebral blood volume, also highly suggestive of a high-grade astrocytoma.

There are two classes of astrocytic tumors: those with narrow zones of infiltration (pilocytic astrocytoma, subependymal giant cell astrocytoma, pleomorphic xanthoastrocytoma) and those with diffuse zones of infiltration. According to the WHO classification, infiltrating astrocytic tumors may be divided into three subtypes: low-grade astrocytoma, anaplastic astrocytoma, and GBM. The histologic criteria for these subdivisions depend on the cellular density, number of mitoses, presence of necrosis, nuclear and cytoplasmic pleomorphism, and vascular endothelial proliferation. GBM typically has all of these histologic features, whereas low-grade astrocytomas may only demonstrate minimal increased cellularity and cellular pleomorphism. The presence of necrosis and vascular endothelial proliferation in particular favors GBM.

Histologically, anaplastic astrocytomas have features that are between those of a low-grade astrocytoma and those of GBM. On imaging, they typically show heterogeneous enhancement; however, the enhancement pattern may vary from avid and nodular to minimal (as in this case). Necrosis is much less common than that seen in the more malignant GBM. Anaplastic astrocytomas are highly malignant, with an average survival time of 2.5 years after diagnosis.

Notes

(handwritten notes)
- edema
- enhancement
- necrosis
- hemorrhage
-

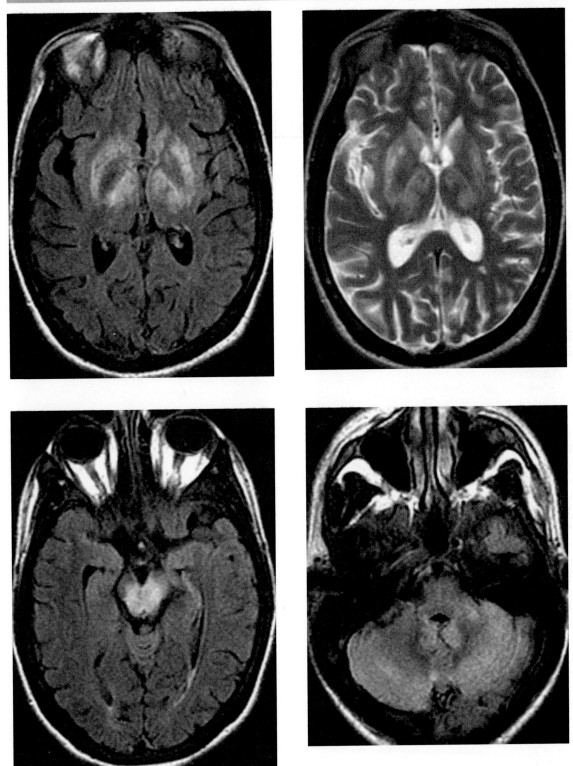

1. Huntington's disease affects what nuclei in the basal ganglia?

2. What neurodegenerative disease is caused by progressive loss of dopaminergic neurons?

3. What would ophthalmologic examination show in this patient?

4. This patient has very low levels of what circulating serum protein?

CASE 182

Wilson's Disease

1. The caudate and putamen.

2. Parkinson's disease.

3. Kayser-Fleischer rings (copper deposition in Descemet's membrane of the cornea). This is present in approximately 80% of patients. Wilson's disease is also associated with "sunflower cataracts," brown or green pigmentation of the anterior and posterior lens capsule.

4. Ceruloplasmin.

References

Akhan O, Akpinar, Oto A, et al: Unusual findings in Wilson's disease, *Eur Radiol* 12(Suppl 3):S66–S69, 2002.

van Wassenaer-van Hall HN, van den Heuvel AG, Algra A, Hoogenrad TU, Mali WP: Wilson's disease: findings at MR imaging and CT of the brain with clinical correlation, *Radiology* 198:531–536, 1996.

Cross-Reference

Neuroradiology: THE REQUISITES, 2nd ed, pp 392–394.

Comment

Wilson's disease (hepatolenticular degeneration) is an autosomal recessive hereditary disease that results from abnormal metabolism of copper caused by deficiency of its carrier protein, ceruloplasmin. As a result, there is extensive abnormal deposition of copper in multiple organ systems (most pronounced in the liver and brain). Although neurologic symptoms may be directly related to copper deposition within the brain parenchyma, they may also be a manifestation of hepatic encephalopathy caused by liver failure. Neurologic signs and symptoms may include a pseudoparkinsonian-like syndrome, with rigidity, gait disturbance, and difficulty with fine motor skills. Dysarthria and progressive cognitive and psychiatric disturbances may also be present. Symptoms usually begin at 10 to 20 years of age, but sometimes do not begin until the age of 30 years and beyond. Presentation before 5 years of age is rare, even though the biochemical defect is present at birth. Treatment of Wilson's disease is with D-penicillamine (chelation therapy).

On MR imaging, the most common finding may be atrophy. Regions of abnormal T2W signal intensity in particular are noted to involve the deep gray matter of the basal ganglia and the thalami, as well as the white matter. In particular, the putamen of the lentiform nucleus and the caudate are involved. In addition to signal abnormality, atrophy of the caudate nuclei may be present. Regions of T2W hypointensity have also been noted in the basal ganglia and have been attributed either to the paramagnetic effects of copper or possibly to associated iron deposition. Abnormalities on MR imaging may also be present in the brainstem and in the white matter of the cerebellum, as in this case. The diagnosis is made by laboratory analysis in which there are elevated copper levels within the urine as well as low serum ceruloplasmin levels.

Notes

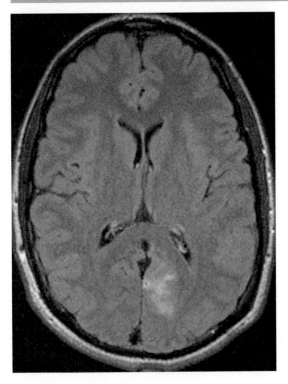 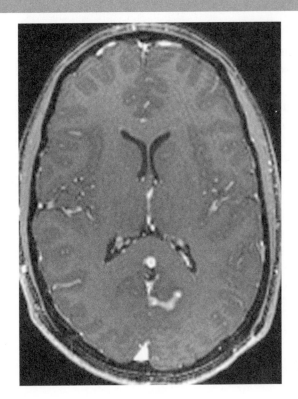

1. What are the imaging findings?

2. What is the differential diagnosis in this young patient?

3. What was this patient's clinical presentation?

4. What is the most common location of a pleomorphic xanthoastrocytoma?

Pleomorphic Xanthoastrocytoma

1. There is high signal intensity in the superficial medial left occipital lobe, with avid leptomeningeal enhancement.

2. The differential diagnosis of a cortically based mass with meningeal involvement includes an inflammatory lesion, granulomatous disease (sarcoid), lymphoma, metastases, and primary brain tumors, including oligodendroglioma and pleomorphic xanthoastrocytoma.

3. Seizures.

4. The temporal lobe.

Reference

Tien RD, Cardenas CA, Rajagopalan S: Pleomorphic xanthoastrocytoma of the brain: MR findings in six patients, *AJR Am J Roentgenol* 169:1287–1290, 1992.

Cross-Reference

Neuroradiology: THE REQUISITES, 2nd ed, pp 135, 141.

Comment

Pleomorphic xanthoastrocytomas are rare primary brain tumors that likely arise from astrocytes. They typically present in children and young adults, as in this case, and they occur with equal frequency in boys and girls. They occur most commonly in the temporal lobe and frequently present with a history of seizures. They then occur in decreasing order of frequency in the parietal, occipital, and frontal lobes. These tumors may be well demarcated, with avid enhancement, and approximately one third have cystic changes. These tend to be superficial, cortically based tumors that may have leptomeningeal enhancement as a result of direct invasion of the meninges and peritumoral edema, as in this case. The differential diagnosis of a cortically based enhancing mass with meningeal involvement includes an inflammatory mass, granulomatous disease (sarcoid), lymphoma, metastases, meningioma, and primary brain tumors, including oligodendroglioma and pleomorphic xanthoastrocytoma.

On histologic examination, fusiform cells arranged in a storiform pattern are intermixed with areas of marked pleomorphism of astrocytes. Microscopic features include dense cellular areas with hyperchromatic pleomorphic cells that may be multinucleated, a reticulin network, perivascular lymphocytes, and lipidization of astrocytes. Treatment is usually surgical resection. Peritumoral edema and leptomeningeal enhancement have been associated with a higher rate of recurrence.

Notes

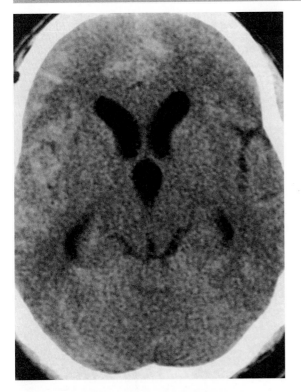

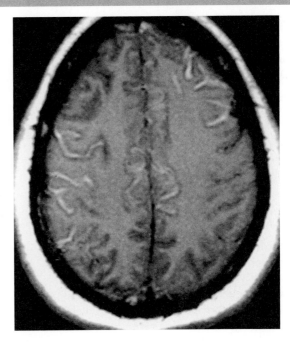

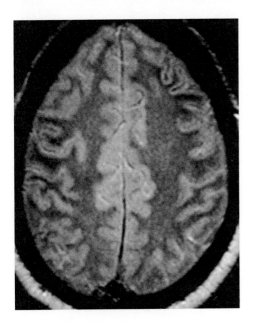

1. What are causes of high density or intensity in the subarachnoid spaces on unenhanced CT or FLAIR MR imaging, respectively?

2. What is the first-line imaging modality in the evaluation of suspected nontraumatic subarachnoid hemorrhage?

3. Why is melanoma sometimes noted to be hyperintense on T1W images and hypointense on T2W images?

4. What are the diagnostic criteria for primary leptomeningeal melanosis?

Primary Leptomeningeal Melanosis

1. Acute subarachnoid hemorrhage, iodinated contrast material (as is seen after myelography), and a proteinaceous exudate, as is seen in meningitis.

2. Unenhanced head CT.

3. Paramagnetic effects of melanin.

4. Demonstration of the proliferation of melanocytes within the meninges, absence of cutaneous or ocular melanoma, and absence of systemic metastases.

References

Byrd SE, Reyes-Mugica M, Darling CF, Chou P, Tomita T: MR of leptomeningeal melanosis in children, *Eur J Radiol* 20:93–99, 1995.

Hayashi M, Maeda M, Majji T, et al: Diffuse leptomeningeal hyperintensity on fluid attenuated inversion recovery MR images in neurocutaneous melanosis, *AJNR Am J Neuroradiol* 25:138–141, 2004.

Cross-Reference

Neuroradiology: THE REQUISITES, 2nd ed, p 105.

Comment

Leptomeningeal melanosis refers to an increase in the number of melanocytes in the leptomeninges. Melanoblasts (precursors to melanocytes) are derived from the neural crest. Proliferation of melanocytes along the leptomeninges may be seen in a variety of forms, including primary leptomeningeal melanosis, primary leptomeningeal melanoma, and metastatic melanoma. Metastatic melanoma is the most common cause of such proliferation.

The diagnosis of primary leptomeningeal melanosis can be made when the following criteria are met: (1) there is a proliferation of melanocytes within the meninges or melanocytosis (high melanocyte count in the CSF); (2) there is no cutaneous or ocular melanoma; and (3) an extensive workup, including a bone scan as well as CT of the chest, abdomen, and pelvis, shows no metastatic lesions. Primary CNS melanocytic proliferation carries a poor prognosis. Patients may present with signs of increased intracranial pressure, seizures, and cranial neuropathies. Leptomeningeal melanosis may be benign or malignant. When malignant, there is characteristically invasion of the adjacent brain or the spinal cord.

Because melanocytosis in the CSF may be associated with a high protein content, unenhanced CT may show a hyperdense exudate in the subarachnoid spaces that may be mistaken for acute hemorrhage. On MR imaging, unenhanced T1W and FLAIR images may show hyperintense lesions along the leptomeninges within the subarachnoid spaces. Involved leptomeninges and brain may show regions of T2W hypointensity because of the paramagnetic effects of melanin. Involved leptomeninges show prominent enhancement.

Leptomeningeal melanosis associated with cutaneous nevi is referred to as neurocutaneous melanosis and is classified as a phakomatosis. These patients typically have multiple congenital hyperpigmented or giant hairy pigmented cutaneous nevi. Malignant transformation of meningeal melanosis may occur in as many as 50% of patients and often presents with seizures when the intracranial compartment is involved because of invasion. Leptomeningeal melanosis responds poorly to radiation and chemotherapy. Reported cases suggest that intrathecal recombinant interleukin-2 may provide a more promising response.

Notes

— leptomeningeal melanosis

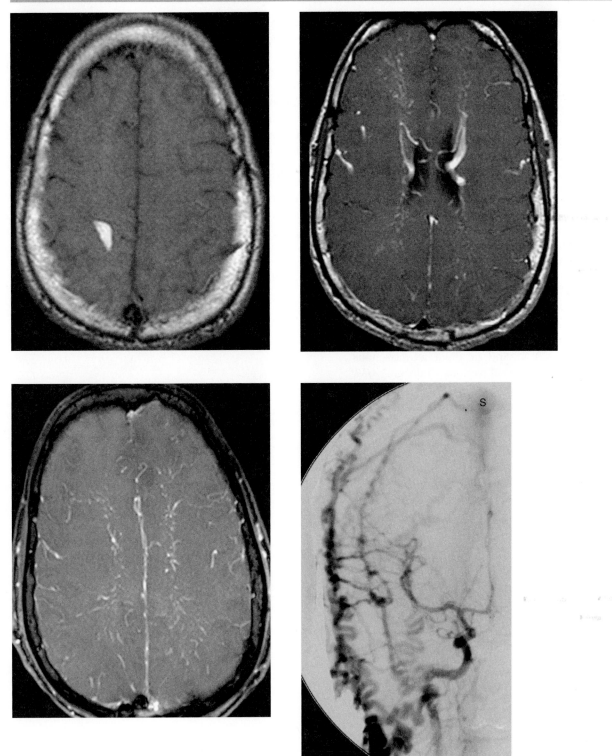

1. What are the findings on the MR images?

2. What are the findings on the right common carotid artery injection from the conventional arteriogram, and what is the diagnosis?

3. What are proposed mechanisms for the development of these lesions?

4. What types of intracranial hemorrhage may be associated with these lesions?

Dural Arteriovenous Fistula—Part I

1. There is hyperintensity on the unenhanced axial T1W image in the right parietal lobe, consistent with a subacute hemorrhage. The enhanced T1W images show bilaterally symmetric prominent cortical veins and enhancement in the deep white matter along the medullary veins.

2. There are enlarged external carotid artery branches feeding the superior sagittal sinus(es) that fill(s) during the arterial phase, consistent with a dural arteriovenous fistula (DAVF).

3. Venous thrombosis is the most widely accepted etiology; however, these lesions may also be seen as a consequence of trauma, surgery, or venous hypertension without venous thrombosis.

4. Intraparenchymal or subarachnoid hemorrhage.

Reference

Willinski R, Terbrugge K, Montanera W, et al: Venous congestion: an MR finding in dural arteriovenous malformations with cortical venous drainage, *AJNR Am J Neuroradiol* 15:1501–1507, 1994.

Cross-Reference

Neuroradiology: THE REQUISITES, 2nd ed, pp 237–238.

Comment

Dural arteriovenous malformations (DAVMs) and fistulas account for approximately 12% of all intracranial vascular malformations. More than half occur in the posterior fossa, and they may be categorized based on the dural venous sinus involved by the vascular abnormality. These vascular malformations most commonly involve the sigmoid or transverse sinuses, accounting for as many as 70% of all of these lesions. The cavernous sinus is the next most common site for DAVMs and DAVFs, representing approximately 10% to 15% of these lesions.

Most dural vascular malformations present clinically in older adults. They are believed to be acquired lesions that typically arise as a consequence of dural venous sinus thrombosis. As a result, a collateral network of vessels develops, including enlargement of normally present microscopic arteriovenous shunts within the dura. In addition, as arteriovenous shunting increases, venous hypertension develops. In certain DAVMs, venous hypertension may result in retrograde filling of leptomeningeal or cortical veins that communicate with the involved sinus, as in this case. In such cases, rupture of the enlarged venous collaterals may occur. Approximately 10% to 15% of DAVMs are associated with intracranial hemorrhage, which is usually intraparenchymal or subarachnoid. Hemorrhage is associated with lesions in which there is development of dilated leptomeningeal veins. DAVMs and DAVFs that drain strictly to the dural venous sinuses are not usually associated with hemorrhage.

It is important to recognize that DAVMS and DAVFs are difficult to diagnose on CT and MR imaging. Imaging findings may include venous thrombosis, dilated cortical veins, or intracranial hemorrhage. However, imaging findings may be normal, and a high index of suspicion is required.

Notes

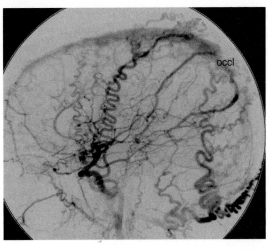

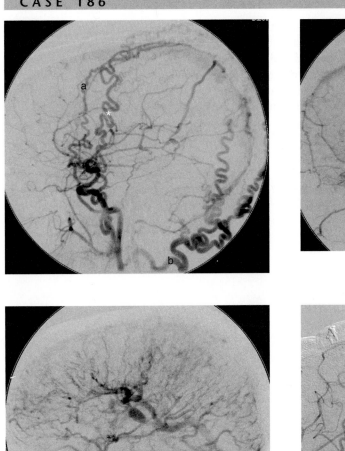

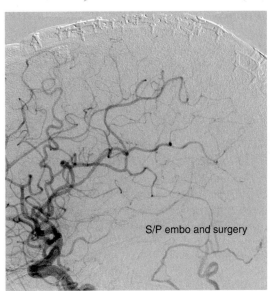

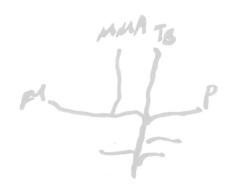

1. What anatomic structures do a, *, and b represent?

2. With dural arteriovenous malformation (DAVMs) hemorrhage is more commonly associated with what type of venous drainage?

3. DAVMs most commonly involve what dural venous sinuses?

4. What is the typical clinical presentation of these patients?

Dural Arteriovenous Fistula—Part II

1. The middle meningeal, superficial temporal, and occipital artery branches from the external carotid artery, respectively.

2. Those with leptomeningeal or cortical venous drainage. Those whose drainage is isolated to the dural venous sinuses have a much lower rate of hemorrhage.

3. The sigmoid and transverse sinuses.

4. Symptoms of DAVMs depend on their size and location as well as the venous sinuses involved. Symptoms may be related to elevated intracranial pressure and may include headaches, tinnitus, and subarachnoid or parenchymal hemorrhage.

Reference

Hurst RW, Bagley LJ, Galetta S, et al: Dementia resulting from dural arteriovenous fistulas: the pathologic findings of venous hypertensive encephalopathy, *AJNR Am J Neuroradiol* 19:1267–1273, 1998.

Cross-Reference

Neuroradiology: THE REQUISITES, 2nd ed, pp 237–238.

Comment

The right common carotid injection shows that the external artery branches fill ahead of the right anterior and middle cerebral arteries, consistent with excessive flow to the external carotid circulation. There is a dural fistula with the superior sagittal sinus that is supplied by multiple feeders, including the middle meningeal, superficial temporal, occipital, and posterior auricular arteries. The superior sagittal sinus is interrupted or occluded at the posterior two thirds (*occl*), with arteriovenous shunting into the anterior and posterior components of the superior sagittal sinus around the obstruction. There is retrograde filling into enlarged cortical and medullary veins in both cerebral hemispheres on the delayed venous phase. Delayed drainage does occur into an enlarged deep venous system that drains into the transverse and sigmoid sinuses. Left common carotid arteriography showed similar findings.

The superficial temporal, middle meningeal, and occipital artery feeders to the dural nidus were embolized using endovascular techniques, with significant occlusion of the nidus. Subsequently, surgery was performed. Angiography performed after embolization and surgery showed excellent treatment of the DAVM or fistula, with a normal-appearing angiogram.

This patient presented with progressive dementia, a less common presentation of DAVM. The dementia syndrome (venous hypertensive encephalopathy) is secondary to elevated intracranial venous pressure with associated diminished cerebral perfusion. This type of dementia is potentially reversible, as it was in this case, after endovascular embolization and neurosurgical resection. This patient experienced significant return of cognitive function.

Notes

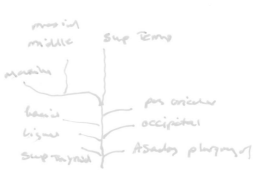

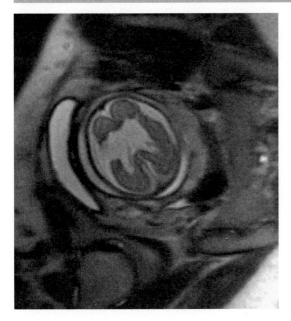
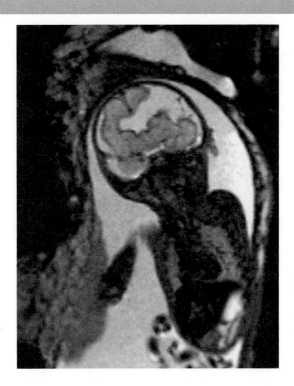

1. What type of study is this?

2. What is the diagnosis?

3. This finding, in combination with absence of the septum pellucidum and optic nerve hypoplasia, is consistent with what diagnosis?

4. What associated migrational abnormality is typically seen in the adjacent cortex?

Fetal Schizencephaly

1. Fetal MR imaging.

2. Open-lipped schizencephaly diagnosed on fetal MR. The first image is a HASTE sequence; the second image is an echoplanar susceptibility sequence.

3. Septo-optic dysplasia.

4. Polymicrogyria.

References

Ceccherini AF, Twining P, Varied S: Schizencephaly: antenatal detection using ultrasound, *Clin Radiol* 54:620–622, 1999.

Glenn OA, Barkovich J: Magnetic resonance imaging of the fetal brain and spine: an increasingly important tool in prenatal diagnosis: part 2, *AJNR Am J Neuroradiol* 27:1807–1814, 2006.

Cross-Reference

Neuroradiology: THE REQUISITES, 2nd ed, pp 423–425.

Comment

Fetal MR imaging is an increasingly available technique used to evaluate the fetal neural axis. Ultrafast T2W sequences, parallel imaging, and new coil designs have allowed fetal MR imaging to be used to evaluate processes that cannot be evaluated by other imaging techniques. Fetal MR allows assessment of in vivo brain development and early diagnosis of congenital abnormalities inadequately evaluated by prenatal sonography. It has been especially useful in the evaluation of sonographically diagnosed ventriculomegaly, suspected abnormalities of the corpus callosum, and posterior fossa lesions.

Schizencephaly is a migrational abnormality that results from an injury to the germinal matrix and causes failure of normal migration and neuronal differentiation. This anomaly is thought to be the result of an in utero watershed ischemic event leading to damage not only to the germinal matrix but also to the radial glial fibers along which the neurons normally migrate from the germinal region to their final destination in the cortex. As a result, schizencephaly extends from the ventricular surface to the subarachnoid surface of the brain and is lined by dysplastic gray matter. Usually, there is a CSF cleft between the layers of gray matter. When the CSF cleft is large and gaping, it is referred to as "open-lip" schizencephaly. When the layers of gray matter are in apposition or when there is only a thin layer of CSF between them, the condition is referred to as "closed-lip" schizencephaly.

Up to 25% to 50% of patients with schizencephaly have septo-optic dysplasia. Patients with migrational anomalies usually present with a seizure disorder. Depending on the size of the migrational abnormality, there may also be focal neurologic deficits, such as hemiparesis. MR imaging is the imaging modality of choice to assess these abnormalities. Closed-lip schizencephaly, when the gray matter layers are apposed, may be difficult to detect. A small ventricular "dimple" or diverticulum may be a clue to the diagnosis and should prompt a close search for closed-lip schizencephaly. Other conditions that may cause dimpling of the ventricle are previous injuries, such as periventricular ischemia or infection.

Notes

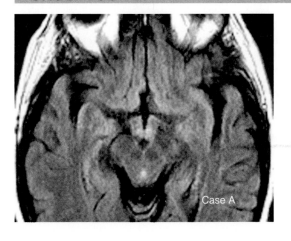

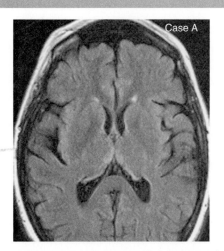

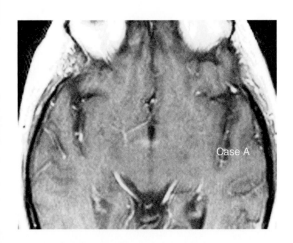

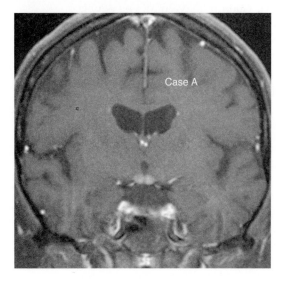

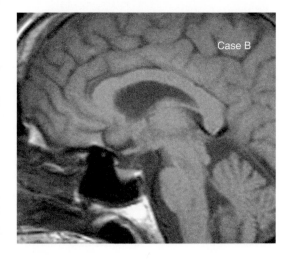

1. What are the imaging findings in Case A?

2. What is the best diagnosis?

3. What is the cause of this entity?

4. What vascular abnormalities can result in bithalamic signal alteration?

Wernicke Encephalopathy

1. There is FLAIR high signal intensity and enhancement in the mamillary bodies as well as T2W and FLAIR high signal intensity in the medial thalami.

2. Wernicke encephalopathy.

3. Thiamine deficiency, usually in the setting of chronic alcoholism.

4. Venous ischemia or infarction (due to deep vein thrombosis) and infarct of the artery of Percheron (a single vascular pedicle that supplies the paramedian thalamic arteries).

References

Mascalchi M, Belli G, Guerrini L, Nistri M, Del Seppia I, Villari N: Proton MR spectroscopy of Wernicke encephalopathy, *AJNR Am J Neuroradiol* 23:1803–1806, 2002.

Weidauer S, Nichtweiss M, Lanfermann H, Zanella FE: Wernicke encephalopathy: MR findings and clinical presentation, *Eur Radiol* 13:1001–1009, 2003.

Cross-Reference

Neuroradiology: THE REQUISITES, 2nd ed, pp 357, 396–397.

Comment

These cases show many of the radiologic findings seen in Wernicke encephalopathy. Case A shows FLAIR high signal intensity and enhancement in the mamillary bodies and FLAIR high signal intensity in the medial thalami. Wernicke encephalopathy is typically associated with generalized cerebral cortical and cerebellar vermial atrophy. In addition, specific deep structures are involved and are best assessed with MR imaging, which is more sensitive than CT in evaluating the small structures involved in this entity. Abnormal T2W and FLAIR hyperintensity is seen in the mamillary bodies (in essentially all patients), and may also be seen in the hypothalamus, periaqueductal gray matter, and medial thalami. Imaging findings are often bilaterally symmetric. In the acute setting, there may be mild swelling associated with the signal alteration, and enhancement has also been reported, as is seen in Case A. Resolution of the signal alterations after treatment with thiamine has been reported. In the late stages, atrophy (particularly of the mammillary bodies) may be the main finding, as is seen in Case B.

Wernicke encephalopathy is related to thiamine deficiency and is found most commonly in chronic alcoholism; however, this vitamin deficiency may also be present in other conditions that result in chronic malnutrition, such as anorexia nervosa, prolonged infectious or febrile conditions, and hyperemesis gravidarum. Wernicke syndrome has also been reported in association with long-term parenteral therapy. Wernicke encephalopathy clinically manifests with tremors, ocular symptoms (nystagmus and gaze paralysis), confusion, delusions, and ataxia; in contrast, Korsakoff psychosis is manifested by retrograde amnesia and difficulty acquiring new information. The two sometimes occur together.

Notes

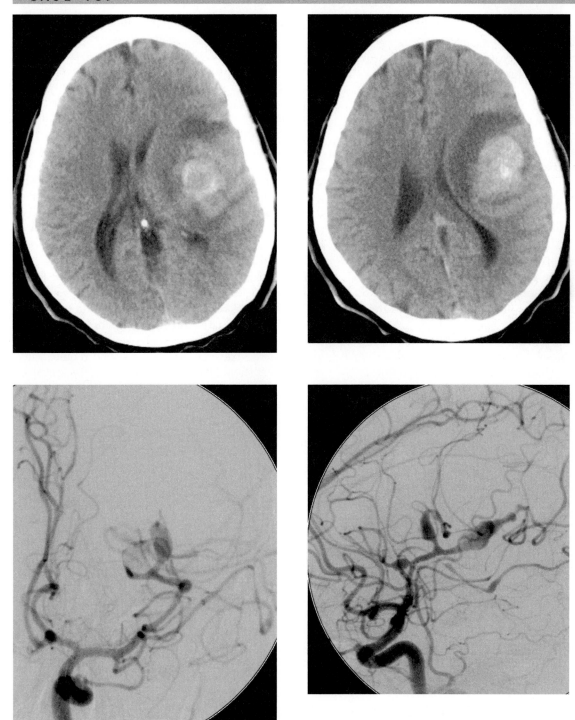

1. What types of aneurysm typically arise from the distal cerebral arteries?

2. What is the most common site of intracranial mycotic aneurysms?

3. How often are infectious aneurysms multiple?

4. How often do septic emboli occur in patients with subacute bacterial endocarditis?

Ruptured Mycotic Aneurysm

1. Mycotic aneurysms, traumatic aneurysms, and aneurysms arising from invasion of the arterial wall by tumor emboli (atrial myxoma).

2. The distal branches of the middle cerebral artery (75%–80% of cases), reflecting the embolic origin of these lesions.

3. In 20% of cases, They have a greater propensity to bleed than other aneurysms.

4. Septic emboli occur in 4% of patients with subacute bacterial endocarditis.

References

Cloft HJ, Kallmes DF, Jensen ME, Lanzino G, Dion JE: Endovascular treatment of ruptured, peripheral cerebral aneurysms: parent artery occlusion with short Guglielmi detachable coils, *AJNR Am J Neuroradiol* 20:308–310, 1999.

Loevner LA, Ting TY, Hurst RW, Goldberg H, Schut L: Spontaneous thrombosis of a basilar artery traumatic aneurysm in a child, *AJNR Am J Neuroradiol* 19: 386–388, 1998.

Cross-Reference

Neuroradiology: THE REQUISITES, 2nd ed, pp 224, 287, 289.

Comment

Up to 15% of patients with acute subarachnoid hemorrhage die before reaching the hospital. The incidence of aneurysmal rebleeding occurs at a rate of approximately 2% per day in the first 2 weeks after the initial hemorrhage. There are several issues that the angiographer must address. These include identifying the vessel from which the aneurysm arises, the size of the aneurysm, the presence or absence of an aneurysm neck, the orientation of the aneurysm, and the anatomy of the circle of Willis. A search for multiple aneurysms is necessary. If there is more than one aneurysm, it is necessary to try to determine which aneurysm bled.

A mycotic aneurysm results from an infectious process that involves the arterial wall. *Streptococcus viridans* and *Staphylococcus aureus* are the most common pathogens. These aneurysms may be caused by a septic embolus that causes inflammatory destruction of the arterial wall, beginning with the endothelial surface. Infected embolic material also reaches the adventitia through the vasa vasorum. Inflammation then disrupts the adventitia and muscularis, resulting in aneurysmal dilation. Mycotic aneurysms are estimated to account for 2% to 3% of all intracranial aneurysms. They have an increased incidence in the setting of drug abuse and in a spectrum of immunocompromised states. The thoracic aorta is reported to be the most common site of mycotic aneurysms. Intracranial mycotic aneurysms are less common. They occur with greater frequency in children and are often found on vessels distal to the circle of Willis. They frequently present with a cerebral hematoma, as in this case of middle cerebral artery mycotic aneurysm. Mycotic aneurysms generally have a fusiform morphologic appearance and are usually very friable. Therefore, treatment is difficult or risky. Most cases are treated emergently with antibiotics, which are continued for 4 to 6 weeks. Serial angiography helps to document the effectiveness of medical therapy. Even if aneurysms seem to be shrinking, they may subsequently grow, and new ones may form.

Delayed clipping or coiling may be more feasible; indications include subarachnoid hemorrhage, increasing size of the aneurysm during treatment with antibiotics (this is controversial), and failure of the aneurysm to shrink after 4 to 6 weeks of antibiotic treatment. Patients with subacute bacterial endocarditis who require valve replacement should have bioprosthetic (ie, tissue) valves instead of mechanical valves to eliminate the need for risky anticoagulation therapy.

Notes

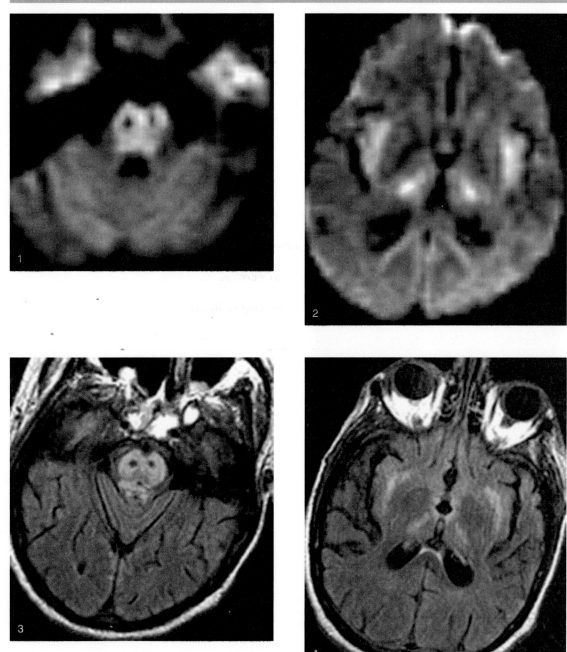

1. What anatomic structures are relatively spared in the pons?

2. What extrapontine structures are involved in this case?

3. This condition is frequently associated with overzealous correction of what electrolyte abnormality?

4. What type of patients typically present with this disorder?

Osmotic Demyelination

1. Descending corticospinal tracts.

2. The deep gray matter (thalami, lentiform nuclei) and deep white matter, including the tracts around the corpus striatum (external and internal capsules). The cerebellum may also be involved.

3. Hyponatremia.

4. Alcoholics and the malnourished.

Reference

Sterns RH, Riggs JE, Schochette SS Jr: Osmotic demyelination syndrome following correction of hyponatremia, *N Engl J Med* 314:1535–1542, 1986.

Cross-Reference

Neuroradiology: THE REQUISITES, 2nd ed, pp 355–356.

Comment

Osmotic demyelination may be seen in underlying systemic processes that have a predilection for electrolyte abnormalities. It is most commonly seen in alcoholics and in chronically debilitated and malnourished patients after rapid correction of hyponatremia. It is not the low serum level but rather the rapidity with which it is corrected that is believed to be responsible for this disorder. Overzealous correction of serum sodium levels may be followed by acute or subacute clinical deterioration, including change in mental status, coma, quadriparesis, extrapyramidal signs, and if unrecognized, death. This process not uncommonly involves extrapontine structures, as in this case. Pathologically, demyelination is noted without a significant inflammatory response, with relative sparing of axons. There is an associated reactive astrocytosis.

When osmotic demyelination is localized only in the pons (central pontine myelinolysis), it is characterized by hyperintensity on T2W images in the central pons, with relative sparing of the peripheral pons. The corticospinal tracts are usually spared. In this case, the first two images are diffusion-weighted images obtained in the acute setting. They show restricted diffusion (hyperintensity) in the regions of acute demyelination in the pons and extrapontine structures involved. The two FLAIR images obtained 1 week later show signal abnormality in the regions of previously noted restricted diffusion (the hyperintensity seen on the diffusion-weighted images resolved). Usually, osmotic demyelination is not associated with enhancement or significant mass effect.

When osmotic demyelination is localized only to the pons, the radiologic diagnosis is usually easy. However, if there is pontine and extrapontine involvement or involvement only in extrapontine structures, the differential diagnosis is somewhat broad, including other demyelinating disorders, encephalitis, and ischemia.

Notes

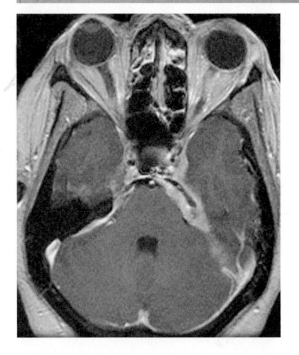

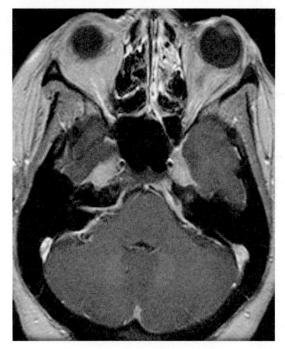

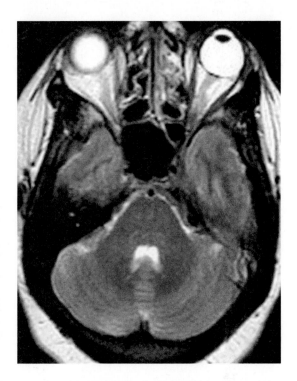

1. The abnormalities noted in this case involve predominantly what structure?

2. What is the differential diagnosis?

3. What is the classic presentation of Rosai-Dorfman disease?

4. What percentage of patients with Rosai-Dorfman disease have intracranial involvement?

CASE 191

Rosai-Dorfman Disease—Benign Sinus Histiocytosis

1. The meninges, with extensive dural-based disease. Meckel's cave is also involved bilaterally.

2. Sarcoid, lymphoma, meningiomatosis, metastases, sinus histiocytosis (letting the zebra with red stripes out of the zoo!). There is diffuse dural enhancement, with corresponding T2W hypointensity of the involved dura.

3. Massive, painless cervical lymphadenopathy.

4. Approximately 5%.

Reference

Wu M, Anderson AE, Kahn LB: A report of intracranial Rosai-Dorfman disease with literature review, *Ann Diagn Pathol* 5:96–102, 2001.

Cross-Reference

Neuroradiology: THE REQUISITES, 2nd ed, p 684.

Comment

Rosai-Dorfman disease, also known as benign sinus histiocytosis, is a rare disorder in which there is overproduction and accumulation of histiocytes within the lymph nodes. The pathogenesis is unknown, but it may represent an autoimmune disease or a reaction to an infectious agent. Classically, it causes significant painless cervical lymphadenopathy. It may also cause nasal obstruction and enlargement of the palatine tonsils. Extranodal involvement occurs in one-third of cases and may involve the skin, orbit, upper respiratory tract, testes, kidneys, and gastrointestinal tract. The CNS is rarely involved, with approximately 5% of patients with this disease having intracranial manifestations. In approximately two thirds of patients with CNS involvement, the presentation is limited to the brain and spinal cord without lymphadenopathy, as in this case. The typical age of presentation is between 20 and 40 years. Symptoms vary based on the location of involvement.

Intracranial disease may present with headaches, cranial nerve palsies (as in this case), and seizures. More than 90% of patients with CNS disease have involvement of the leptomeninges, with a predominant radiologic presentation of dural-based enhancing masses. It may result in vasogenic edema of the underlying brain parenchyma. On histopathologic evaluation, Rosai-Dorfman disease of the meninges is similar to that in the lymph nodes. The dura is thickened and fibrotic, resulting in its hypointensity on T2W, and it contains inflammatory cells, with a predominance of lymphocytes and plasma cells. Interspersed are pale histiocytes with vacuolated cytoplasm.

The differential diagnosis includes granulomatous disease, such as sarcoid, lymphoma (Hodgkin's disease), and Langerhans' histiocytosis. When the mass is isolated, it may closely resemble a meningioma.

Meningeal Rosai-Dorfman disease is primarily treated with surgical resection. Disease progression after surgery is reportedly uncommon. Progressive disease occurs most often when there is multiple-organ involvement. In such cases, as well as in cases like this one, where there is diffuse meningeal involvement, other therapies, including steroids, vincristine, cyclophosphamide (Cytoxan), and radiation, have had variable success.

Notes

Rosai Dorfman,
- Massive LN
-

Sarcoid / TB
lymphoma
meningioel carinomes
histiocytosis

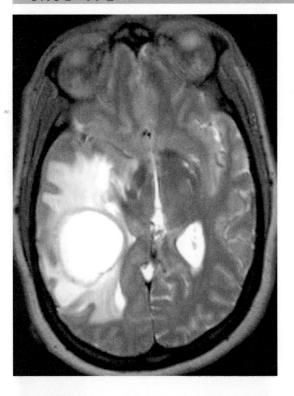

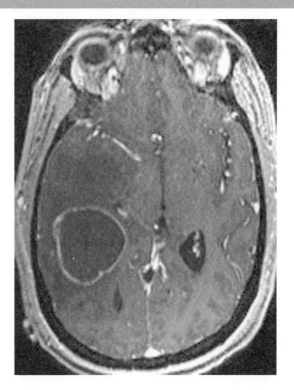

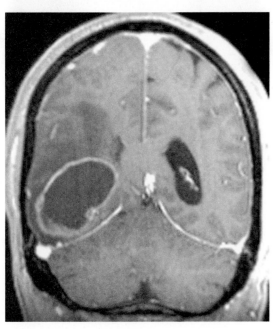

1. What is the main differential diagnosis?

2. What MR imaging sequence would be most useful in establishing the diagnosis of a brain abscess?

3. How often are brain metastases solitary lesions?

4. What histologic cell type of metastatic disease is frequently associated with cystic necrotic metastases?

CASE 192

Cystic Necrotic Brain Mass—Part I

1. Brain abscess, metastatic disease, and primary glial neoplasm.

2. Diffusion-weighted imaging.

3. Approximately 30% to 50% of patients with brain metastases have isolated lesions on imaging.

4. Adenocarcinomas.

30—50% solitary mets

Reference

Kim YJ, Chang KH, Song IC, et al: Brain abscesses and necrotic or cystic brain tumor: discrimination with signal intensity on diffusion weighted MR imaging, *Am J Roentgenol* 171:1487–1490, 1998.

Cross-Reference

Neuroradiology: THE REQUISITES, 2nd ed, pp 16–17, 109, 113, 148–152.

Comment

The differential diagnosis of a single ring-enhancing lesion with prominent associated vasogenic edema includes metastatic disease, a brain abscess, and a high-grade primary glial neoplasm. Less common causes of large ring-enhancing lesions include demyelination and resolving hematoma. Advanced MR imaging techniques, such as diffusion-weighted imaging, spectroscopy, and perfusion imaging, can sometimes be helpful in distinguishing among these. Abscesses may show cytosolic amino acids, including alanine and valine, as well as other metabolites, such as lactate and pyruvate, which are end-products of bacterial metabolism. However, some necrotic tumors may have spectra with many of these features (lactate, amino acids).

Diffusion-weighted MR imaging provides information about the diffusional properties of water in the brain related to the local cellular microenvironment. The central cavity of a brain abscess frequently has restricted diffusion (restricted mobility of water protons) as a result of several factors, including, but not limited to, the cellularity and viscosity of pus, as well as the presence of large molecules, such as fibrinogen. It is important to recognize, however, that abscesses evolve over time on treatment, and so do their imaging characteristics. Changes in their signal characteristics on diffusion-weighted imaging are related to increases in free water and associated changes in the viscosity of the fluid, different bacteria, and the concentration of inflammatory cells.

Notes

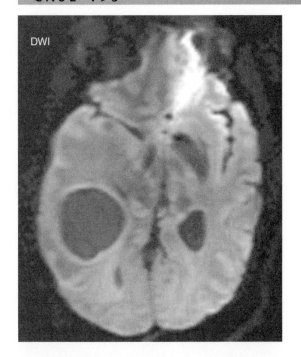

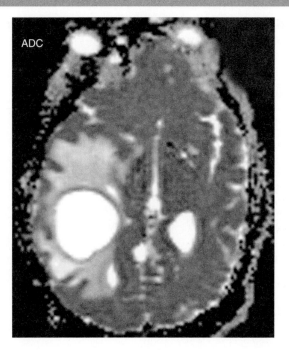

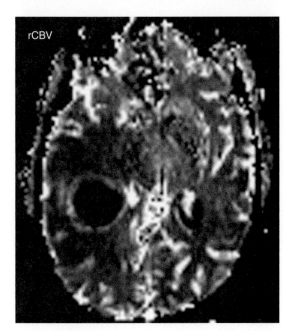

1. Using the diffusion-weighted and corresponding apparent diffusion coefficient (ADC) map, what diagnosis is likely to be eliminated in this case?

2. What does ADC correspond to?

3. What does the perfusion regional cerebral blood volume show?

4. What type of adenocarcinoma has been reported to show restricted diffusion?

Cystic Necrotic Brain Mass—Part II—Metastatic Adenocarcinoma of the Lung

Notes

1. Brain abscess. If untreated, these lesions often show restricted diffusion (hyperintensity on diffusion-weighted imaging, with corresponding low signal intensity on ADC map).

2. ADC is a quantity corresponding to a matrix of tensor vectors in various directions.

3. Elevated flow in the peripheral capsule of the necrotic mass.

4. Metastatic mucinous adenocarcinoma. The presence of mucin may contribute to restricted diffusion.

Reference

Desprechins B, Stadnik T, Koerts G, Shabana W, Breucq C, Osteaux M: Use of diffusion-weighted MR imaging in differential diagnosis between intracerebral necrotic tumors and cerebral abscesses, *AJNR Am J Neuroradiol* 20:1252–1257, 1999.

Cross-Reference

Neuroradiology: THE REQUISITES, 2nd ed, pp 16–17, 109, 113, 148–152.

Comment

Adenocarcinoma of the lung is the most common type of lung cancer and accounts for 30% to 35% of primary lung tumors. The most common source of brain metastasis is cancer of the lung. Other primary cancers that can metastasize to the brain include breast, kidney, melanoma, and cancers of the gastrointestinal tract (eg, stomach, colon, rectum).

The treatment of brain metastases depends on several factors, such as the tumor of origin (ie, adenocarcinoma of the lung), the number and location of the lesions within the brain, and the extent of cancer in places other than the brain. Most patients are given steroids, such as dexamethasone (Decadron), to treat brain swelling. Patients may also take an antiseizure medication if they have seizures as a symptom. Systemic chemotherapy does not reach or treat brain tumors. Radiation therapy is a cornerstone of treatment of brain metastases. The standard approach with brain metastases of any origin is to decide whether the tumor can be removed. MR imaging is helpful in determining the number and location of tumors. Surgical resection of the dominant lesion, followed by irradiation, is common. Stereotactic radiation, sometimes referred to as stereotactic radiosurgery, may be performed in which irradiation is precisely targeted to the site of brain metastases.

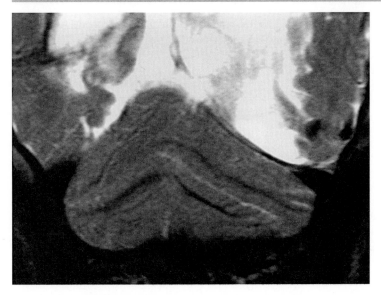

1. What structure is absent?

2. In this condition, what other posterior fossa abnormalities are present?

3. What other posterior fossa anomalies are associated with vermian dysgenesis or agenesis?

4. Among Dandy-Walker malformations, Joubert's syndrome, and rhombencephalosynapsis, which is associated with agenesis of the corpus callosum?

Rhombencephalosynapsis

1. The cerebellar vermis.

2. Fusion anomalies of the cerebellar hemispheres, colliculi, middle cerebellar peduncles, and dentate nuclei.

3. Dandy-Walker malformation and Joubert's syndrome.

4. Dandy-Walker malformation.

References

Montull C, Mercader JM, Peri J, Martinez FM, Bonaventura I: Neuroradiological and clinical findings in rhomboencephalosynapsis, *Neuroradiology* 42:272–274, 2000.

Utsunomiya H, Takano K, Ogasawara T, et al: Rhomboencephalosynapsis: cerebellar embryogenesis, *AJNR Am J Neuroradiol* 19:547–549, 1998.

Cross-Reference

Neuroradiology: THE REQUISITES, 2nd ed, p 436.

Comment

Rhombencephalosynapsis is an anomaly of the cerebellar vermis that is agenetic or hypoplastic. There is fusion of the cerebellar hemispheres, with variable fusion of other posterior fossa structures, including the middle cerebellar peduncles, cerebellar dentate nuclei, and superior and inferior colliculi. In the cerebellar hemispheres, the orientation of the folia is disorganized. They are usually transverse in configuration, extending across the midline without intervening vermis. MR imaging typically shows an absent or severely hypoplastic vermis, with fusion of the cerebellar hemispheres. There is usually posterior pointing of the fourth ventricle. Associated supratentorial anomalies include partial or complete absence of the septum pellucidum, a hypoplastic anterior commissure, ex vacuo enlargement of the ventricular system related to surrounding volume loss of the brain parenchyma, and fusion of the thalami. Hypertelorism and migrational anomalies have also been reported with this condition. The clinical presentation is more commonly related to the associated supratentorial anomalies.

Joubert's syndrome, another dysplasia of the posterior fossa contents, is characterized by severe hypoplasia or aplasia of the cerebellar vermis. It has a characteristic imaging appearance, including a "bat-wing" configuration of the fourth ventricle, as well as a horizontal orientation of the superior cerebellar peduncles. Unlike rhombencephalosynapsis, the cerebellar hemispheres are apposed in the midline, but are not fused. Associated supratentorial anomalies are uncommon.

Notes

splint colliculi

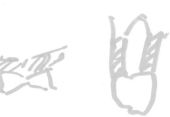

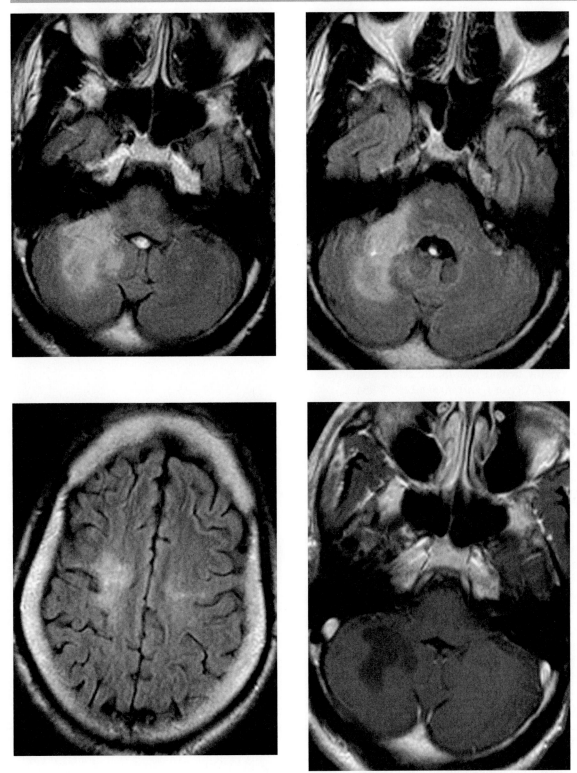

1. What is the differential diagnosis in this immunocompromised patient?

2. What imaging findings favor progressive multifocal leukoencephalopathy (PML)?

3. What are common MR imaging findings in HIV demyelination and cytomegalovirus (CMV) infection?

4. What is the infectious agent responsible for PML?

Progressive Multifocal Leukoencephalopathy

1. Demyelination related to CMV, PML, lymphoma, and direct HIV infection.

2. Asymmetric white matter involvement, subcortical and deep white matter involvement, and the absence of mass effect and enhancement.

3. These two direct viral infections of the white matter most commonly have periventricular T2W hyperintensity, which is bilateral and frequently symmetric.

4. The papovavirus (J-C virus).

References

Mader I, Herrlinger U, Klose U, Schmidt F, Kuker W: Progressive multifocal leukoencephalopathy: analysis of lesion development with diffusion-weighted MRI, *Neuroradiology* 45:717–721, 2003.

Thurnher MM, Post MJ, Rieger A, Kleibl-Popov C, Loewe C, Schindler E: Initial and follow-up MR imaging findings in AIDS-related progressive multifocal leukoencephalopathy treated with highly active anti-retroviral therapy, *AJNR Am J Neuroradiol* 22:977–984, 2001.

Cross-Reference

Neuroradiology: THE REQUISITES, 2nd ed, pp 347–348, 352.

Comment

Before the AIDS epidemic, PML was largely seen in a spectrum of immunocompromised patients, including those with hematologic malignancies (leukemia and lymphoma), those who had undergone organ transplantation, patients taking immunosuppressive drugs, and those with autoimmune disorders. However, over the last few decades, the majority of cases of PML have been noted in patients with HIV infection. Progressive multifocal leukoencephalopathy is caused by infection of the oligodendrocytes with a papovavirus (JC virus). Histologically, multifocal regions of demyelination involve the subcortical U-fibers.

The clinical presentation of PML includes focal neurologic deficits (hemiparesis), visual symptoms, and especially progressive cognitive decline. The infection is rapidly progressive, with continued neurologic decline, CNS demyelination, and death usually occurring within 6 months to a year from the onset of symptoms.

MR imaging is far more sensitive than CT in defining the number and extent of lesions in PML. On CT, PML usually appears as focal regions of hypodensity within the white matter, usually without mass effect or enhancement. On MR imaging, increased T2W signal intensity with associated T1W hypointensity is noted in the involved white matter. PML has a predilection to involve the subcortical white matter, although the deep white matter is also commonly involved. There is a slight preference for involvement of the parietal and occipital white matter, but any area of the brain may be affected, including the cerebellum, as in this case. Although single focal lesions may be seen, multifocal lesions typically occur and may or may not be bilaterally symmetric in distribution. Unilateral multifocal distribution may also occur. Mass effect or enhancement is less common in PML, occurring in 5% to 10% of cases.

Notes

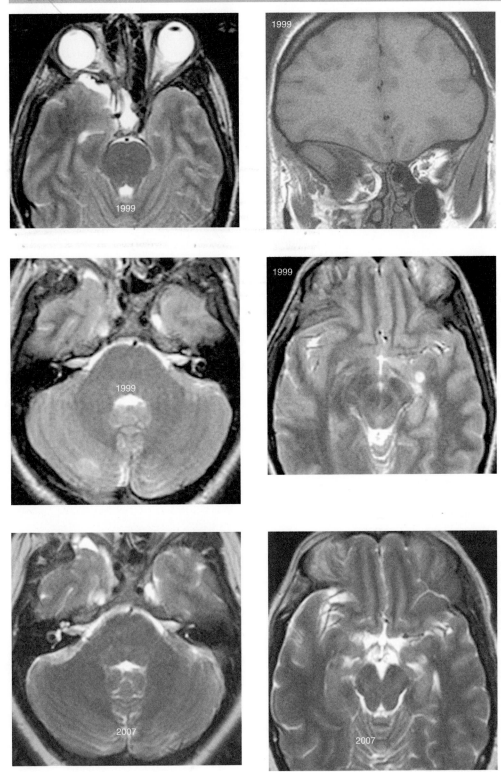

1. What structure is missing, and what does this result in?

2. What is the diagnosis?

3. This entity is associated with what central tumors?

4. What characteristic abnormalities of the spine are seen with this entity?

Sphenoid Dysplasia and Brain Dysplasia—Neurofibromatosis Type 1 (von Recklinghausen's Disease)

1. The right greater wing of the sphenoid bone is absent, resulting in an <u>encephalocele</u> involving the base of the skull (sphenoid sinus) and orbit.

2. Neurofibromatosis type 1.

3. Pilocytic astrocytomas of the visual pathway as well as astrocytomas of the brain (brainstem, cerebellum, and cerebrum).

4. Lateral thoracic meningocele and dural ectasia with vertebral dysplasia.

Reference

Itoh T, Magnaldi S, White RM, et al: Neurofibromatosis type 1: the evolution of deep gray and white matter MR abnormalities, *AJNR Am J Neuroradiol* 15:1513–1519, 1994.

Cross-Reference

Neuroradiology: THE REQUISITES, 2nd ed, pp 426–427, 449–450.

Comment

There is still some controversy over what the hyperintense lesions on T2W imaging represent in patients with neurofibromatosis type 1. These lesions are frequently located in the peduncles or deep gray matter of the cerebellum, the basal ganglia, the white matter of the cerebral hemispheres, and the brainstem, especially the pons. Some of the lesions may be mildly hyperintense on unenhanced T1W imaging. In this case, such lesions are seen in the right cerebellum and medial left temporal lobe on images obtained in 1999. On a follow-up study in 2007, the cerebellar lesion has resolved and the left temporal lobe lesion is smaller. Heterotopias and hamartomas have been suggested as the cause of these T2W hyperintense foci. Heterotopias are related to anomalous migration of gray matter, whereas hamartomas represent nonneoplastic proliferation of normal brain tissue in abnormal locations. The pathologic literature has described gliosis and vacuolar and spongiotic change. Myelin vacuolization in areas of dysplastic white matter seems to be commonly suggested. These lesions typically appear during the first decade of life, and may regress over time. If there is growth or enhancement of one of these foci, the possibility of an astrocytoma must be considered. Astrocytomas are seen with an increased incidence in neurofibromatosis type 1. It is believed by many (but not all) that these are separate lesions and that they do not arise from regions of dysplastic brain.

The primary manifestation of mesodermal dysplasia is hypoplasia or absence of the greater wing of the sphenoid bone. This may present with encephaloceles, as in this case, or with pulsatile exophthalmos. Buphthalmos is seen with increased frequency in neurofibromatosis type 1, and it refers to an enlarged globe caused by increased intraocular pressure secondary to obstruction of the canal of Schlemm from a mass or membranes composed of aberrant mesodermal tissue.

Neurofibromatosis type 1 can be diagnosed when two or more of the following criteria are present: a first-degree relative with neurofibromatosis type 1, one plexiform neurofibroma or two or more neurofibromas of any type, six or more café-au-lait spots, two or more Lisch nodules (iris hamartomas), axillary or inguinal freckling, optic pathway glioma, or a characteristic bone abnormality (dysplasia of the greater wing of the sphenoid, overgrowth of a digit or limb, pseudarthrosis, lateral thoracic meningocele, dural ectasia with vertebral dysplasia).

Notes   glioma

hamartoma

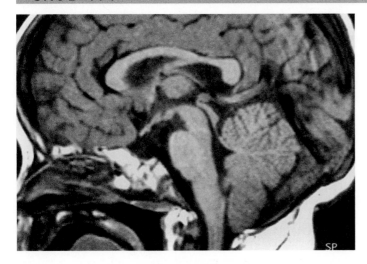 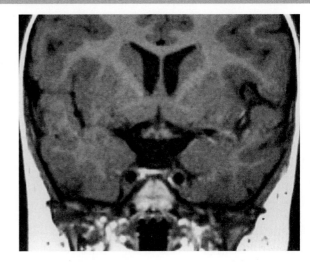

1. What are the imaging findings in this patient?

2. What is the normal signal intensity of the posterior gland (neurohypophysis) on unenhanced T1W imaging?

3. When is the posterior pituitary normally not hyperintense on unenhanced T1W imaging?

4. What is the characteristic MR imaging finding of an ectopic posterior pituitary gland?

Panhypopituitarism with Absence of the Infundibulum

1. Absence of the pituitary stalk, absent or diminutive anterior lobe, and absence of the normal posterior pituitary "bright" spot.

2. Hyperintense to white matter.

3. During pregnancy and the first 3 months of life.

4. High signal intensity at the apex or median eminence of the pituitary stalk is characteristic of an ectopic posterior pituitary gland.

References

Caruso RD, Postel GC, McDonald CS, et al: High signal on T1-weighted MR images of the head: a pictorial essay, *Clin Imaging* 25:312–319, 2001.

Saeki N, Hayasaka M, Murai H, et al: Posterior pituitary bright spot in large adenomas: MR assessment of its disappearance or relocation along the stalk, *Radiology* 226: 359–365, 2003.

Cross-Reference

Neuroradiology: THE REQUISITES, 2nd ed, pp 539–541.

Comment

This case shows an absent or diminutive anterior pituitary lobe, absence of the pituitary stalk, and absence of the normal posterior pituitary "bright" spot in the pituitary sella. The normal neurohypophysis is of high signal intensity on unenhanced T1W images; however, the exact etiology of this is debated, with explanations including vasopressin, phospholipid, and neurophysin stored in neurosecretory granules of the posterior pituitary gland. High signal intensity at the apex or median eminence of the pituitary stalk is characteristic of an ectopic posterior pituitary gland. The differential diagnosis of high signal intensity along the apex of the stalk at the floor of the third ventricle includes a tuber cinereum lipoma or fat in the marrow of the tip of the dorsum sella. In the latter two conditions, the normal posterior pituitary "bright" spot in the sella is present. Disappearance of the "hyperintensity" on fat-suppressed imaging could also confirm the presence of fat (lipoma or marrow). Absence of the normal posterior pituitary high signal intensity may be seen in Langerhans' cell histiocytosis and hemosiderosis.

The neurohypophysis is ectopic in a subset of patients with pituitary dwarfism. Specifically, low growth hormone levels associated with other pituitary hormonal deficiencies may be accompanied by an ectopic posterior pituitary gland and absence of the infundibulum on MR imaging. Failure of development of the infundibulum and posterior pituitary gland may be an isolated condition or may be part of a larger brain anomaly. It is believed that an ectopic posterior pituitary gland is related to an injury to the pituitary infundibulum, which normally transmits hormonal mediators from the hypothalamus to the neurohypophysis through a rich venous plexus. An ectopic posterior pituitary gland has also been associated with traumatic transection of the pituitary stalk.

Notes

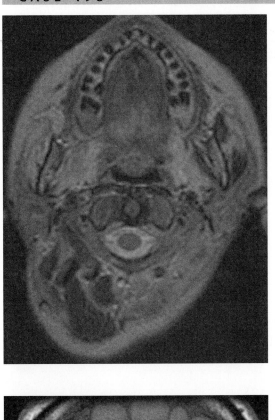
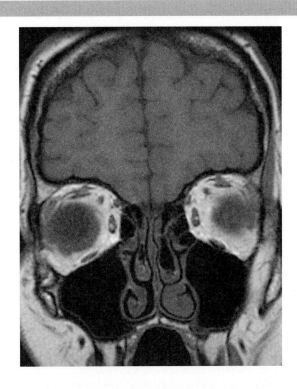
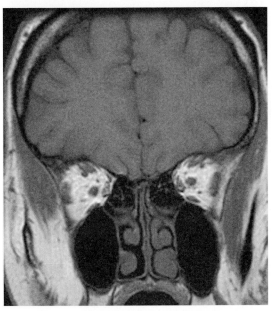
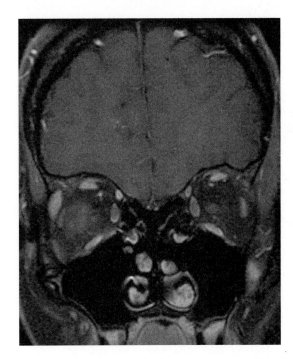

1. What are the imaging findings?

2. What is the telltale laboratory finding in Leigh disease?

3. What organs are especially affected in Kearns-Sayre syndrome?

4. Which mitochondrial defect is associated with stroke-like episodes?

Progressive External Ophthalmoplegia Syndrome—due to Mitochondrial Defect

1. There is extensive atrophy of the muscles of mastication, with the right side affected more than the left. There is also atrophy of the left suboccipital and neck muscles, as well as atrophy of the extraocular muscles, most notably, the medial rectii, which show fatty replacement.

2. Metabolic acidosis with elevated lactate levels. Leigh disease is likely due to an enzyme deficiency associated with pyruvate breakdown.

3. The orbits (chronic progressive ophthalmoplegia, weakness and atrophy of the extraocular muscles, retinitis pigmentosa) and the heart (cardiac conduction defects and cardiomyopathy).

4. MELAS.

Reference

Carlow TJ, Depper MH, Orrison WW Jr: MR of extraocular muscles in chronic progressive external ophthalmoplegia, *AJNR Am J Neuroradiol* 19:95–99, 1998.

Cross-Reference

Neuroradiology: THE REQUISITES, 2nd ed, pp 24, 401–403.

Comment

This patient presented with external ophthalmoplegia syndrome that was progressive over a 20-year period. The patient also had dysphagia and vertigo. Chronic progressive external ophthalmoplegia (CPEO) is a disorder characterized by slowly progressive paralysis of the extraocular muscles. It is usually bilateral and symmetrical. The ciliary and iris muscles are not involved. CPEO is the most frequent manifestation of mitochondrial myopathies. CPEO in association with mutations in mitochondrial DNA may occur in the absence of any other clinical sign, but usually, it is associated with skeletal muscle weakness. This patient's extensive evaluation was notable for a mutation in a region of a nuclear-encoded gene that encodes a DNA polymerase involved in mitochondrial gene maintenance. The mutation is in a gene that has been implicated in these syndromes, and it is in a region where pathogenic mutations have been identified. The region is highly conserved from fruit flies to humans. All of these factors make it likely to be a pathogenic mutation. These mutations are usually associated with DNA depletion syndromes, in which there is less DNA overall in the mitochondria. The treatment is limited and involves a "mitochondrial cocktail": vitamin C, vitamin E, coenzyme Q10, creatine, carnitine, riboflavin, pantothenate, thiamine, and lipoic acid.

The differential diagnosis includes other progressive external ophthalmoplegia syndromes, such as SANDO and Kearns-Sayre, as well as ocular pharyngeal dystrophy and myasthenia gravis. Kearns-Sayre syndrome is a mitochondrial myopathy in which the onset of CPEO occurs before 20 years of age and pigmentary retinopathy occurs as well. Kearns-Sayre syndrome also is associated with cardiac conduction defects, elevated cerebrospinal fluid protein, and a cerebellar syndrome.

Notes

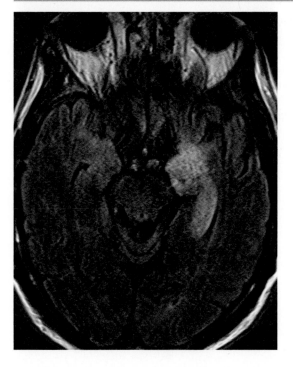
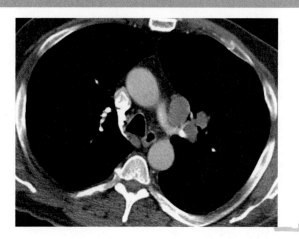

1. What is the differential diagnosis?

2. What are the two most common sites of involvement in CNS paraneoplastic syndromes?

3. What structures are most commonly involved in limbic encephalitis?

4. What malignancy is most commonly associated with this entity?

Limbic Encephalitis—Paraneoplastic Syndrome (Small Cell Lung Carcinoma)

1. Limbic encephalitis, viral encephalitis (herpes), seizures, and carbon monoxide intoxication (when the globus pallidus is also involved).

2. The medial temporal lobes (limbic encephalitis) and cerebellum.

3. The hippocampal formations, amygdala, and insula. The gyri may also be involved.

4. Small cell carcinoma of the lung.

References

Aguirre-Cruz L, Charuel JL, Carpentier AF, et al: Clinical relevance of non-neuronal auto-antibodies in patients with anti-Hu or anti-Yo paraneoplastic diseases, *J Neurooncol* 71:39–41, 2005.

Ances BM, Vitaliani R, Taylor RA, et al: Treatment-responsive limbic encephalitis identified by neuropil antibodies: MRI and PET correlates, *Brain* 128:1764–1777, 2005.

Cross-Reference

Neuroradiology: THE REQUISITES, 2nd ed, pp 152–154.

Comment

Paraneoplastic syndromes affecting the CNS represent a spectrum of neurologic manifestations that are associated with extracranial cancers, but are not the result of direct invasion of the CNS by tumor. They occur in fewer than 1% of patients with cancer; however, in 33% to 50% of patients with a paraneoplastic syndrome, the syndrome develops before the diagnosis of systemic neoplasm. Such syndromes include limbic encephalopathy, cerebellar degeneration, opsoclonus or myoclonus, retinal degeneration, Lambert-Eaton myasthenic syndrome, and myelopathy. Lung cancer, particularly small cell carcinoma, is the most common malignancy associated with neurologic paraneoplastic syndromes. However, these syndromes may be seen in ovarian carcinoma, testicular germ cell tumors, gastrointestinal cancer, Hodgkin's disease, breast cancer, and neuroblastoma in children. The cause of paraneoplastic syndromes is unknown; however, the most widely accepted theory is that they occur as a result of an autoimmune disorder. Circulating autoantibodies have been identified in several paraneoplastic syndromes. Anti-Yo is specific to paraneoplastic cerebellar degeneration associated with breast and ovarian cancer, and anti-Hu is most often associated with paraneoplastic limbic encephalitis.

Paraneoplastic limbic encephalitis may present with a change in mental status, personality changes, and memory impairment. CT may be unremarkable. On MR imaging, high signal intensity may be identified in the medial temporal lobes on T2W and FLAIR images. Mild enhancement may occur. Involvement of the hypothalamus may also be noted. On pathologic evaluation, nonspecific inflammatory changes and cellular infiltrates are identified without the presence of tumor or viral inclusions. Treatment of the primary malignancy may result in improvement of the neurologic symptoms.

Notes

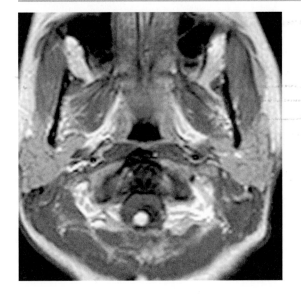
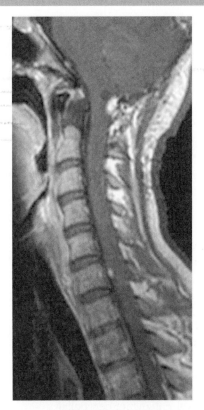
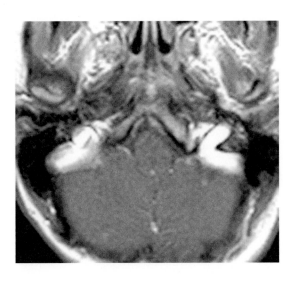
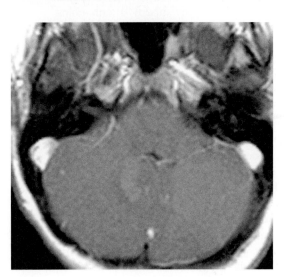

1. What is the most common cause of multiple cerebellar masses in adults?

2. What neoplasms may present as a cystic mass with an enhancing mural nodule?

3. What finding makes the diagnosis of pilocytic astrocytoma highly unlikely?

4. In what anatomic region is the lesion at the craniovertebral junction located?

von Hippel-Lindau Disease

1. Metastases.

2. Pilocytic astrocytoma, hemangioblastoma, and metastases.

3. The multiplicity of lesions (pilocytic astrocytomas are usually isolated neoplasms in children).

4. The area postrema (vomiting center) along the dorsal surface of the medulla oblongata at the caudal end of the fourth ventricle.

Reference

Slater A, Moore NR, Huson SM: The natural history of cerebellar hemangioblastomas in von Hippel-Lindau disease, *AJNR Am J Neuroradiol* 24:1570–1574, 2003.

Cross-Reference

Neuroradiology: THE REQUISITES, 2nd ed, pp 456–457.

Comment

This case shows a cystic mass with a solid enhancing mural nodule in the region of the area postrema of the medulla, as well as multiple small enhancing cerebellar lesions. Also noted is one of many superficial enhancing nodules along the pial surface of the spinal cord. Because this patient is an adult and the lesions are multiple, juvenile pilocytic astrocytoma is not a consideration. The differential diagnosis includes multiple hemangioblastomas seen in von Hippel-Lindau disease and, less likely, metastatic disease.

Although von Hippel-Lindau disease is a neurocutaneous syndrome, neurocutaneous is a misnomer in that there are no cutaneous manifestations. The hallmark lesion is the hemangioblastoma. Approximately 20% of patients with hemangioblastomas have von Hippel-Lindau disease. Conversely, up to 45% of patients with von Hippel-Lindau disease have CNS hemangioblastomas. In von Hippel-Lindau disease, these neoplasms are multiple in at least 40% of cases. Hemangioblastomas occur most commonly in the cerebellum and retina, although they may also arise in the brainstem (especially the medulla), the spinal cord, and (rarely) the cerebrum and viscera outside of the CNS. In addition to CNS lesions, patients with von Hippel-Lindau disease also have a spectrum of findings in other organs. Cysts in the pancreas occur in the majority of patients, but cysts may also be seen in the kidneys, liver, and epididymis in men and ovaries in women. Renal cell carcinomas are common and are different from garden variety renal cell adenocarcinoma in that in von Hippel-Lindau disease they are frequently bilateral, small, and less malignant. There is an approximately tenfold increase in the incidence of pheochromocytomas in these patients. Polycythemia related to the production of erythropoietin by the hemangioblastomas is not uncommon. Diagnostic criteria for von Hippel-Lindau disease include more than one CNS or retinal hemangioblastoma; a CNS hemangioblastoma and at least one visceral abnormality; and a family history of von Hippel-Lindau disease and at least one of the visceral manifestations.

Notes

POS
El craniocervical junction

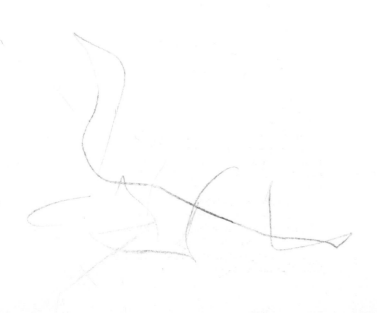